D1340290

Reproductive ageing

THF

RCOG PRESS

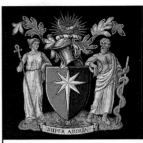

Since 1973 the Royal College of Obstetricians and Gynaecologists has regularly convened Study Groups to address important growth areas within obstetrics and gynaecology. An international group of eminent clinicians and scientists from various disciplines is invited to present the results of recent research and to take part in in-depth discussions. The resulting volume, containing enhanced versions of the papers presented, is published within a few months of the meeting and provides a summary of the subject that is both authoritative and up to date.

SOME PREVIOUS STUDY GROUP PUBLICATIONS AVAILABLE

The Placenta: Basic Science and Clinical Practice
Edited by JCP Kingdom, ERM Jauniaux and PMS O'Brien

Disorders of the Menstrual Cycle
Edited by PMS O'Brien, IT Cameron and AB MacLean

Infection and Pregnancy
Edited by AB MacLean, L Regan and D Carrington

Pain in Obstetrics and Gynaecology
Edited by A MacLean, R Stones and S Thornton

Incontinence in Women
Edited by AB MacLean and L Cardozo

Maternal Morbidity and Mortality
Edited by AB MacLean and J Neilson

Lower Genital Tract Neoplasia
Edited by Allan B MacLean, Albert Singer and Hilary Critchley

Pre-eclampsia
Edited by Hilary Critchley, Allan MacLean, Lucilla Poston and James Walker

Preterm Birth
Edited by Hilary Critchley, Phillip Bennett and Steven Thornton

Menopause and Hormone Replacement
Edited by Hilary Critchley, Ailsa Gebbie and Valerie Beral

Implantation and Early Development
Edited by Hilary Critchley, Iain Cameron and Stephen Smith

Contraception and Contraceptive Use
Edited by Anna Glasier, Kaye Wellings and Hilary Critchley

Multiple Pregnancy
Edited by Mark Kilby, Phil Baker, Hilary Critchley and David Field

Heart Disease and Pregnancy
Edited by Philip J Steer, Michael A Gatzoulis and Philip Baker

Teenage Pregnancy and Reproductive Health
Edited by Philip Baker, Kate Guthrie, Cindy Hutchinson, Roslyn Kane and Kaye Wellings

Obesity and Reproductive Health
Edited by Philip Baker, Adam Balen, Lucilla Poston and Naveed Sattar

Renal Disease in Pregnancy
Edited by John M Davison, Catherine Nelson-Piercy, Sean Kehoe and Philip Baker

Cancer and Reproductive Health
Edited by Sean Kehoe, Eric Jauniaux, Pierre Martin-Hirsch and Philip Savage

Reproductive ageing

Edited by

Susan Bewley, William Ledger and
Dimitrios Nikolaou

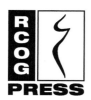

Sean Kehoe MD FRCOG
Convenor of Study Groups, Lead Consultant in Gynaecological Oncology, Oxford Gynaecological Cancer Centre, John Radcliffe Hospital, Headington, Oxford OX3 9DU

Susan Bewley MD MA FRCOG
Consultant Obstetrician / Maternal Fetal Medicine, Guy's & St Thomas' NHS Foundation Trust, Women's Services, 10th Floor North Wing, St Thomas' Hospital, Westminster Bridge Rd, London SE1 7EH

William Leigh Ledger MA DPhil FRCOG
Professor, Jessop Wing, Royal Hallamshire Hospital, Sheffield S10 2SF

Dimitrios Nikolaou MD MRCOG
Consultant Gynaecologist and Specialist in Reproductive Medicine and Surgery, Ovarian Ageing and Fertility Clinic, Assisted Conception Unit, 4th Floor, Chelsea and Westminster Hospital, 369 Fulham Road, London SW10 9NH

The Editors would like to thank Mr Douglas Gibb and Merck Serono for their unrestricted grant in support of the recording and transcription of the discussants' comments. These appear at the end of each section and, we think, explore and broaden the authors' contributions.

Published by the **RCOG Press** at the Royal College of Obstetricians and Gynaecologists, 27 Sussex Place, Regent's Park, London NW1 4RG

www.rcog.org.uk

Registered charity no. 213280

First published 2009

ISBN 978-1-906985-13-4

Cover image: poppy seed head, courtesy of Kenneth Stirling, Victoria, Australia

RCOG Editor: Andrew Welsh
Original design by Karl Harrington, FiSH Books, London
Typesetting by Andrew Welsh
Index by Liza Furnival, Medical Indexing Ltd
Printed by Henry Ling Ltd, The Dorset Press, Dorchester DT1 1HD

Contents

SECTION 3   PREGNANCY: THE AGEING MOTHER AND MEDICAL NEEDS

SECTION 4   THE OUTCOMES: CHILDREN AND MOTHERS

SECTION 5   FUTURE FERTILITY INSURANCE: SCREENING, CRYOPRESERVATION OR EGG DONORS?

SECTION 6   SEX BEYOND AND AFTER FERTILITY

Participants

David Barlow
Executive Dean of Medicine and Professor of Reproductive Medicine, University of Glasgow, Wolfson Medical School Building, University Avenue, Glasgow G12 8QQ

Susan Bewley
Consultant Obstetrician / Maternal Fetal Medicine, Guy's & St Thomas' NHS Foundation Trust, Women's Services, 10th Floor North Wing, St Thomas' Hospital, Westminster Bridge Rd, London SE1 7EH

Siladitya Bhattacharya
Professor of Reproductive Medicine and Head, Section of Applied Clinical Sciences, Division of Applied Health Sciences, School of Medicine and Dentistry, University of Aberdeen, Aberdeen Maternity Hospital, Cornhill Road, Aberdeen AB25 2ZD

Beverley Botting
Government Statistician, Office for National Statistics, 1 Myddelton Street London EC1R 1UW at the time of the Study Group meeting; now Survey Outreach Officer, National Centre for Social Research, 35 Northampton Square, London EC1V 0AX

Peter Braude
Head of Department of Women's Health, King's College London, School of Medicine, Guy's, King's and St Thomas' Hospitals, 10th Floor North Wing, St Thomas' Hospital, Westminster Bridge Road, London SE1 7EH

Kate Brian
Author and trustee of Infertility Network UK (INUK). katebrian@mac.com.

Catherine Coulson
Associate Specialist in Psychosexual and Reproductive Medicine, Reproductive Medicine Clinic, St Michael's Hospital, Southwell Street, Bristol BS8 2EG

Melanie Davies
Consultant Gynaecologist, Reproductive Medicine Unit, University College London Hospitals, Euston Road, London NW1

Mandish K Dhanjal
Consultant Obstetrician and Gynaecologist, Queen Charlotte's and Chelsea Hospital, Imperial College Healthcare NHS Trust, Du Cane Road, London W12 0HS

Donna Dickenson
Emeritus Professor of Medical Ethics and Humanities, University of London and Honorary Senior Research Fellow, University of Bristol

Roger Gosden
Professor and Director of Research in Reproductive Biology, Center for Reproductive Medicine and Infertility, Weill Medical College of Cornell University, 1305 York Avenue (7th floor), New York, NY 10021, USA

Berkeley Greenwood
Political Adviser to the National Infertility Awareness Campaign (NIAC) and Senior Consulting Director, Portcullis Public Affairs, St James House, 13 Kensington Square, London W8 5HD

Stephen G Hillier
Professor of Reproductive Endocrinology, Centre for Reproductive Biology, The
University of Edinburgh, The Queen's Medical Research Institute, 47 Little France
Crescent, Edinburgh EH16 4TJ

Stijn Hoorens
Senior Analyst, RAND Europe, 37 Square de Meeus, B-1000 Brussels, Belgium

Sean Kehoe
Convenor of Study Groups, Lead Consultant in Gynaecological Oncology, Oxford
Gynaecological Cancer Centre, John Radcliffe Hospital, Headington, Oxford OX3 9DU

Anna Kenyon
Clinical Lecturer/Sub-specialty Trainee in Maternal and Fetal Medicine, Fetal Medicine
Unit, Elizabeth Garrett Anderson Wing, University College Hospital, 235 Euston Road,
London NW1 2BU

William Ledger
Professor, Jessop Wing, Royal Hallamshire Hospital, Sheffield S10 2SF

Diana Mansour
Associate Medical Director, NHS Newcastle and North Tyneside, Community Services,
New Croft Centre, Sexual Health Services, Market Street (East), Newcastle upon Tyne
NE1 6ND

Finbarr Martin
Consultant Geriatrician, Elderly Care Unit, St Thomas' Hospital, Westminster Bridge
Road, London SE1 7EH

Gita Mishra
Senior Research Scientist, MRC Unit for Lifelong Health and Ageing, Royal Free and
University College Medical School Department of Epidemiology and Public Health, 33
Bedford Place, London WC1B 5JU

Dimitrios Nikolaou
Consultant Gynaecologist and Specialist in Reproductive Medicine and Surgery,
Ovarian Ageing and Fertility Clinic, Assisted Conception Unit, 4th Floor, Chelsea and
Westminster Hospital, 369 Fulham Road, London SW10 9NH

Helen Picton
Chair in Reproduction and Early Development, The Reproduction and Early
Development Research Group, Leeds Institute of Genetics, Health and Therapeutics,
University of Leeds, The Light Laboratories, Clarendon Way, Leeds LS2 9JT

Jane Preston
Senior Lecturer, King's College London, Pharmaceutical Sciences Research Division,
Hodgkin Building, Guy's Campus, London SE1 1UL

Gordon CS Smith
Professor and Head of Department of Obstetrics and Gynaecology, University of
Cambridge, Box 223, The Rosie Hospital, Robinson Way, Cambridge CB2 0SW

Alastair Sutcliffe
Senior Lecturer in Paediatrics and Honorary Consultant Paediatrician, General and
Adolescent Unit, Institute of Child Health, University College London, 30 Guilford
Street, London WC1N 1EH

Herman Tournaye
Senior Medical Director, Centre for Reproductive Medicine, Universitair Ziekenhuis Vrije Universiteit Brussel, 101, Laarbeeklaan, Brussels B-1090, Belgium

Maya Unnithan
Reader in Social Anthropology, Department of Anthropology, ARTSC, University of Sussex, Falmer, Brighton BN1 9SJ

Zoe Williams
Journalist, The Guardian, Kings Place, 90 York Way, London N1 9GU

Additional contributors

Yasmin Baki
Paediatric Registrar, Department of Paediatrics, University College Hospital, 235 Euston Road, London NW1 2BV

Emma Chambers
Research Fellow, The Reproduction and Early Development Research Group, Leeds Institute of Genetics, Health and Therapeutics, University of Leeds, The Light Laboratories, Clarendon Way, Leeds LS2 9JT

Rachel Cooper
Career Development Fellow, MRC Unit for Lifelong Health and Ageing, Royal Free and University College Medical School Department of Epidemiology and Public Health, 33 Bedford Place, London WC1B 5JU

Ahmed Gibreel
Research Fellow, Division of Applied Health Sciences, School of Medicine and Dentistry, University of Aberdeen, Aberdeen Maternity Hospital, Cornhill Road, Aberdeen AB25 2ZD

Abha Maheshwari
Clinical Lecturer and Subspeciality Trainee in Reproductive Medicine, Division of Applied Health Sciences, School of Medicine and Dentistry, University of Aberdeen, Aberdeen Maternity Hospital, Cornhill Road, Aberdeen AB25 2ZD

Lucinda Veeck Gosden
Director of Clinical Embryology and Associate Professor, Center for Reproductive Medicine and Infertility, Weill Medical College of Cornell University, 1305 York Avenue (7th floor), New York, NY 10021, USA

DECLARATIONS OF PERSONAL INTEREST

All contributors to the Study Group were invited to make a specific Declaration of Interest in relation to the subject of the Study Group. This was undertaken and all contributors complied with this request. David Barlow has received sponsorship or paid consultancy work from Novo Nordisk, PregLem Pfizer and Wyeth. He holds shares of nominal value in PregLem. He is the Dean of Medicine at Glasgow University, which receives grants from a wide range of companies. He is an officer or member of the British Menopause Society, the National Osteoporosis Society, the European Menopause and Andropause Society and the RCOG. He was Editor-in-Chief of the journal *Human Reproduction* until 2007. Susan Bewley was paid for consultancy work in 2008 by RAND Organisation and is a member of the Medical Defence Union (MDU) Council and the National Childbirth Trust. She receives small royalties as editor of the OUP textbook *Training in Obstetrics and Gynaecology*. Peter Braude's department receives financial support from Merck Serono, Organon and Hologic. He is a consultant to or member of the Advisory Committee on the Safety of Blood, Tissues and Organs (SaBTO), the Human Fertilisation and Embryology Authority (HFEA) and the Multiple Births Stakeholder Group. His department holds four patents related to premature labour. Kate Brian is a member of the board of trustees of Infertility Network UK (INUK) and is the author of *The Complete Guide to Female Fertility* and *The Complete Guide to IVF*. Catherine Coulson's department has received educational grants from Organon and Merck Serono and she is a consultant to the British Society of Psychosomatic Obstetrics, Gynaecology and Andrology. She is a Member of the Institute of Psychosexual Medicine and a member of the British Fertility Society. Melanie Davies is lead investigator for a research project sponsored by Organon. She has received limited editorial fees for two books that are in print. Roger Gosden has occasionally received honoraria for conference lectures. His department has received grants for research from EMD Serono and Ferring Pharmaceuticals and he is an unpaid consultant for Fertile Hope (New York) and for the Diamond Foundation, which are both non-profit organisations. Berkeley Greenwood is a consultant to the National Infertility Awareness Campaign (NIAC), which receives sponsorship from commercial organisations. Stephen Hillier has in the past received lecture fees or honoraria from Serono, Organon and Ferring. He has authored two patents but does not own them now. Stijn Hoorens has declared that RAND Europe has received research grants from Ferring Pharmaceuticals and Organon. RAND Europe has policies and contractual arrangements to safeguard the independence and objectivity of its research. Sean Kehoe has acted as an adviser for Sanofi Pasteur and received support to attend educational meetings. He is a council member of the British Gynaecological Cancer Society, a member of the NCRI Ovarian Subgroup and the British Society For Colposcopy and Cervical Pathology, a spokesperson for WOW, a trustee for OVACOME and an editorial board member of *BJOG*, the *European Journal of Obstetrics and Gynaecology* and the *European Journal of Surgical Oncology*. William Ledger has received honoraria for lecturing/teaching from Schering Plough and Amirall. His department receives research funding for commercial studies from Akzo Nobel, Ferring, Schering Plough and Ipsen. He is a consultant to Verity – the PCOS charity, the National Infertility Awareness Campaign and the Pituitary Foundation. He has received payment for work as an Editorial Board Member of *Obstetrics, Gynaecology and Reproductive Medicine*. Dimitrios Nikolaou has been sponsored by Ferring and Serono to attend scientific meetings (less than £5,000 per year). His wife has some shares in Pfizer. His unit is sponsored for research by Ferring and Serono. Helen Picton's research group has received funding for research from industry for clinical trials and basic research. None of these projects would constitute a conflict of interest on this topic. She is the current chair of the Society for Reproduction and Fertility, which is a basic science society as well as a charity. Lucinda Veeck Gosden's department has received grants for research from EMD Serono and Ferring Pharmaceuticals. Herman Tournaye's department receives financial support from all major gonadotrophin companies (Ferring, Serono, Organon).

Infertility and miscarriage

Such hope.
And then the rain
Comes again.

I am angry,
I am frustrated,
I cry,
I am frustrated with the world,
But most of all,
I am frustrated with myself,
Although doctors frustrate me
A great deal.

In my head
I know I am not to blame,
In my heart,
I don't know who else there is.

Involutary childlessness
Is like walking around
With an invisible limb missing.

When I leave my fertile years behind me
Will I finally be able to let it all go?
Or will the next generation
Appear to haunt me still?

Treatment

Courage is not
The absence of fear,
But rather
The ability to act
In the face of it

They say,
Infertility is as stressful
As cancer.
How many people know that?

Stereotypes

I am not a mother,
But nor am I
A career woman
Or over fourty,
But if I was,
Should I be judged
For using my brain, my talents
And forging a successful career?
Should I be criticised
For finding unsuccessful relationships
And for not finding Mr Right?
After all, it takes two
To make a baby and create a family.
And some people genuinely believe
That stability and life experience
Are factors in bringing up children,
Contrary to popular opinion,
Not all women consciously think
I'll be OK, no matter what,
Let me choose where the kids will fit in,
There's always the easy option of
Fertility Treatment and IVF
With their gilt-edged guarantees.
I can always buy
An egg, sperm, embryo, a baby.
No. It is not thoughlessness that delays
The decision to have a family,
Far from it,
For the majority, it is life.

Darwin and his gene pool suck.
All I can hope
Is that evolution adapts,
And men start having babies too,
Which will not only benefit infertile women,
But also the work place, society
And the world in general.

Afterwards

I chase
Single magpies
Out of the garden

© Kate Bentley

Preface

Ageing can be welcomed, endured or feared but it remains inevitable. Obstetricians and gynaecologists are uniquely placed to see and to alleviate the complications of diseases of pregnancy and the reproductive organs. They have to be knowlegeable and skilled in their broad or subspecialist expert areas in order to provide high-quality medical services to women. They have an understanding of how age affects biology and disease, particularly when the population is ageing and in an era of deferred childbearing. They also have to respect and understand the complex lives that women lead and the diverse families and communities they come from, and be sensitive to the impact that obstetric and gynaecological problems may have. Our histories, examinations, tests, diagnoses and prognoses can threaten the core of a woman's identity and her fertility, sexuality, family and life experiences. Doctors have to avoid stereotypes and empathise with and listen to their patients but cannot always 'walk in another's shoes'. The poems opposite distil some of the private pain and public pleas of women experiencing the adverse effects of reproductive ageing.

Since 1973, the RCOG has regularly convened Study Groups to address important topics in our specialty. Ageing and reproductive ageing affect us all as individuals and as society. Obstetricians and gynaecologists are witnesses to the impact of reproductive ageing and to some of the fears, misinformation and misapprehensions that the general public have. One purpose of the Study Group was to raise awareness of the societal trends and implications. Practitioners, academics and informed lay contributors from around the world were brought together to look at the current situation and available evidence. The wider importance of the subject to the whole of society is emphasised by the contributions in this volume from experts from other disciplines, both within and outside medicine. Reproductive ageing has effects on individual and public health, now and in generations to come. It is experienced differently by different cultures, by the voluntarily and involuntarily childless and by those responsible for organising health services. Although women are healthier than ever, biology can still determine destiny and the decline in fertility and rise in complications with age remain. Scientists can understand but cannot yet control or reverse the processes of ageing, even as they contribute to the means of alleviating the suffering that it may bring. This volume gathers together a diverse but timely set of contributions in order to inform Members and Fellows of the RCOG, interested healthcare and research workers and the general public.

We are greatly indebted to the participants who provided their manuscripts on time and who worked so hard during the Study Group. As always, the RCOG staff made the behind-the-scenes work run smoothly and contributed to the success of the meeting. In particular, we would like to thank Jessica Letters, Andrew Welsh and Jane Moody. The Study Group participants wanted to celebrate the positive aspects of ageing, not stigmatise older women. We enjoyed ourselves and hope that those who read the book, and especially the stimulating discussions, will do so too.

Susan Bewley
William Ledger
Dimitrios Nikolaou
Sean Kehoe

Section 1

Background to ageing and demographics

Chapter 1
Ageing: what is it and why does it happen?

Finbarr Martin and Jane Preston

Introduction

The world faces unprecedented challenges and opportunities from an ageing population. In health care, this is resulting in a transition from the dominance of acute illnesses and infections to that of chronic and degenerative conditions. Clinical recognition of this is hardly new. Hippocrates noted common age-associated medical conditions and Aristotle even offered a theory of ageing based on loss of heat. Remarkably, our current concepts of ageing are also bound up with combustion – cellular respiration. The emergence of old age as the focus of a medical specialty was prompted by the growth of older populations living in urban poverty in Paris[1] and, later, New York and London. Now that the expectation of growing old is commonplace in developed countries and is very rapidly spreading worldwide, it is beginning to influence attitudes and behaviour throughout life. In this chapter we address briefly several issues.

- What is population ageing, and why and how does it occur?
- The genetics and evolution of ageing – has ageing evolved?
- What distinguishes ageing from disease?
- What are the cellular and molecular processes involved with ageing of somatic cells?
- How do germ cells differ from somatic cells?
- How does menopause fit in with evolution of ageing?

Population ageing – why and how?

The demographic transition

The transition from populations with a great preponderance of the young into the current pattern typical of developed countries can be understood as a series of stages. The classic pattern of this demographic transition starts from a steady-state 'young' population with typically high fertility rates and high mortality rates throughout the lifespan. Only a minority of individuals reach old age, so the population shape has a broad base and narrow apex, like a pyramid. The first change is a decline in death rates, particularly in infancy. For example, deaths occurring under the age of 5 years, as a proportion of all deaths occurring in England and Wales, fell from 37% in 1901 to 0.6% by 2000 and, during the same period, death after the age of 75 years rose from

12% to 64%.[2] As a result, a male born in England and Wales in 2006 is estimated to have a 91% chance of reaching age 65 years and a female a 94% chance. The resultant changes in life expectancy since the mid-19th century are shown in Table 1.1. Thus, there are more people from the broad base, the young, that survive into older age. At this stage, the fertility rate remains high. The pyramid retains the broad base but with a wider apex, the population grows and the proportion and absolute numbers of older people increase. Subsequently, fertility rates decline. In England and Wales, for example, the fertility rate remained at over four per woman for the two centuries from 1700 until nearly the start of the 20th century,[3] before falling below two per woman by the 1930s, the rate which currently remains.[4] As a result, the pyramid base narrows and begins to resemble the shape of a broad pillar. Mortality rates continue to decline, so the proportion of older people rises further. However, as the smaller birth cohorts work through, many decades later the absolute numbers of older people may fall again. In this classic model, the new steady state has a higher overall population but lower fertility rates and low death rates throughout the lifespan until advanced ages, and radically changed relative proportions of different age groups.

There are, of course, numerous factors that modify this pattern. The post-World War II 'baby boom' is one example. Most members of this much larger birth cohort are surviving into older age, producing the current rapid rise in the numbers and proportion of older people in the UK. They will be followed by smaller cohorts and therefore there will be a dramatic reduction in the proportion of adults of working age (Figure 1.1). In recent decades, these trends have been further exaggerated by significant improvements in life expectancy for people having already reaching age 65 years, an increase of nearly 4 years for men and women since 1981 (Figure 1.2). In 2008, for the first time, there were more pensioners in the UK than those aged under 16 years. In addition, significant variation exists. The extremes of life expectancy in the UK in 2007 are 83.7 years for residents of Kensington and Chelsea (London) and 70.8 years for their fellow citizens in Glasgow (Scotland). Most of the difference is explicable by socio-economic factors, operating throughout the lifespan.

Worldwide, the most notable variation in this demographic transition is the speed at which it occurs. Demographers encapsulate the rate of population ageing by estimating the years taken for a doubling from 7% to 14% of the number of people aged 65 years or over as a proportion of the total population. In early industrialised European countries, this was typically in the region of 50 years or more. In contrast, this takes about half that time or less in the later developing countries; for example, 21 years from 2011 to 2032 is the current estimate for Brazil.

Table 1.1   Expectation of life at birth for England and Wales, 1838–54 to 2008; data from the Office for National Statistics[32,33]

Year(s)	Males	Females
1838–54	40	42
1901–10	49	52
1950–52	66	72
2007	77	81
2008 (estimate)	76.37	81.46

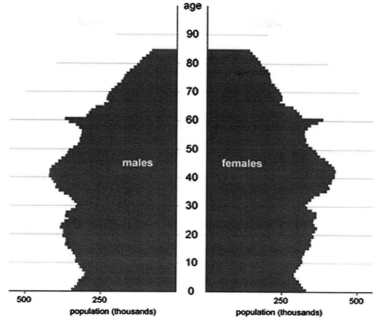

Figure 1.1   Age structure of England and Wales, mid-2007; data from the Office for National Statistics[4]

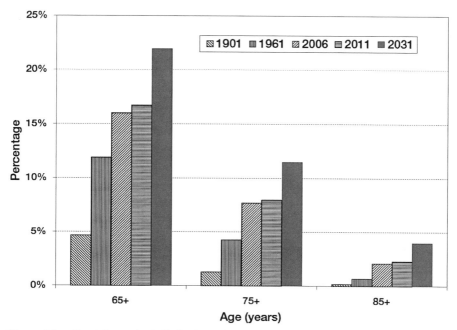

Figure 1.2   Population ageing in England and Wales from 1901 to 1961[34] and projections from 2006 to 2031[35]; data from House magazine[34] and the Government Actuary's Department[35]

Why have mortality rates declined?

The reduction in mortality rates is largely a story of improved public health through increasing availability of clean water, sanitation and adequate foods at key life stages, and through reductions of accidental deaths. Healthier cohorts, related to better gestational nutrition, is a possible mechanism for the continuing improvements in life expectancy as low birth weight is associated with higher rates and earlier onset of cardiovascular diseases, diabetes and hypertension.[5] Post-war improvements in housing, welfare and medical care during old age have also contributed significantly towards the end of this period of transition. The decline in fertility follows falls in mortality rates for socio-economic and cultural reasons, and these may be changing further in modern society.

Implications of ageing populations on the health of older people

The dramatic survival changes in recent decades have prompted debate in the gerontological literature on whether the added years of life would be characterised by increasing age-related disability or whether, conversely, there would also be a delay of the average age of onset of disabling conditions. This idea has been termed the compression of morbidity.[6] Various possible scenarios exist. There may be an increase in the survival rates of sick people, which would result in longer periods of morbidity for individuals and an increased population prevalence of disability. Social and medical advances may control the progression of chronic diseases, thus delaying death but not necessarily the disability resulting from these conditions. Improvement of the health status of new cohorts of older people, associated with more advantageous early life experiences (and perhaps improved health behaviours) would perhaps result in a compression of morbidity. Finally, if age-related frailty is an inevitable development in the absence of specific diseases, there would be the emergence of very old and frail populations, which would result in expansion of morbidity. It is probable that all these factors are operating currently, so projections of healthy life expectancy become problematic. However, evidence from the UK suggests that only about half of the extension of life expectancy for older people in the past two decades has been extra life in good health.

The genetics and evolution of ageing

When low death rates are followed by a sharp acceleration at a stage we have come to regard as 'old age', it produces a rectangularisation of the life survival curve (Figure 1.3). If death occurred randomly from birth onwards, with age (time since birth) playing no part in the likelihood of death, the result would be a life survival curve with an exponential shape. Something like this has probably been the majority situation during animal life on earth. The rectangularisation suggests that we are now observing a 'natural life span', as a result of species-specific longevity. Only in later phases of animal evolution, most particularly with primates and domesticated or farmed animals, have we seen this rectangularisation and thus confronted ageing as a significant issue.

Not all organisms age. A single-cell organism such as *Escherichia coli* reproduces by division without having undergone the range of ageing changes seen in multicellular organisms. As more complex life forms have evolved, ageing has appeared. Although an estimated two-thirds of the genome have some effect on ageing changes, a number of factors point to the central role of relatively few genes in the determination of

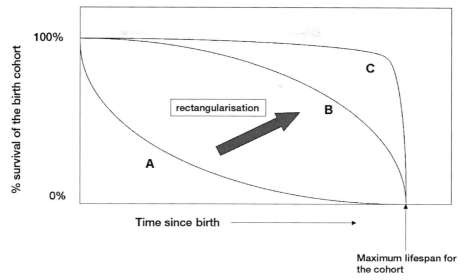

Figure 1.3   Different patterns of cohort ageing: **A** represents the survival curve for most animals in the wild, with time since birth having little or no influence on death rate; **B** is the survival curve pattern for domesticated animals and human populations that is typical of developed countries in recent centuries, with time since birth influencing death rate but still with many 'premature' deaths; **C** is the idealised survival curve to represent ageing societies, with most individuals reaching old age before death; this is typical of current developed countries

the maximum lifespan. Longevity is species specific and closely related species with substantial genetic similarity can have markedly different longevity if their natural habitat or habitus differ. Fast-ageing 'progeria' syndromes such as Werner syndrome, which is due to genetic mutation, produces a dramatic and visible acceleration of ageing, with life expectancy of about 40 years, but the genetic change is sufficiently specific not to prevent normal intrauterine development and infancy. We know from these genetically based fast-ageing syndromes and from animal studies that there are multiple genes that can adversely affect ageing. However, while genes may be powerful agents of maximum potential, it is important to note that twin studies suggest that only about 25% of the explanation for long-lived families is genetic.[7] The rest is due to shared environmental exposures.

Has ageing evolved?

Most animals in the wild, like humans until a few hundred years ago, live no more than 50% of their potential lifespan. This maximum potential survival was thus achieved by inheritance through the reproduction of relatively young animals and not as a result of selective survival and successful reproduction of long-lived animals. In this sense, the maximum potential lifespan has exerted little or no direct evolutionary pressure. On the contrary, it must have developed as an indirect result of evolutionary pressures on other characteristics. To put it another way, natural selection has favoured genotypes that produce (i) fitness to successfully reproduce during young adulthood and (ii) a phenotype that ages and has a maximum lifespan built in. Ageing has thus not evolved 'for itself' but as a consequence of other characteristics being preferentially selected under evolutionary pressures.

Central to understanding this dichotomy is the fact that tissues in multicellular animals show specialisation, with separation of the tissues concerned with maintaining life now (the soma) from the tissues concerned with propagation of the species through inheritance (the germ line). The biological activity resulting in the molecular, cellular and tissue 'ageing' changes described below may sooner or later impair cellular or organ function and survival. There is thus evolutionary pressure to develop ways of preventing or overcoming these deleterious changes but only in so far as they impede the fitness of the animal. In evolutionary terms, the fitness of an animal is its ability to produce offspring. When the risk of 'premature' death is high, this means producing viable offspring soon after reaching maturity. In conditions of finite environmental resources such as food, the evolution of form and function capable of reaching this fitness involves a number of compromises in the best use of biological energy. In Kirkwood's 'disposable soma' theory, the separation of the germ line from other cells in the body has allowed the selection of mechanisms for specific accurate preservation of the germ line but at the expense of the biological adaptability needed to preserve the soma.[8] Since the soma and the genetic material in the cells of the soma are not available for inheritance, preserving them for immortality in the face of inevitable death through predation, accident or deprivation would be energy wasted.

Development, ageing and disease

The stages of the lifespan of mammals can be distinguished as (i) fertilisation and birth, (ii) infancy to sexual maturity and (iii) adult reproductive life through to death, which may include a distinct post-reproductive phase. The molecular changes that are commonly regarded as ageing, and which will be described below in more detail, do not begin at a defined stage but seem to develop gradually. There is no evidence of an overall switch or controlling clock governing the pace of changes observed over time in various cells, tissues and physiological systems. The leading biogerontologist Strehler[9] proposed that the term 'ageing' should be reserved for those changes that occur gradually and universally, that are intrinsic in origin and that are detrimental to life. Universality must allow for some variability between members of a species. To show that biological changes are gradual is challenging. Most natural phenomena exhibit episodic changes, even if underlying processes are gradual. Life consists of an organism's biological interaction with the environment, so 'intrinsic' can only sensibly imply that the changes do not depend upon particular non-essential environmental factors. Below, we discuss some of these changes that could credibly contribute to death or disease but the relationship for others is not established. If we therefore limit the term 'ageing' to those changes for which such causality has been established, we would have a severely restricting definition. The current consensus in biological gerontology is to view ageing as those changes that deviate from the state presumed to be advantageous at the stage of optimal reproductive capacity. This makes sense from an evolutionary viewpoint.

Employing this broader approach to ageing, Rowe and Khan[10] drew attention to the difference between those older people without apparent disease and who remain independent until sudden death at advanced age and those people who clearly suffer one or a series of potentially avoidable degenerative or involutional diseases resulting in frailty and dependency. Both groups must surely be subject to degrees of ageing change: the difference is the result of the complex and cumulative interaction between genes, ageing-related molecular damage and environmental factors. The simple view that we can strictly distinguish degenerative diseases from ageing is no longer tenable.

Ageing of the soma – cellular and molecular processes

At the molecular level, it is clear that damage to all cellular components accumulates with increasing age. Some of these changes occur whether in the test tube or in the living cell; for example, the progressive increase in cross-links between the strands in a collagen molecule. Others occur as a product of biological activity, such as cell division. Recent findings have supported integration of the long-standing and apparently conflicting theories that favoured either programmed ageing or wear and tear as the underlying explanations.

Of central importance in current thinking is the integrity of DNA. This macromolecule is inherently unstable. Spontaneous changes include base alteration and single-strand or double-strand breaks and are seen at increasing rates with ageing.[11] Added to this is damage caused by deleterious agents, such as reactive oxygen species (ROS). The most common ROS in mammals are the superoxide anion, hydrogen peroxide, the hydroxyl radical and the nitric oxide radical. They arise from a variety of sources, primarily the mitochondria that form superoxide free radical anions alongside ATP in the vital process of oxidative phosphorylation. Other sources of ROS include the macrophages, particularly during chronic infections, the peroxisomes involved in lipid degradation and cytochrome P450 involved in drug detoxification.

Interaction of ROS with DNA, both mitochondrial and nuclear, can result in breaks in the sugar–phosphate backbone, resulting in mutations or deletions. A variety of effects may result, including transformation into an immortal cell line – a step on the route to a neoplastic tumour. The outcome of ROS-induced damage in the vascular system endothelial cells is production of adhesion molecules by dying cells that attract neutrophils and macrophages in a local inflammatory reaction releasing hydrogen peroxide. This additional ROS load further damages the compromised cell as well as the extracellular matrix and surrounding cells, resulting in a cascade of oxidative stress.[12.]

The free radical theory of ageing based on ROS-induced damage has received more attention than any other aspect of biogerontology. Although an attractive rationale for somatic ageing, not to mention the basis for a large industry promoting antioxidants, its prominence as the cause of ageing is now being questioned. Although ROS are estimated to 'hit' genomic DNA around 10 000 times each day, it seems that these random events are usually balanced by effective DNA repair enzymes, which are largely able to negate the negative consequences of damage.[13] Furthermore, interventions to modify antioxidant activity, such as studies using transgenic mice adapted to enhance the exogenous antioxidants superoxide dismutase and catalase, have not shown improvements in life expectancy.[14] Although epidemiological studies on humans have suggested a protective effect of a high dietary intake of antioxidants against visual cataract, memory loss and vascular damage, prospective clinical trials have been largely negative. Nevertheless, oxidative stress is still an important avenue for research into specific age-related disease states such as neurodegeneration and cardiovascular disease.

However, the importance of effective DNA maintenance remains and is illustrated by the fast-ageing progeria syndromes. People with Werner syndrome display damaged DNA due to lack of helicase required for DNA repair and mRNA formation. In

Hutchinson–Gilford progeria syndrome, DNA replication does not take place, owing to alterations in the nuclear envelope. In both cases, rapid progression to an aged phenotype results in extremely premature death from ostensibly 'old-age' related disorders.

The effectiveness of DNA repair correlates reasonably well with species lifespan. Short-lived mammals such as the mouse and shrew have around one-fifth the rate of DNA repair compared with humans. According to the disposable soma theory, evolution has favoured strategies that devote energy and resources to enable the soma to attain reproductive fitness with the germ line safe from damage. There are indeed several features evident in the germ cell line, for example the ovary, that may result in enhanced protection for the genetic material compared with those present in the cells of other tissues. It would be expected from this theory that the cellular mechanisms to protect the soma from damage would be better developed in species likely to live longer. Thus, those adapted to their environment in such a way as to experience a lower rate of predatory or accidental deaths, for example primates, would differ in their anti-ageing mechanisms from species demonstrating an almost exponential survival curve such as the mouse. In neither case then would the effects of ageing be prominent. Available evidence confirms this prediction.[15]

Cell senescence and loss of telomeres

Two particular aspects of DNA damage have received much attention over the past decade: loss of telomeric ends of nuclear DNA and mutations to mitochondrial DNA. In the early 1960s, Hayflick and Moorhead[16] made the observation that cells in culture could undergo only a limited number of cell divisions (subsequently termed the 'Hayflick limit'). Further research showed that cultured fibroblasts from old donors could undergo fewer cell divisions than those from young donors, that cells frozen for extended periods could 'remember' how many divisions they had left and, more recently, that senescent cells that had stopped dividing could be identified *in vivo*. These studies, and others, pointed to a biological clock capable of counting the number of cell divisions and whose possible function was to prevent cancer, allowing the animal to reach healthy reproductive maturity, with the trade-off being limited cellular replication. The site of this clock is now largely held to be the telomere end regions of DNA, the repeat sequences of nuclear DNA that cap both ends of chromosomes and that shorten with each cell division. Telomeres are particularly vulnerable to free radical attack because they contain a short region of single-strand DNA and have few specific repair enzymes in the majority of somatic cells. People with Werner syndrome demonstrate shortened telomeres.[17]

In addition to free radical damage, portions of telomeres are lost during normal DNA replication and after several cell divisions (around 100 in humans) the telomere is eroded to such an extent that the cell enters replicative senescence and is no longer able to divide. This process is speeded up either by high exposure to oxidative stress or in rapidly dividing cells such as lymphocytes in response to infection or vascular endothelium in response to damage. Detection of senescent cells *in vivo* poses technical difficulties but studies have implicated them in the cornea, blood vessels and skin. It is suggested that senescent cells have a role in tissue ageing because of the limited regenerative potential of tissues containing large numbers of senescent cells. This would be important for cells with a naturally high turnover, such as the immune system, and in response to damage, such as in turbulent or branched regions of the vascular system and skin or eye wounding; evidence is accumulating that this holds true.[18.]

Mitochondrial DNA (mtDNA) sustains damage both from mutation and from oxidative stress from ROS. DNA point mutations and deletions occur at a ten-fold higher rate in mtDNA compared with nuclear DNA. The mitochondria are particularly susceptible to DNA damage as their DNA repair mechanisms are also less efficient than in the nucleus. These facts underpin the mitochondrial theory of ageing, which suggests that mtDNA mutation and mitochondrial damage result in a progressive impairment to the cell's ATP production.[19] Damage accumulates over time and may be passed on to daughter cells. As ATP production declines it becomes insufficient for effective holistic maintenance and cells begin to die. In addition, as mitochondria become damaged, excess free radicals are thought to be released, damaging proteins and lipids throughout the rest of the cell. Brain tissue is particularly vulnerable to the effects of sustained mitochondrial damage and reduced ATP availability, with affected cells dying by apoptosis or the fatal excitotoxicity cascade in those cells with N-methyl-D-aspartic acid receptors, such as in the hippocampus dentate gyrus.

Another aspect of spontaneous and random damage that warrants attention is the damage caused by free sugars. Spontaneous chemical reactions between sugars such as glucose and fructose and any proteins they encounter (especially lysine-rich proteins) give rise to the formation of glycated aggregates.[20] In mature form, these 'advanced glycation end products' (AGEs) cannot be degraded by cellular proteasomes and therefore gradually accumulate in all tissues. This mechanism is used clinically as glycated haemoglobin (HbA$_{1c}$) reflects the ambient glucose concentration exposed to the red cells. The same process results in AGE-induced increased stiffness of the protein elements in vasculature, ligaments and lung, and thickening of cellular basement membrane in the kidney. The result is reduced function in all affected tissue.

Given the detrimental effects of both oxidative stress and AGEs, it is perhaps not surprising that recent research on animal longevity provides tantalising links between the two processes. In the micoscopic worm *Caenorhabditis elegans*, which is used as a model of ageing, mutation of genes for insulin-receptor subunits and the associated downstream intracellular messengers has resulted in the doubling of the worm's maximum lifespan and has illustrated a link between glucose metabolism and ageing. Furthermore, mammals reared under conditions of caloric restriction (the only intervention known to consistently increase mammalian maximum life- and health-spans) produce fewer mitochondrial ROS.

AGE production and the associated damage is greater if ambient plasma glucose levels are exceptionally high. This has led some researchers to consider diabetes as an accelerated model for this aspect of ageing.

Neuroendocrine theories of ageing, in particular involving insulin signalling, have moved the emphasis back towards genomic events with the discovery of the *sir2* (silent information regulator) gene regulating insulin production, DNA repair and protein synthesis.[21] Overexpression of *sir2* in simple animals such as the nematode worm can almost double maximum lifespan and the mammalian variants (*SIRT1–7*) have roles in neuronal survival, pancreatic cell survival, insulin secretion, altered gluconeogenesis and enhanced ATP production.[22] It remains to be seen whether manipulation of these genes can enhance human health and survival but the broad role of 'sirtuins' in fundamental aspects of metabolic control and homeostasis suggest that these are promising targets for the future.

Germ cell ageing

Unlike the soma, the germ line is required to be effectively immortal. So the question arises, how can these cells escape or slow down changes that are affecting the rest of the body? At the DNA level, germ cells have an additional battery of maintenance enzymes. Together with stem cells, they express the enzyme telomerase, which effectively replaces lost or damaged telomeres and so maintains maximal telomere length. They also contain highly efficient repair enzymes for the remainder of the DNA, ensuring genomic stability for longer than somatic cells.[23] In addition, there is cell selection at progressive stages for example primordial germ cells, gametogenesis and inter-gamete competition. However, the process is not perfect and aneuploidies (any deviation from an exact multiple of the haploid number of chromosomes) are detected in about 5% of oocytes from women aged 30 years and increase exponentially to over one-half of all oocytes from women in their mid-40s.[24]

The menopause and ageing theory

The existence of the menopause at what has seemed to be an invariable stage of life, about 50 years of age, could be regarded as evidence for programmed ageing. But what do we know about the evolutionary events that may have led to menopause and does this have any bearing on longevity? Will increased longevity affect fecundity? The disposable soma theory would predict that increased longevity would ultimately lead to reduced fecundity and this seemingly counterintuitive suggestion is indeed supported by comparison with various animal species. Short-lived animals with short reproductive lifespans (such as mice, rats and rabbits) have considerably more offspring compared with long-lived species with long reproductive lifespans (such as elephants and primates). But what about the relationship in human populations?

For current Western populations, estimated maximum longevity (not average lifespan) is increasing at a rate of just over 1 year per decade. This coincides with an observed increase in the age of menopause by approximately 0.6–1 year per decade in two cohorts that have been studied.[25,26] Since maximum longevity does not appear to be reaching a plateau, will age at menopause continue to correlate with longevity and therefore occur at later ages in the future? This might be possible if the processes that contribute to longevity (improved cell maintenance and repair) also contribute to improved maintenance of the germ line and thus increase the chances of successful pregnancy at older ages. Conversely, will the known prenatal effects on ovum development predominate, so that the longevity and menopausal age become more dissociated? What will be the overall effect on fecundity of an increase in the reproductive lifespan because of an earlier menarche or a later menopause?

Theories about the relationship of longevity to the menopause have considered whether this relationship is adaptive or not. An important contribution to increased human lifespan is thought to be the development of increased brain size some 0.5–1.5 million years ago.[27] Increased cognitive power would have conferred survival advantages through predator avoidance, more sophisticated and successful food-gathering strategies and development of complex societies. At the same time, giving birth would have become riskier for the mother, and the infant would have been born premature compared with other primates, thus requiring a prolonged period of nurturing and maternal investment. Adaptive evolutionary theories suggest that an early menopause protects mothers from the increased risks of late childbearing and the children are more likely to survive. This is the basis of the 'mother' effect, which suggests that menopause is a positive adaptation. By extension, the 'grandmother' hypothesis suggests that menopause allows older mothers to care for their adult daughters while they are having their children and so older women contribute to successful rearing of their grandchildren. This idea is supported by data from

Canada using birth and death records from the late 1800s, which show that long-lived grandmothers had more grandchildren and that rates of grandmother mortality accelerated when their daughters reached the end of their reproductive lifespan.[28]

In contrast, non-adaptive strategies have been suggested based on the disposable soma theory; that is, that increased lifespan favours increased cell maintenance but at the expense of reproduction. The menopause is therefore a by-product of longevity.[29] Investigating this proposition is complicated by lack of good historical records from which trends in births, deaths and ages at menopause can be drawn and by the difficulty of accounting for other important influences on death rates such as socio-economic factors. However, data from Finnish populations between 1679 and 1839 suggest that longevity correlates positively with late age at last childbirth, which is taken as a proxy for late menopause.[30] This would seem to argue against the non-adaptive theories since longevity should correlate with reduced fecundity. In another study,[31] the strongest influence on child survival in a Gambian population was found to be the presence of a grandmother during the first 1–2 years of life. The analysis of this population lends support to the adaptive 'grandmother' hypothesis. However, the authors also suggest that it is consistent with the non-adaptive disposable soma theory of ageing since an early menopause could release resources for cell maintenance and therefore longevity. For future womanhood, these issues remain unresolved.

References

1. Charcot JM. *Clinical Lectures on Senile and Chronic Diseases*. London: New Sydenham Society; 1881.
2. Grundy E. The epidemiology of aging. In: Tallis R, Fillit H, Brocklehurst JC, editors. *Brocklehurst's Textbook of Geriatric Medicine and Gerontology*. 5th ed. London: Churchill Livingstone; 1998. p. 1–17.
3. Wrigley EA, Schofield RS. English population history from family reconstitution: summary results 1600–1799. *Popul Stud (Camb)* 1983;37:157–84.
4. Office for National Statistics. Various reports [www.statistics.gov.uk/].
5. Barker DJ. The developmental origins of adult disease. *J Am Coll Nutr* 2004;23(6 Suppl):588S–95S.
6. Fries JF. Aging, natural death, and the compression of morbidity. *N Engl J Med* 1980;303:130–5.
7. Cournil A, Kirkwood TB. If you would live long, choose your parents well. *Trends Genet* 2001;17:233–5.
8. Kirkwood TB, Rose MR. Evolution of senescence: late survival sacrificed for reproduction. *Philos Trans R Soc Lond B Biol Sci* 1991;332:15–24.
9. Strehler BL. *Time, Cells and Life*. New York and London: Academic Press; 1964.
10. Rowe JW, Kahn RL. Human aging: usual and successful. *Science* 1987;237:143–9.
11. Gaubatz JW, Tan BH. Aging affects the levels of DNA damage in postmitotic cells. *Ann N Y Acad Sci* 1994;719:97–107.
12. Giacomoni PU, D'Alessio P. Skin ageing: the relevance of antioxidants. In: Rattan SIS, Toussaint O, editors. *Molecular Gerontology. Research Status and Strategies*. New York: Plenum Press; 1996. p. 177–92.
13. Lombard DB, Chua KF, Mostoslavsky R, Franco S, Gostissa M, Alt FW. DNA repair, genome stability, and aging. *Cell* 2005;120:497–512.
14. Muller FL, Lustgarten MS, Jang Y, Richardson A, Van Remmen H. Trends in oxidative aging theories. *J Free Radic Biol Med* 2007;43:477–503.
15. Holliday R. *Understanding Ageing*. Cambridge: Cambridge University Press; 1995.
16. Hayflick L, Moorhead PS. The serial cultivation of human diploid cell strains. *Exp Cell Res* 1961;25:585–621.
17. Passos JF, Saretzki G, von Zglinicki T. DNA damage in telomeres and mitochondria during cellular senescence: is there a connection? *Nucleic Acids Res* 2007;35:7505–13.

18. Faragher RGA, Kipling D. How might replicative senescence contribute to human ageing? *Bioessays* 1998;20:985–91.

19. Pang CY, Ma YS, Wei YU. MtDNA mutations, functional decline and turnover of mitochondria in aging. *Front Biosci* 2008; 13:3661–75.

20. Baynes JW. The role of AGEs in aging: causation or correlation. *Exp Gerontol* 2001;36:1527–37.

21. Pallàs M, Verdaguer E, Tajes M, Gutierrez-Cuesta J, Camins A. Modulation of sirtuins: new targets for antiageing. *Recent Pat CNS Drug Discov* 2008;3:61–9.

22. Haigis MC, Guarente LP. Mammalian sirtuins – emerging roles in physiology, aging, and calorie restriction. *Genes Dev* 2006;20:2913–21.

23. Kirkwood TBL. Sex and ageing. *Exp Gerontol* 2001;36:413–18.

24. Pellestor F, Andréo B, Arnal F, Humeau C, Demaille J. Maternal aging and chromosomal abnormalities: new data drawn from *in vitro* unfertilized human oocytes. *Hum Genet* 2003;112:195–203.

25. Rödström K, Bengtsson C, Milsom I, Lissner L, Sundh V, Bjoürkelund C. Evidence for a secular trend in menopausal age: a population study of women in Gothenburg. *Menopause* 2003;10:538–43.

26. Nichols HB, Trentham-Dietz A, Hampton JM, Titus-Ernstoff L, Egan KM, Willett WC, *et al.* From menarche to menopause: trends among US Women born from 1912 to 1969. *Am J Epidemiol* 2006;164:1003–11.

27. Kirkwood TB. Understanding ageing from an evolutionary perspective. *J Intern Med* 2008;263:117–27.

28. Lahdenperä M, Lummaa V, Helle S, Tremblay M, Russell AF. Fitness benefits of prolonged post-reproductive lifespan in women. *Nature* 2004;428:178–81.

29. Wu JM, Zelinski MB, Ingram DK, Ottinger MA. Ovarian aging and menopause: current theories, hypotheses, and research models. *Exp Biol Med (Maywood)* 2005;230:818–28.

30. Helle S, Lummaa V, Jokela J. Are reproductive and somatic senescence coupled in humans? Late, but not early, reproduction correlated with longevity in historical Sami women. *Proc Biol Sci* 2005;272:29–37.

31. Shanley DP, Sear R, Mace R, Kirkwood TB. Testing evolutionary theories of menopause. *Proc Biol Sci* 2007;274:2943–9.

32. Office for National Statistics. *Mortality Statistics: General. Review of the Registrar General on Deaths in England and Wales, 1997*, Series DH1 no. 30. London: The Stationery Office; 1999.

33. Office for National Statistics. News release, 30 October 2008.

34. *House* magazine, 24 June 1991, table on p. 19.

35. Government Actuary's Department. 2006-based national population projections [www.gad.gov.uk/].

Chapter 2
Culture and reproductive ageing

Maya Unnithan

Introduction

Reproductive ageing is a contextual process that is made meaningful through cultural construction (notions of the body, morality and appropriate reproductive behaviour) and gendered experience (of individual women and men to physiological change and in terms of the social expectations that accompany them). It cannot be de-contextualised.

The relevance of a cultural and anthropological perspective is that it focuses on the lived experience of ageing and the associated diverse meanings that inform people's health-seeking behaviour in response to it. It is ethnographic in the sense of being characterised as the first-hand study of a specific community, not necessarily located in the same place. The focus is on obtaining diverse local perceptions through the intense engagement of the researcher in the life worlds of members of the community. The ethnographic example is the basis upon which theoretical and comparative generalisations are then made. An ethnographic perspective on the ways in which ageing is conceptualised, experienced and acted upon is important as it facilitates an emic (actor-centred) and interpretive understanding beyond the insights provided by statistics and data on prevalence. Such an analysis is critical in the sense that it is able to provide explanations as to why the statistics are as they are.

Cultural studies on reproduction and ageing tend to focus on three key issues:

- the body and diverse meanings attributed to bodily processes (how does procreation take place, who 'owns' the body)
- morality/religion (what is appropriate reproductive behaviour)
- social hierarchy/power (who has more reproductive work, responsibility and entitlement).

The various ways in which these aspects combine lead to differences but also similarities across cultures. Equally, there are variations within groups sharing the same broad cultural framework on the basis of wealth, education and strength of belief, for example.

New theoretical social science perspectives of the body (as an agent in its own world construction) are critical to understanding how the body can be a site that both represents cultural expectation and influences the processes that shape it. The body has increasingly become the focus of intense social science research as it provides key insights into the practice and experience of institutionalised power over individuals as well as in the control and management of human populations.[1-3] The reproductive body is, for example, regarded as symbolic of societal norms and values at the same time as it represents societal forms of control.[2,4,5] Anthropological work on the body has shown it to be a means of understanding individual, familial and cultural anxieties to do with reproduction, ageing and death. The ageing or post-reproductive body has been linked to societal concerns about the care of the elderly[6] or of a rampant modernity.[7] In some contexts, the act of birthing or the expenditure of reproductive energy is itself linked to ageing.[8]

There have been several cultural, anthropologically based studies on reproductive ageing since the 1990s.[8,9] These have been mainly based in the USA, Japan and West Africa. There has, however, been no specific ethnographic study on reproductive ageing in the UK, where anthropological work on human reproduction has tended to focus on the implications of the technologies of assisted conception for ideas of kinship, relatedness and ethics.[4,10-13] The role of reproductive technologies in the creation of new forms of parenthood (genetic, surrogate) and the blurring of generational differences among kin have been of particular interest. Other work of note has focused on the ways in which the advent of biotechnology has changed the meaning of what it is to be biological.[11,14] There is, nevertheless, a major gap in the culturally informed knowledge about reproductive ageing in this country, an important area for contribution by the social sciences.

The next section of this chapter sets out what an ethnographic perspective entails and its significance in understanding reproductive ageing. The following sections discuss the kinds of variation that exist within populations thought to be culturally similar and some of the challenges that the cultural perspectives present to current dominant thinking on reproductive ageing. The final section briefly concludes with a few recommendations for future work and policy.

Reproductive ageing in ethnographic context

In the following lines, I draw on some examples of the ideas and practices to do with the menopause, infertility and childbearing in differing social and cultural contexts to illustrate the importance of an ethnographic perspective.

Ageing and menopause in rural north India

Most rural Rajasthani women across caste believe that it is immoral to engage in reproductive activity once their children have been married, especially when there is a daughter-in-law in the house. In this sense, they tend to experience social regulation of their fertility irrespective of whether their menstrual cycle has ceased. For women, the cessation of menstruation is itself not a ritually or socially marked life-course transition. In fact, there is a noted absence of any discussion of menopausal symptoms or related health-seeking behaviour.[15-18] The physiological symptoms associated with the end of menstrual cycles, such as hot flushes and night sweats noted in Euro-American contexts, are lacking or not considered significant to report. The ages of women undergoing the perimenopause are also difficult to determine as most village-born women are unaware of their precise dates of birth. A clinically based study of rural north Indian women suggests an average age of 44 years for the cessation of menstruation, with a percentage of women reported to have a premature menopause at age 30–34 years (17 million women or 3.1% of the population) and at age 34–39 years (44 million or 8% of the population).[19,20]

Studies on gender, body and ageing in India tend to suggest that any physiological symptoms that could be associated with the end of menstruation tend to be subsumed within wider ideas of ageing: a process where the body becomes 'dry' and 'cold' as opposed to the 'wetness' and 'heat' of more youthful constitutions.[21] Cultural notions of the body suggest that women's bodies cease to be 'hot' (procreative) because they are no longer 'open' (to the passage of reproductive substances) once they experience an absence of their menstrual cycles. This 'closing-off' of the body increases its purity (previously denied because of an association with impure menstrual blood) and is accompanied by an increased social status and authority. Women whose bodies become cold and dry attain male attributes and a related social power. The power associated with ageing is reflected for women in the fewer constraints on their mobility in terms of visits to friends and family and their time spent away from housework in general.

Older men, in the same context, are expected to cease their involvement with household duties and married life altogether and to seek spirituality. For Indian men, reproductive ageing is conceptualised as marking the social transition from householder to ascetic, as set out in the Hindu *shastra*. The ascetic stage of life includes the renunciation of all worldly possessions and passions, including those of sex.

A woman's increase in social status is relative to the declining household authority that she and her husband face as they grow old. Especially in joint family arrangements, the elderly are expected to give up their authority in exchange for care and security provided by their son and daughter-in-law. Married women are expected to provide day-to day care for their parents-in-law whereas adult sons are expected to provide financial support for their parents and any unmarried siblings, and there are similar expectations among Pakistani families at home and in Britain.[22] Contemporary debates in India around ageing are therefore not based so much on the biological symptoms of ageing as they are about social issues: the decline of the joint family and the inability of nuclear families to take care of ageing parents, and the threat that modernisation brings in terms of the respect for the elderly.[7] This is in contrast to the bodily discomfort, related anxieties about sexuality and health and the lower societal esteem that accompany the end-of-menstrual experiences of women in European and North American societies.[2,6]

Reproductive ageing in Japan

Anthropological work on the cessation of menstruation in Japan[6,9] also highlights its embeddedness within wider social processes. The end of menstruation is locally conceptualised as one contributing factor in a wider and gradual ageing process (*konenki*) for women and men aged 45–60 years. For Japanese women, the end of menstruation is regarded as leaving 'stale' blood in the body (an idea commonly found in Sino/Japanese medicine)[23] that causes a number of non-specific symptoms such as dizziness, palpitations, headaches, chilliness, stiff shoulders and a dry mouth.[23] In terms of the conditions as well, there appears to be no clear distinction between the ageing of men and women. Japanese women rarely consult a gynaecologist for ageing-related concerns. In fact, there is a popular understanding that only weak-minded women allow themselves to be disrupted by this life-cycle transition and that women should 'ride-over' *konenki*.[23]

As in the Indian case mentioned above, the debates around women's ageing in Japan are not so much about their health but more about their role as caregivers in an ageing society where both men and women are regarded as moving towards bodily fragility and an inability to contribute to work or care for the family. Unlike India, however, Japan is among the post-industrial countries with a highly developed and relatively accessible medical system. Nevertheless, it is social expectation that orients health-seeking behaviour (or its absence) in the domain of ageing, placing constraints on the resort to technological intervention.

Changing perceptions of menopause in Newfoundland

Research carried out over a 10-year period among a fishing community in Newfoundland has shown how the undermining of public collective life as a consequence of modernisation has led to changing perceptions of the body and a rise in medical perspectives on health and ageing.[24] Folk idioms of nerves and blood dominated local discourse of health in this area in the 1970s. Women's lives were characterised by 'hardship, worry, self-sacrifice and endurance which use up one's nerves'. Worn-out nerves cause problems on 'the change' (word for menopause). The change of life was welcomed by many women as the flushes and heavy bleeding were thought to burn away the impurities that could build up in the blood in the postmenopausal years.

Davis[24] argues that a declining transmission of folk knowledge about the body led to a decline in the value attributed to local knowledge about reproductive ageing. This was replaced by an increasing consultation with medical doctors. Increasingly, reproductive ageing comes to be viewed as related to womb dysfunction and cancer (although not with heart disease or osteoporosis) and as a time for hysterectomy and hormone replacement therapy to combat an estrogen deficiency. Talk about the body in the 1970s, Davis observes, was about everything else but the physical body; in the late 1980s, talk about the body had become talk about the physical body. Davis's findings show how ideas about reproductive ageing shift with the changing nature of interpersonal relations as well as an attendant medicalisation. The common metaphor of nerves and blood used by women to talk about ageing and other bodily conditions in the Newfoundland community she studied became associated with an older out-of-touch generation in a fast urbanising and modernising world. Davis's study especially highlights the fact that the social responses to ageing can differ across generations within a specified cultural context.

Infertility and the extension of reproductive life

Infertility is not a condition restricted to the Western world as it occurs globally. It is widespread, especially in poorer and highly populated countries such as in sub-Saharan Africa, South Asia and the Middle East and it is even prevalent in South East Asia although to a lesser extent (1–2% of the population).[25]

Infertility has in general been a neglected issue for policymakers in resource-poor and highly populated countries, where fertility control is the top priority of state planners.[26,27] Infertility has also been a neglected area of study within the social sciences because of its strong association with physiological pathology (as a disease or organ dysfunction) rather than with its social consequences.[25]

In resource-poor countries where the state does not provide any form of financial security, childlessness has critical consequences for the survival of families and households. In these contexts, the ability to bear children is highly valued for three main reasons:

- the social and economic security it provides
- the related social power and status connected with the wealth in human and physical resources
- social perpetuity (social reproduction of the family and group).

Universal clinical definitions of infertility may have little relevance for those who experience it in different locations around the world. For instance, in some social groups in India, Africa and the Middle East, infertility is culturally defined as the inability of women to produce sons[25,28] or their inability to become pregnant within the first few months of marriage. These definitions point towards the anxieties and related significance placed upon childbearing, a burden faced especially by women in these countries. While infertile men and women both face stigma, it is more strongly associated with women's inability to bear children. Infertile women often face an insecure marriage, either being prone to divorce or having to accept a co-wife. Men's infertility is much more difficult to establish in these contexts, largely because of the threat to their virility and social standing that such aspersions would entail.

The gender differences existing in relation to infertility arise from the differential ways in which the genders are associated with reproduction, their reproductive contribution and related entitlements. In Egypt and also in parts of India, men are regarded as contributing, with their sperm, a fully formed fetus (thus owning their offspring) which is only nurtured with the woman's womb and her blood.[25] Infertility is seen to arise as a defect of nurturance rather than procreation. Such notions serve to reinforce the superiority of men over women, at the same time as the individual woman's 'worth' becomes dependent on her fertility and the quantity and the 'quality' (sex, health) of offspring to which she gives birth. In many societies, infertility is attributed to supernatural causes and therefore divine intervention is regarded as the most efficacious. Attributing causality to an external agent is also helpful in alleviating the blame of infertility from falling solely upon the woman (a notable difference from the association of blame with biological dysfunction associated with infertile bodies in the West).

The tremendous anxiety relating to the infertility of women and the related social implications that this has for their husbands and the wider family is manifest in the great extent to which external intervention is sought for these conditions. Studies on the health-seeking behaviour of infertile women and couples in Africa and South Asia suggest that religious healers are widely sought out. There is an equal resort to medical intervention, often alongside or after consultation with religious healers has taken place.[15,26,29] Paradoxically, the medical provision of infertility services in itself contributes to increasing the incidence of secondary sterility, as most of the providers are unqualified doctors.[27]

Religious ideas also tend to limit the options provided by medical intervention, depending upon what is regarded as a morally acceptable intervention. Inhorn's work on Egypt and Lebanon[30] shows, for example, that with regard to Sunni views on fertility treatment, artificial insemination with the husband's semen is allowed whereas third-party donation of any kind is disallowed (*haram*) as it would be akin to *zina* (adultery or prostitution) and confuse kinship, descent and inheritance. The tie by *nasab*/lineage or relation by blood is considered to be one of God's great gifts to his worshippers.[31] In Shia Islamic interpretations, on the other hand, donated egg and sperm are allowed, although the resulting offspring have no inheritance rights. A largely similar position is found among South Asian families in the UK, although less concern was expressed over donated eggs compared with donated sperm.[32]

Similar concerns to do with incest and adultery emerge in British views on sperm and egg donation.[10,33] Edwards's study[10] in the 1990s of views on *in vitro* fertilisation held by a group of people living in north-west England found that, while there was a fear of incest associated with the anonymous donation of eggs, donations between known or related individuals such as between daughter and mother, or between sister and sister, were problematic in maintaining the appropriate order and authority of social relations between them.

Surrogacy is a medical intervention that appears to have the most social sanction attached to it. All forms of surrogacy, including gestational surrogacy, are disallowed across Shia and Sunni Islam. In the UK as well, surrogacy has been subject to some debate. In 1984, the Warnock report[34] prohibited surrogacy on the grounds that the bonds formed through gestation between mother and child determined motherhood. Surrogacy was considered 'unnatural' in that it interrupted the connection between gestation and birth considered so vital to motherhood. Surrogate arrangements are now among the various fertility treatments recognised by the Human Fertilisation and Embryology Authority to be made especially available to those women who are at medical risk if they become pregnant.[35]

Studies in the USA have shown that surrogacy has become a popular way for infertile couples to have children, with gestational surrogacy (donated ova) preferred over traditional surrogacy, where the ova of the surrogate mother are used.[36,37] This is connected with the increasing tendency to disregard gestation as central to motherhood in favour of maintaining a genetic link with the child. It also enables a wider range of surrogate mothers (from diverse ethnic backgrounds, for example) to be commissioned. Widespread popular science education on gametes and DNA also allows the acceptance of a genetic basis to surrogacy in the USA and UK, although this is yet to be recognised in a legal sense.[38]

There are a number of issues that emerge from such cultural and gender-based understandings of infertility that are of particular relevance to the provision of health services. The examples above highlight why certain groups and individuals seek medical intervention and others primarily seek divine intervention. But the question that arises in a context of limited medical resources is about who has access to such services and how this gets determined; that is, about who is regarded as having a greater need for infertility services and the role that cultural constructions of gender and sex play here. Are men and women equally evaluated in terms of the needs? What about the needs of infertile gay and lesbian couples within the populations discussed above? It is likely, given the heterosexual norms that dominate the ideas of reproduction and parenthood, that infertility may be dismissed as a problem for lesbian and gay individuals. There is a dearth of social science work in the UK that focuses on infertile gay and lesbian couples who desire children and seek treatment.

Ageing at each childbirth in the Gambia

Bledsoe[8] turns our attention to the connections made between reproductive ageing and childbearing by the Gambian women in her area of study. Here, every birth episode is regarded as a traumatic assault on the health of women, whose bodies age as a result. To halt this ageing associated with childbirth, women require a 'recovery period'. Contraceptives are popular, especially with women who have experienced child loss, because they enable women to procure periods of 'recovery' and halt the bodily ageing commonly associated with childbearing among the Gambian communities in Bledsoe's study.[8] The Gambian example shows ageing to be contingent upon obstetric trauma from which recovery or the ability to halt or slow down the process is possible following each episode. This is a very different understanding of ageing from the Western notion of ageing and the ability to reproduce as connected with the passage of time.

Reproductive ageing beyond 'culture': variation within populations

It is important to recognise that 'culture' is not a consensual system of interconnected ideologies, beliefs and practices associated with a specific and homogeneous social group. For the purposes of this discussion, this means that ideas and practices to do with reproduction and ageing are unlikely to be uniformly shared by all members of a group. There are variations that exist within populations who subscribe to the same cultural ideology depending on, for example, their economic and education levels (lower/middle classes), different modes of production and lifestyles (rural/urban), as well as ethnic and religious differences. Class differences are a good example of the variation that can exist within populations, where groups having a similar genetic make-up have different responses to reproductive ageing. So, for example, the desire for an extension to reproductive life through medical intervention may be based on the criteria of a woman's employment and her class-based aspirations.

Economic differentiation/class

In India, it is primarily village-based women who seek an early 'release' from their childbearing. Reversible contraception is rarely used and tubal ligations are popular among women who have achieved the desired sex and number of offspring. Middle and upper middle class women who are employed and are usually town-based, on the other hand, seek to delay and space their children and thus extend their reproductive lives. In contrast to rural women, middle and upper middle class women, especially those who are employed, tend to use contraceptives such as the pill (*mala D*), condoms (*nirodh*), intrauterine devices such as the copper T, or a diaphragm.[39] These women, who live in urban and more nuclear family contexts, seek to balance childrearing with waged employment. Among these women are also those who contemplate an extension to their reproductive lives and the benefits of hormone replacement therapy. The wider contexts of social and economic mobility embedded within middle and upper middle class women's employment thus produces a very different response despite being part of a wider population that places great value on childbearing.

Women in better-off households are able to afford to pay for the latest technologies. *In vitro* fertilisation, for example, is fast gaining popularity in the Middle East, South and South East Asia. It is offered primarily by the private health sector and therefore available mainly to those who are able to pay for such services (in some cases, poorer households have also been found to invest a substantial portion of their household income to secure improved reproductive outcomes).

Body ideals also vary according to class. For example, in certain Middle Eastern and North African societies such as the Tuareg,[40,41] a woman's fat body symbolises the wealth of her husband. Only wealthy households can afford to feed women to such an extent where they cannot participate in household labour processes. Among the Tuareg, where fatness is a socially desirable gender characteristic, obesity in women is not stigmatised. There is no direct connection made between fatness as a means to enhance fertility nor do people consider it to inhibit fertility.[42] However, in populations where fatness is socially undesirable, fat women may find it difficult to obtain partners, thus restricting their role in reproduction.

Economic variation is itself historically contingent. Schneider and Schneider[43] found that the high fertility of peasant (*braccianti*) families in Sicily during the interwar years in Europe was connected to the decline of fertility of the landed gentry (*burghisi*) and their exploitation of peasant women as domestic workers in their households. Busy peasant mothers would wean their babies early and lose the protection of their lactative amenorrhoea against a new conception. The differing reproductive patterns of the two classes can only be understood in terms of their interdependence and the exploitation of one over the other. The example also illustrates how peasant fertility behaviour shifts with the passage of time and was connected with economic independence of the peasantry as in the post-war years in Sicily.

Religious differences and similarities

Notions of procreation may be similar but may also differ across religions and are important in determining local ideas of fertility and reproductive health-seeking behaviour.

In rural Rajasthan, Sunni Muslim and Hindu caste women share ideas of childbearing as a duty to one's family and as a main function of women. Sunni Muslim women have a strong sense of childbearing as destiny (that each woman has a certain number of children 'written' in her fate as it is the will of God) and that it is their duty to carry them to term.[15] The anxieties of being unable to establish one's fertility and the fear of subsequent sterility (borne out by its high prevalence) mean that any form of contraception is approached with unease, even among younger women. It is only older women who contemplate contraception when they achieve the desired number and sex of their children. Older women prefer to terminate their childbearing altogether by recourse to tubal ligation. While both Hindu and Muslim women are desirous of sterilisation, it is approached with greater deliberation by Muslim women, depending on how orthodox the community and/or head of household is in their interpretation of the Quran.

In Islam, the correct action (including in reproductive matters) to be undertaken by devout Muslims is set out in the Quran or *hadith*. Nevertheless, there are differences within Islam depending on the interpretation of these texts. Religious judgements are arrived at by religious leaders through a process of *ijtihad* or the discussion of various interpretations and application of personal and analogous reasoning. This is especially the case when there is an absence or ambiguity in the Quranic instruction, such as to do with medical intervention in reproduction.[31] It is the duty of religious leaders to issue *fatwa*s (non-binding religious opinions) that guide the public as to whether the reproductive intervention they are contemplating is obligatory (*wajib*), recommended (*sunna*), permitted (*mubah/hallal*), disfavoured (*makruh*) or forbidden *(haram)*. The use of all reproductive technologies is not prohibited in Islam, as is popularly believed. In the case of infertility, certain techniques are expressly desired because they make possible the creation of *nasab* (a kin tie) between previously infertile parents and their subsequent babies.[31,44]

Kahn's study[33] on infertility among the ultra-orthodox Jewish community in Israel shows a similar religious accommodation to medical intervention taking place. The Hasidic community there places great value on childbearing and, consequently, women who are unable to do so face social stigma. Their religious doctrine forbids the use of another Jewish man's sperm by an infertile wife (which would be considered adultery, as in Islam). However, the sperm of a non-Jewish donor is acceptable because genetic heritage is considered to be matrilineal and pass through the mother. Thus, *in vitro* fertilisation using specific sperm is religiously sanctioned while religious restrictions apply to such interventions more generally.

Challenges to the dominant paradigm on ageing

Relation of biology to culture

The association of reproductive ageing with each childbearing and birth, as in the Gambian example, underscores a key anthropological understanding of the relationship between biology and culture: it can be non-linear and culture can influence biological ageing, bringing it forward or delaying it. Such a relationship is also evident, although less dramatically, in the case of rural north Indian women who 'age', in that they cease to bear children once they become mothers-in-law, even though they may still be biologically fertile. These ideas challenge the linear relationship between biology and culture that dominates notions of ageing in European and North American societies.

The cross-cultural studies on reproductive ageing in India, Japan and the Gambia as discussed above also show that there is no standard or common physiological experience for women at the end of their menstruation. Physiological end-of-menstruation experiences may further vary depending on an individual's 'local biology'; that is, family genetic history, the effects of a pregnant woman's diet, alcohol consumption, smoking and medication on the female fetus. Menopause then becomes a product of a continuing dialectic between 'biology' and culture, in which both are contingent.[6,9,23]

The relationship between biology and culture is further complicated when we take into consideration that cultural ideas of the body are themselves shaped by scientific understanding, technological breakthroughs, pharmaceutical marketing and media coverage. As Davis's work in Newfoundland[24] demonstrates, cultural understandings of the end of menstruation have become more medicalised for the younger generation. An increasing cultural emphasis on the somatisation or physical manifestation of menopausal symptoms, in the USA and the UK for example, can be related to the promotion of a hormonal consciousness among the lay public, fuelled by the debates around the safety of hormonal replacement therapies.[2,6]

Reproductive ageing and the language of decline in clinical medicine

Martin[2] shows that the depictions of menopause and menstruation in the medical literature are made in a negative sense and are regarded primarily in terms of 'failed reproduction' (menstruation as the failure to produce a fetus). This modern medical description of reproductive processes in terms of failure not only pervades medical thinking on the issue, it dominates cultural understandings of reproduction. Anthropological studies suggest that this can result in feelings of bodily and societal alienation, especially when medical descriptions do not capture women's subjective experiences.

Martin suggests that the negative stereotypes associated with ageing women in the West are a direct product of viewing the body in a specific way – as a hierarchical information processing system. Ageing, as in menopause, represents the atrophy, decline and functionlessness of the body, resulting in the breakdown of its information system and its authority. Such views are well captured in the language of medicine: 'the cause of ovarian decline is the decreasing ability of the ageing ovaries to respond to pituitary gonadotrophins … At every point the systems fails and falters. Follicles "fail to muster the strength" to reach ovulation. As functions fail, so do the members of the system decline …, breasts and genital organs gradually atrophy, "wither" and become "senile". Everywhere there is regression, decline, atrophy, shrinkage, and disturbance.'[2] Martin suggests that these images of broken-down hierarchy and dysfunction induce tremendous anxiety in the technologically advanced (and well-organised) societies in which we live. The kind of break-down images associated with ageing at the same time are suggestive of particular kinds of remedial actions such as hormonal replacement therapies, that need to be undertaken to regain physical control over our bodies.

Given the power that medical language and images exert over popular consciousness, including feelings of wellbeing in the West, Martin suggests that medical texts use positive images of reproductive processes. These could be, for example, a view that menstrual blood is a desired product of the female cycle, that the hypothalamus, the pituitary and the ovaries work together to produce pregnancies but also to avoid them, and that menopause is a 'quieter' level of interaction between them. A more positive language of reproductive ageing may in turn bring psychosocial benefits for women who are anxious about ageing and the loss of social worth (of beauty, sexual desirability, health and the capacity to participate fully in society) that this entails.

It is also worth noting that reproductive ageing and the related language of decline has been primarily associated with women, reinforcing the connection of women with physical ageing and constituting them as 'natural' subjects for medical intervention compared with men (reflected, for example, in the growth of gynaecology as a discipline as contrasted with the underdevelopment of a science of masculinity).[45] The invisibility of the male reproductive body in science and popular consciousness has been challenged in the late 1990s by the emergence of Viagra® (Pfizer) as a treatment for male impotence.[45] As Oudshoorn,[45] among others, suggests, the spectacular demand for Viagra, the fastest selling drug in the USA in the year it was first marketed, points to the concern with declining male fertility and the attempts to defer male ageing. It also points to the fact that men may now suffer social anxieties related to their fertility that are similar to women and, in turn, have a related need for health services.

Summary

Ageing is a lived experience that should be studied in social and cultural terms, beyond the statistics that indicate its prevalence. There is a lack of sufficient understanding of such issues in the UK. It is important to encourage ethnographic and qualitative work on reproductive ageing in the UK that complements the demographic and clinical, quantitative perspectives.

In terms of service provision, it is important to acknowledge and address the economic, social and religious variation within populations sharing the same cultural ideology. It is also important to understand how these change over time. The inequalities in provision of and access to care that are based on different understandings of the role of class, education, region, ethnic or religious differences, or any combination of these, need to be understood and addressed in wider social as well as clinical terms.

Policies should encourage a gender- and sexuality-based perspective on ageing that recognises that the experiences of fertility, infertility and reproductive ageing are products of the unequal relations between the sexes. This will include implementing measures to counter any exclusion that is based on inequalities, for example through encouraging men to undertake equal roles and responsibilities regarding fertility and infertility. The measures should be extended across social groups and consider provision of services to those who may be excluded in gender and sexuality terms, such as men in terms of their reproductive ageing concerns and lesbian and gay couples.

Last but not least, there will be an advantage to promoting positive images of reproductive ageing through medical and popular language and representations and targeting both young and elderly populations, and both women and men.

References

1. Foucault M. *Birth of the Clinic*. London: Tavistock; 1975.
2. Martin E. *The Woman in the Body: A Cultural Analysis of Reproduction*. Boston: Beacon Press; 1987.
3. Scheper-Hughes N, Lock M. The mindful body: a prolegomenon to future work in medical anthropology. *Med Anthropol Q* 1987;1:6–41.
4. Strathern M. *Reproducing the Future: Anthropology, Kinship and the New Reproductive Technologies*. Manchester: Manchester University Press; 1992.
5. Bordo S. *Unbearable Weight: Feminism, Western Culture and the Body*. Berkeley: University of California Press; 1993.
6. Lock M. *Encounters with Aging: Mythologies of Menopause in Japan and N. America*. Berkeley: University of California Press; 1993.
7. Cohen L. *No Aging in India: Alzheimer's, the Bad Family and Other Modern Things*. Berkeley: University of California Press; 1998.
8. Bledsoe C. *Contingent Lives: Fertility, Time and Aging in West Africa*. Chicago: University of Chicago Press; 2002.
9. Lock M. Menopause: Lessons from anthropology. *Psychosom Med* 1998;60:410–19.
10. Edwards J, Franklin S, Hirsch E, Price F, Strathern M, editors. *Technologies of Procreation: Kinship in the Age of Assisted Conception*. London: Routledge; 1993.
11. Franklin S. *Embodied Progress: A Cultural Account of Assisted Conception*. London: Routledge; 1997.
12. Konrad, M. From secrets of life to the life of secrets: tracing genetic kowledge as genealogical ethics in biomedical Britain. *J Roy Anthrop Inst* 2003;9:339–58.
13. Featherstone K, Atkinson P, Bharadwaj A, Clarke A. editors. *Risky Relations: Family, Kinship and the New Genetics*. Oxford: Berg Publishers; 2006.
14. Rose N. *The Politics of Life Itself*. Princeton: Princeton University Press; 2007.
15. Unnithan-Kumar M. Emotion, agency and access to healthcare: women's experiences of reproduction in Jaipur. In: Tremayne S, editor. *Managing Reproductive Life: Cross-cultural Themes in Fertility and Sexuality*. Oxford: Berghahn Books; 2001.
16. Unnithan-Kumar M. Midwives among others: knowledges of healing and the politics of emotions. In: Rozario S, Samuels G, editors. *Daughters of Hariti: Birth and Female Healers in South and Southeast Asia. Theory and Practice in Medical Anthropology and International Health*. London: Routledge; 2002.
17. Unnithan-Kumar M. Reproduction, health, rights: connections and disconnections. In: Mitchell J, Wilson R, editors. *Human Rights in Global Perspective: Anthropology of Rights, Claims and Entitlements*. London: Routledge; 2003.
18. Unnithan-Kumar M. Spirits of the womb: migration, reproductive choice and healing in Rajasthan. *Contrib Indian Sociol* 2003;37:16–188.
19. Singh A, Arora AK. Profile of menopausal women in rural North India. *Climacteric* 2005;8;177–84.
20. Institute of Social and Economic Change. Report on Pre-Mature Menopause. *Times of India*, 23 January 2007.
21. Lamb S. *White Saris and Sweet Mangos: Aging, Gender and Body in North India*. Berkeley: University of California Press; 2000.
22. Shaw A. British Pakistani elderly without children: an invisible minority. In. Kraeger P, Schroder-Butterfill E, editors. *Ageing without Children*. Oxford: Berghahn Books; 2004. p. 198–223.
23. Lock M. The final disruption? Biopolitics of post reproductive life. In: Inhorn M, editor. *Reproductive Disruptions*. Oxford: Berghahn Books; 2007. p. 200–25
24. Davis D. Blood and nerves revisited: menopause and the privatisation of the body in a Newfoundland post industrial fishery. *Med Anthropol Q* 1997;11:3–20.
25. Inhorn M, Van Balen F. *Infertility around the Globe*. Berkeley: University of California Press; 2002.
26. Kielman K. Barren ground: contesting identities of infertile women. In: Lock M, Kaufert P, editors. *Pragmatic Women and Body Politics*. Cambridge: Cambridge University Press; 1998. p. 127–64.
27. Unnithan-Kumar M, editor. *Reproductive Agency, Medicine and the State: Cultural Transformations in Childbearing*. Oxford: Berghahn Books; 2004.

28. Patel T. *Fertility Behaviour: Population and Society in Rajasthan*. Delhi: Oxford University Press, 1994.

29. Cornwall A. Looking for a child: enduring and surviving infertility in Ado-Ado, SW Nigeria. In: Tremayne S, editor. *Managing Reproductive Life*. Oxford: Berghahn, 2001. p. 140–57

30. Inhorn M. *Quest For Conception: Gender, Infertlity and Egyptian Medical Traditions*. Philadelphia: University of Pennsylvania Press; 1994.

31. Inhorn M. *Local Babies and Global Science: Gender, Religion and In Vitro Fertilisation in Egypt*. New York: Routledge; 2003.

32. Culley L, Hudson N. *Public Perceptions of Gamete Donation in British South Asian Communities*. Leicester: Economic and Social Research Council; 2006.

33. Kahn S. *Reproducing Jews: A Cultural Account of Assisted Conception in Israel*. Durham, NC: Duke University Press; 2000.

34. Warnock, M. *Report of the Committee of Inquiry into Human Fertilisation and Embryology*. London: HMSO; 1984.

35. Human Fertilisation and Embryology Authority. *IVF and Other Fertility Treatments Explained*. London: HFEA; 2008 [www.hfea.gov.uk/356.html].

36. Ragone H. The gift of life: surrogate motherhood, gamete donation and constructions of altruism. In: Layne L, editor. *Transformative Motherhood*. New York: NYU Press; 1999.

37. Ragone H. How race is being transfigured by gestational surrogacy. In: Ragone H, Winddance Twine F, editors. *Ideologies and Technologies of Motherhood*. London: Routledge; 2000. p. 56–76

38. Cots-UK (Childlessness Overcome through Surrogacy). *Is Surrogacy Legal in the UK?* Lairg: Cots-UK; 2008 [www.surrogacy.org.uk/FAQ1.htm].

39. International Institute for Population Sciences (IIPS) and ORC Macro. *National Family Health Survey (NFHS-2), India, 1998–99: Rajasthan*. Mumbai: IIPS; 2001.

40. Poppenhoe, R. *Feeding Desire: Fatness, Beauty and Sexuality among a Saharan People*. London: Routledge; 2004.

41. Walenkowitz, S. *Women with Great Weight: Fatness, Reproduction and Gender Dynamics in Tuareg Society*. Oxford: Berghahn (in press).

42. Randall S. Fat and fertility, mobility and slaves: long term perspectives on Tuareg obesity and reproduction. In: Unnithan-Kumar M, Tremayne S, editors. *Fatness and the Maternal Body: Women's Experiences of Corporeality and the Shaping of Social Policy*. Oxford: Berghahn Books (in press).

43. Schneider P, Schneider J. High fertility and poverty in Sicily: beyond the culture vs rationality debate. In: Greehalgh S, editor. *Situating Fertility*. Cambridge: Cambridge University Press; 1995. p. 179–202.

44. Tremayne S. Not All Muslims are Luddites. *Anthropol Today* 2006;22:1–2.

45. Oudshoorn N. *The Male Pill: A Biography of a Technology in the Making*. Durham, NC: Duke University Press; 2003.

Chapter 3
Ageing

Discussion

Peter Braude: I have always believed that women go into menopause because they live too long. The issue is whether the climacteric and the postmenopause years are physiological. It seems to me that menopause is a pathological phenomenon and should be dealt with as such. Therefore saying that 'we don't want HRT' or 'we need HRT' is fallacious because it is not based on understanding physiology.

Jane Preston: It is interesting that you say that. Humans are not alone in having some kind of climacteric, although we have the longest post-reproductive lifespan of all the animals. Some other primates do seem to have a short period of cessation of fertility towards the end of life. The suggestion is that the animal has to achieve a certain length of lifespan in order for that to be seen. With increasing lifespan, primates gradually do show that increase in the post-reproductive lifespan. If any of them were to live close to our age then the suggestion is that menopause would happen. Whether it is pathology or not, I don't know. Data from women who have late menopause suggest they have better health fitness afterwards. That is, they live longer and appear to be healthier. One of the theories is about the need for grandmothers to be available to nurture their children.

Peter Braude: But what happens in primates – gorillas, chimpanzees and so on? Don't the older ageing females tend to get hounded out of packs?

Jane Preston: Not that I have come across, but I don't know.

Siladitya Bhattacharya: You mentioned the association between longevity and late age at childbirth. Could you elaborate upon fertility and longevity?

Jane Preston: Yes. It is very difficult to study – that is the main factor. You need very good data going back over two to three hundred years with dates of birth, deaths and marriage and you have to correct for husband, age at marriage, etc. But there are data to suggest that there is an inverse link between fertility and longevity from information on Northern European aristocrats in the 1500s to 1800s.[1] Women who lived into their 80s had fewer children than their counterparts. There are problems with that data as this is a very select group. Within the other study that I mentioned,[2] which uses a much broader data group within a rural community, there didn't seem to be any change in fertility or fecundity (the number of children that were born), even though women had later menopause. In some of these groups, women didn't have more children within their extended fertile period so they weren't becoming more fecund during that time, but equally they didn't show any drop in fecundity.

Diana Mansour: This may be a political question but I was fascinated by your slide showing the 1970s and 1990s and the effect of social class on longevity. Eyeballing the figures, it seems to be worsening. Could you comment?

Jane Preston: The differential is probably to do with the larger financial gap between social classes 1 and 5 but I am not a demographer so I can't go into that particularly.

Roger Gosden: Following on Peter Braude's comment about the nature and evolution of menopause, our attitudes to it, and perhaps treatment of it, are influenced by whether we think it is physiological or pathological. I happen to hold the same view as Peter on this, although some well-known nonmedical authorities such as Germaine Greer[3] have a completely different view. I would like to point out a paradox. As you rightly point out, everything about ageing that we understand from animal models, and from looking at human populations, suggests that the menopause hasn't evolved as a result of some killer gene. We don't have group selection in evolution according to current evolutionary dogma. We see ageing as being a non-adaptive process by which repair mechanisms and other mechanisms just fail to be supportive at a sufficient level to keep us going a bit longer. It's a trade-off. Now, when we come to the theories such as the mother hypothesis and grandmother hypothesis which have been discussed endlessly, we have here uniquely adaptive theories – completely different to the rest of ageing and I find this rather odd. I don't find the evidence (some of which is mathematical) consistent with some of the animal data – field studies in lions and things like that – where people looked to see whether the grandmother looked after the young and so there'd be a kin selection process. I wondered what your view was about this dichotomy – between menopause being adaptive and evolved for good, whereas everything else about ageing has evolved because evolutionary selection pressure was blind to it.

Jane Preston: Yes, there has been major criticism of both menopause theory and the grandmother hypothesis precisely because they are adaptive: the menopause confers some advantage on the offspring so this is an adaptive response whereas ageing is just a by-product of us having early offspring because we would die out if we didn't. It is a build-up of detriment that has not evolved down. The real proponents of the 'disposable soma' theory are Tom Kirkwood's group who've looked at non-adaptive explanations for menopause.[4] Essentially, the argument is based on a trade-off between fertility and longevity but there is no solid explanation for why it occurs at one particular time in the life course. They have tried to model what happens to population growth if the menopause occurs later. In some populations, it seems that the growth of the population actually declines when the menopause is later – if one accepts the assumptions of their models. When the menopause happens later, populations are predicted to shrink in size, so there is an optimum age for menopause, which correlates with when the population is maximised. We didn't come to a conclusion in the chapter because there is much more research needed. I agree with you that all ageing theories are non-adaptive and ageing is a by-product of what has gone on earlier. It is therefore difficult to see how menopause can be adaptive and be linked to ageing, let alone to be adaptive and to skip a generation, which is unkown in other biological systems.

Donna Dickenson: I want to ask about the correlation between longevity and age of last child. Perhaps I missed something but the pool would not include those that died having their last child early, so the correlation is perhaps a bit doubtful?

Jane Preston: The correlation would be doubtful if mothers were included who died having their last child early because they would have reduced longevity and early age of last childbirth. The study could identify those who died having their last child so those data were not included. Even without that, there was still a correlation between age at last childbirth and longevity.[2]

Melanie Davies: This association that we find between late menopause and longevity is surely no surprise. The same factors that promote late menopause promote healthy ageing and a long life: which are being born into a higher social class, good childhood nutrition and so on.

Jane Preston: Those are the social and economic factors we know about. We didn't necessarily know them from biology. Menopause is essentially a composite between germ cell ageing (ageing of the ovaries) and the whole of the rest of the body ageing. It didn't necessarily hold from biological theory that menopause should go one way or the other. This is why it has been an area of great interest. But, yes, it makes intuitive sense that menopause should increase as longevity increases.

Roger Gosden: Maya, you said many interesting things. One you didn't mention was the judgements of the courts, which is perhaps a specialised aspect that is reflective of society. You mentioned surrogacy, for example. I think you were implying that IVF surrogacy has been preferred to gestational surrogacy because of the genetic line. There are other examples where the courts in this country, and in the USA, have made judgements which very much reflect their attachment to the importance of the genetic line. This also applies to posthumous insemination cases as well as the recent pertinent court judgement in New York. I was wondering whether this attitude of the court is reflective of the society it comes from? We know that way back in the Old Testament there was a precedent, in a way, with Abraham, Sarah and Hagar. Who was the genetic link? And that was chosen through Sarah, his wife. So this genetic element is emphasised in all sorts of different ways. I wonder if you could explain why we seem to attach so much importance to it now, if I am correct in that assumption.

Maya Unnithan: My response would be that what is actually happening is that the way we conceptualise biology is becoming more 'geneticised'. The important thing, in terms of lay people, is to maintain a biological connection. Therefore the genetic relation becomes more important. Work done by Helena Ragone[5] in the USA looked at lots of different kinds of surrogacy arrangement. What she shows, really interestingly, is that it also allows different groups of people, surrogate mothers, to participate. For instance, you would have black women acting as surrogate mothers [for white women]. Because if you could see that, you know it is this genetic link. It is not the gestation that creates the child, but it is coming through a kind of transferred material; linking the child in some way more closely towards the commissioning parents. There are a number of reasons here why a particular view of biology is becoming important. It allows particular kinds of relationship to carry on. In this case it establishes a link between commissioning parents and their offspring. We're actually blocking out anything the surrogate mother has to contribute. At the end of the day – and this may be controversial – legal ideas also come from some kind of cultural basis. I think the patriarchal family gets reflected in it as well. You see that within Islam. You see it also within so-called secular politics

Donna Dickenson: I agree with this point. It is very interesting to use the word 'biological' as if that were 'not genetic'. The surrogate or gestational mother is also doing something biological. Indeed, in UK law, the biological takes precedence in the sense that the gestational mother is the legal mother. This contrasts with the Baby M case* where there was a dispute between the commissioning couple and the surrogate mother who wished to retain the child. The New Jersey Court actually said that the husband could not pay for what was already his. So the baby was already his by virtue of his genetic input. That ownership model does seem to me to rely on a genetic basis and it also influenced subsequent jurisprudence.

Maya Unnithan: It is the ownership of the mother that is more difficult to establish …

Donna Dickenson: … because she could be either genetic or gestational?

Maya Unnithan: That is right. Motherhood is fragmented across social, nurturing, genetic, surrogate, etc.

Donna Dickenson: Motherhood is not only genetic, but the courts are privileging the genetic – which you might say is privileging men.

William Ledger: A fascinating talk, Maya, with lots of interesting areas to explore. The Japanese concept of *konenki* is perhaps a realistic way of people dealing with ageing in their society. Perhaps it is more healthy than the current Western model that ageing is bad and we must all strive to remain ever young. As Japan is becoming more open to Western ideas through the internet, television, pharmaceutical company marketing, etc., I wonder whether there is evidence that the concept of *konenki* is disappearing and being replaced by Western ideas that ageing is evil and menopause is a change for the worse. Do you have any information on this?

Maya Unnithan: The main person whose work would answer your question is Margaret Lock.[6] She has done a lot of work comparing what is happening in Japan and in the USA. What she has found is that this is not the case. In fact, it is the other way. It is being more reinforced in Japan. Even the groups of Japanese who are in the USA seem to continue to follow the ideas of *konenki*. She has also investigated it in terms of things such as organ donation, when the body is considered to be brain-dead. Clinicians within Japan do not make those decisions of shutting off the machine. The medical culture in Japan is also different. It is not just people's ideas but also medical culture itself which is very different. I don't know whether I answered your question but you see that the interesting thing, despite all the technology, is that it is not changing people's minds.

Susan Bewley: You say that the Japanese maintain their views and yet in Newfoundland there was an example of a very rapid change in views. What kind of cultural resilience is there, or what are the differences that make one population vulnerable to change? Maybe it is a good thing to be susceptible to change. Do anthropologists have a view on why views change rapidly or not?

Maya Unnithan: I hide behind the standard explanation that it is a combination of a number of factors, at least that's what Davis says in the Newfoundland case.[7] This is a small community in which she has been able to track changes over time. What she found was that values are linked to changes in the economy. So, in a sense, it follows

---

* In the Baby M case, the lower court held that the father, William Stern, already had sole rights over the child and that the contract with the 'surrogate' mother, Mary Beth Whitehead, merely covered her 'willingness to be impregnated and carry his child to term.' In awarding custody to the genetic father and his wife, Judge Sorkow went on to say that Stern had not made a contract for the sale or surrender of his child because 'he cannot purchase what is already his.' *In the matter of Baby M*, 217 N.J. Supr. 313 (1987), affirmed in part and reversed in part, 109 N.J. 396 (1988).

the earlier question about how you would expect *konenki* to gradually decrease. But that has not happened in Japan and I will not answer that. [laughter]

Susan Bewley: As we all age and find ourselves disconnected from youth, we can finish wondering how disconnected we will be from the next generation, and whether such things differ from one country to another. Thank you very much.

References

1. Westendorp RG, Kirkwood TB. Human longevity at the cost of reproductive success. *Nature* 1998;396:743–6.
2. Helle S, Lummaa V, Jokela J. Are reproductive and somatic senescence coupled in humans? Late, but not early, reproduction correlated with longevity in historical Sami women. *Proc Biol Sci* 2005;272:29–37.
3. Greer G. *The Change: Women, Aging and the Menopause*. London: Hamish Hamilton; 1991.
4. Shanley DP, Sear R, Mace R, Kirkwood TB. Testing evolutionary theories of menopause. *Proc Biol Sci* 2007;274:2943–9.
5. Ragone H. How race is being transfigured by gestational surrogacy. In: Ragone H, Winddance Twine F, editors. *Ideologies and Technologies of Motherhood*. London: Routledge; 2000. p. 56–76
6. Lock M. *Encounters with Aging: Mythologies of Menopause in Japan and North America*. Berkeley: University of California Press; 1993.
7. Davis D. Blood and nerves revisited: menopause and the privatisation of the body in a Newfoundland post industrial fishery. *Med Anthropol Q* 1997;11:3–20.

Chapter 4

What has happened to reproduction in the 20th century?

Beverley Botting

Introduction

This chapter presents trends in a variety of reproductive measures. It looks mainly at the second half of the 20th century and the first few years of the 21st century. Where possible, age differences in the trends are examined.

Much of the data refer to births. For this chapter, the main data source is birth registration data as given by the parents or informant to the local registration service. It has been a legal requirement to register births since 1837 but these data are only computerised and available for analysis from 1963 onwards. Most of the data refer to England and Wales because data for Scotland and Northern Ireland are handled separately in their respective countries but, where possible, data are given for Great Britain or the UK.

Number of births and total fertility rate

The total fertility rate (TFR) is the average number of children a woman would have if she experienced the age-specific fertility rates for a particular year throughout her childbearing life. It is a useful measure of the current level of fertility as it can be used to examine both changes in fertility over time and between populations by removing the effect of different age distributions. However, changes in the timing of childbearing between generations can distort the TFR so, for example, if women are delaying their childbearing to older ages, as in England and Wales during the 1980s and 1990s, the TFR is likely to underestimate eventual average family size.

The number of live births and TFR both fluctuated throughout the 20th century, with very sharp peaks at the end of both World Wars (Figure 4.1). Live births peaked at near post-war levels again in 1964, when the figure was 875 972 in England and Wales, but since then lower numbers have been seen. The lowest recorded annual number of births in the 20th century was 569 259, in 1977. In 2001, births reached a low of 594 634. There were 690 013 live births in England and Wales in 2007. This was an increase of 3.0% on the 2006 figure of 669 601, the sixth successive annual percentage rise in live births since 2001. The number of live births in 2007 reached the highest level since 1991.

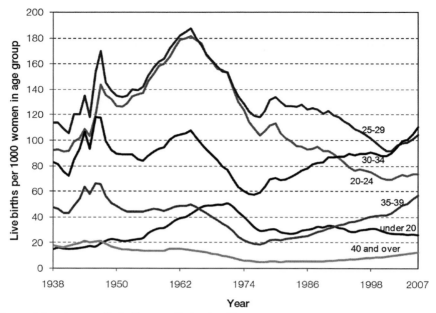

Figure 4.1   Age-specific fertility rates, England and Wales, 1938–2007

The UK TFR has increased each year since 2001, when it dropped to a record low of 1.63. The current level of fertility is relatively high compared with that seen during the 1980s and 1990s. However, the TFR was considerably higher in the 1960s, peaking at 2.95 children per woman in 1964, the height of the 'baby boom'.

The past 5 years have seen rising fertility in all four parts of the UK. Northern Ireland continued to have the highest TFR in 2007 (2.02 children per woman), while Scotland's fertility remained lower (1.73). The TFRs in England (1.92) and Wales (1.90) were close to the UK average.

In 2007, the TFR for England and Wales was 1.92 children per woman, an increase of 3% from 2006 (1.86) and consistent with a comparable increase in the number of live births. The TFR was last higher 34 years previously in 1973 when it was 2.00. The increase in the number of births since the upturn in 2002 reflects a rise in underlying fertility rates and an overall rise in population, whereas the rise in births seen in the 1980s was due mainly to the changing age distribution of the female population rather than a rise in fertility (Figure 4.1).[1]

Age pattern of fertility

The fertility of UK women in their 30s and 40s has shown an increase over the past three decades (Figure 4.1). In 1977, women aged 25–29 years were twice as likely to give birth as women aged 30–34 years. However, in 2007, women aged 30–34 years had the highest fertility of any age group.[1] Women in their 20s have experienced small increases in fertility between 2002 and 2007. This represents a reversal of the trend of falling fertility at these younger ages during the 1980s and 1990s.

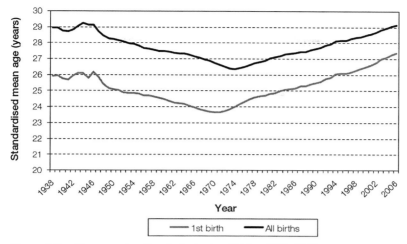

Figure 4.2   Mean age of mothers in England and Wales, 1938–2006

Because fertility is currently rising faster among women aged 30 years or over than among younger women, the average age at childbearing has continued to increase slowly (Figure 4.2). The mean age for giving birth in the UK was 29.3 years in 2007, compared with 28.6 years in 2001.

Multiple births

In 2006 in England and Wales, 9992 women gave birth to twins, 138 to triplets and seven to quadruplets. These maternities included both live births and stillbirths. The multiple maternity rate rose to 15.3 maternities with multiple births per 1000 women giving birth in 2006, compared with 14.9 in 2005 (Figure 4.3). This represents an 11% increase since 1996 when the rate was 13.8. Women aged 40 years or over experienced the highest multiple maternity rate at 25.6 and also the largest increase in this rate.

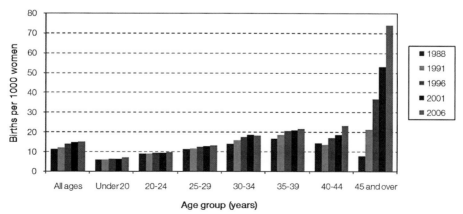

Figure 4.3   Multiple birth rates by mother's age, England and Wales, 1988–2006; data include both live births and stillbirths

Multiple birth rates for women aged 45 years or over showed a nine-fold increase between 1988 and 2006. In contrast, in 1996, the highest multiple maternity rate was for women aged 35–39 years.

Fertility treatment is thought to be one of the main factors behind the increasing number of multiple births in the UK. In 1978, 11 941 babies were born as part of a multiple birth but in 2003, 18 395 babies were born as part of a multiple birth. Babies born as part of a multiple birth are at greater risk of mortality and morbidity. Data collected about babies born as a result of *in vitro* fertilisation (IVF)[2] showed that 126 IVF babies die each year as a consequence of having been born in a multiple birth and of these 51 are stillbirths, 42 are deaths in the first week of life and 33 are deaths later in the first year of life. These figures do not include miscarriage or fetal reduction.

Abortion

The peak ages for abortion are in the 20–24 and 16–19 year age groups. Older women, aged 35–44 years and aged 45 years or over, only make a small contribution to the overall abortion rates.

Conceptions

Conception statistics include both terminations of pregnancy by legal abortion and maternities in which one or more live births or stillbirths occur. Maternities that result in more than one live birth or stillbirth are counted only once. Numbers of miscarriages and illegal abortions are not available so are not included in official conception statistics. Conception statistics are based on year of conception, so conceptions in 2006 resulted in births or abortions in 2006 or 2007.

There were an estimated 870 000 conceptions in England and Wales in 2006, compared with 841 800 in 2005, an increase of 3%. The overall conception rate rose by 3% between 2005 and 2006 from 76.0 to 78.3 conceptions per 1000 women aged 15–44 years. The rate for women aged 40 years or over increased fastest, by 7%, from 11.5 per 1000 women aged 40–44 years in 2005 to 12.3 in 2006. During the same period, the under-18 rate fell from 41.4 to 40.9 conceptions per 1000 girls aged 15–17 years.[3]

In 2006, conception rates increased steadily by age for women aged under 30 years and then decreased with age. The rate was highest for women aged 25–29 years, at 129.5 per 1000 women in that age group. As in previous years, nearly four-fifths of all conceptions resulted in a maternity. Conceptions outside marriage increased from 49% in 1996 to 56% in 2006. Much of this increase was in conceptions where both the maternity and conception were outside marriage but the birth was registered by both parents. The conception rate for girls aged 13–15 years remained at 7.8 conceptions per 1000 girls in that age group.

Childlessness

Figure 4.4 shows the tendency to delay childbirth for women in more recent generations. Women born in 1940 and 1930 tended to start childbearing early and had on average 0.3 more children than earlier and later generations of women. Women born in 1950 started childbearing earlier but then had lower rates of childbearing than those born in 1930 and 1940 once they reached their mid- to late 20s.

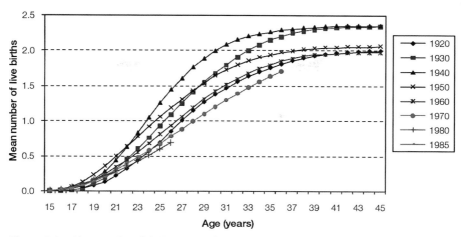

Figure 4.4   Mean number of children by age for different cohorts of women born from 1920 to 1985 in England and Wales

Women born in 1960 tended to follow similar childbearing patterns to those born in 1920 and their completed fertility was at a level similar to women born in 1950. Later generations had fewer children on average by their mid-20s, but higher rates in the future at older ages may mean their completed fertility rates are at a similar level to earlier cohorts.

Figure 4.5 shows the proportion of women who remained childless at the end of their childbearing years. Some women may be voluntarily childless whereas others may have wanted children but been unable to conceive or were not in a relationship.

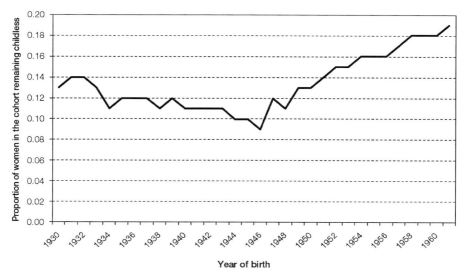

Figure 4.5   Proportion of women in England and Wales born between 1930 and 1960 who remained childless

Age at first intercourse

The past half-century has seen distinct changes in sexual behaviour and these changes have been considerably more marked among women than men. Analysing data from the 1990 and 2000 National Survey of Sexual Attitudes and Lifestyles, Wellings[4] observed a series of significant trends in sexual activity. There has been a continued reduction in the age at which sexual intercourse first took place together with an increase in the proportion of young people who had sexual intercourse before the age of consent. For men and women reaching sexual maturity in the 1950s, the average age at first intercourse was 20 and 21 years, respectively; by the mid-1990s, it was age 16 years for both sexes.

In addition, the proportion of young people who were sexually active before the age of 16 has increased. At the end of the 20th century, a quarter of young women had intercourse before the age of consent compared with less than 1% of those becoming sexually active in the 1950s. The gap between the sexes also narrowed over time and, by the 1990s, the gap had closed.

Contraception

In 2006/07, the majority (76%) of women aged under 50 years were using at least one method of contraception according to the Office for National Statistics (ONS) national household Omnibus survey.[5] This percentage included women who were using at least one non-surgical method (56%) and women who were sterilised or whose partners had had a vasectomy (20%). As in previous years, the contraceptive pill was the most popular method of contraception (27%), followed closely by the male condom (22%). Partner sterilisation (11%) and self-sterilisation (9%) were the next most popular methods. Other methods of contraception used included the intrauterine device (IUD) (4%), withdrawal (3%) and hormonal injection (3%). Two percent of women used the hormonal intrauterine system (IUS). One in four women (24%) was not currently using a method of contraception, of whom just over 50% (13% of all women) were not engaged in a sexual relationship with someone of the opposite sex. The percentages using different forms of contraception and the overall percentage using at least one method showed little change over the 7 years that the Omnibus survey has monitored usage.

In 2006/07, the youngest women were the least likely to be using contraception: just under two-thirds (63%) of women aged 16–19 years were using at least one method of contraception compared with about three-quarters (73–84%) of those in other age groups. Among those who were using at least one form of surgical or non-surgical contraception, the percentage using the pill decreased steadily with age, from 64% among women aged 20–24 years to 11% of those aged 45–49 years. Use of the male condom was also more prevalent among younger women, decreasing from just under 50% of those aged 16–24 years to 16% among those aged 45–49 years. Reliance on hormonal injections or implants as a method of preventing pregnancy showed a similar pattern, with use of these methods being more common among younger women. Conversely, older women who were using contraception were more likely than younger women to rely on surgical methods. Nearly 1 in 3 (30%) women aged 40–44 years reported having a partner who had undergone a vasectomy compared with fewer than 1 in 100 women aged 20–24 years. Female sterilisation was also more common among older women.

Age at menopause

There is wide variation in the age at which natural menopause occurs. In 1992, in the UK, the median age was estimated to be 51.7 years.[6] More recent estimates have been made from the Medical Research Council's National Survey of Health and Development, a birth cohort study, based on a nationally representative cohort of 1583 British women born in March 1946.[7] Women were followed up annually through the menopause until age 57 years.

Conclusion

Fertility rates are now highest for women aged 30–34 years and the mean age at birth is at the highest level for 60 years. Multiple birth rates have continued to increase and, in 2006, women aged 40 years or over experienced the highest multiple maternity rate at 25.6 per 1000 women giving birth in that age group, and also the largest increase in this rate. Multiple birth rates for women aged 45 years or over showed a nine-fold increase between 1988 and 2006. The pill and male condom are the most popular forms of contraception but, for women aged 40 years or over, sterilisation is the most popular form.

References

1. Office for National Statistics. *Birth Statistics: Births and Patterns of Family Building England and Wales (FM1)*. London: ONS; 2008 [www.statistics.gov.uk/STATBASE/Product.asp?vlnk=5768].
2. Oakley L, Doyle P. Predicting the impact of in vitro fertilisation and other forms of assisted conception on perinatal and infant mortality in England and Wales: examining the role of multiplicity. *BJOG* 2006;113:738–41.
3. Office for National Statistics. *Conception Statistics, England and Wales*. London: ONS; 2007 [www.statistics.gov.uk/StatBase/Product.asp?vlnk=15055&More=Y].
4. Wellings K. *Seven Deadly Sins*. Swindon: Economic and Social Research Council; 2005.
5. Office for National Statistics. *Contraception and Sexual Health 2006/07*. Omnibus Survey Report no. 33. London: ONS; 2007.
6. McKinley SM, Brambilla DJ, Posner JG. The normal menopause transition. *Maturitas* 1992;14:102–15.
7. Mishra G, Hardy R, Kuh D. Are the effects of risk factors for timing of menopause modified by age? Results from a British birth cohort study *Menopause* 2007;14:717–24.

Chapter 5
Trends in fertility: what does the 20th century tell us about the 21st?

Stijn Hoorens

Introduction

In the 1970s, the European press was full of dire predictions of overpopulation. Over the past 300 years, the world's population had increased around ten-fold. Particularly alarming was the publication of *The Limits to Growth*[1] by the Club of Rome in 1972, which outlined the Malthusian concerns of the consequences of exponential population growth. In the year of its publication, global average fertility rate was 4.5, a rate that implied the doubling of a population in 36 years. At the same time, life expectancy had increased by nearly 30 years over the previous century, causing the mortality rates to drop across the globe. As a consequence of population growth at previously unprecedented rates, the authors predicted the end of economic growth before the end of the century.

Since the publication of *The Limits to Growth*, the world's population has (as precisely predicted) nearly doubled in size. However, the tables seem to have turned: in Europe and parts of Asia we are now concerned with birth shortages and consequential population ageing. Birth rates are falling worldwide and family sizes are shrinking. The total fertility rate (TFR) is now less than the replacement level of 2.1 children per woman in every member state in the European Union (EU), childlessness is becoming more common and the average age at which women have their first child is nearing 30 years. As a result, European populations are either growing very slowly or even starting to shrink. Furthermore, these low fertility rates also accelerate the ageing of populations. Consequently, by 2040, one in four Europeans will be aged 65 years or over, up from one in eight in 1990.

Three determinants of change

The size and age structure of a population is determined by three factors: fertility, mortality and immigration. Regarding mortality risk by age, Europe has witnessed significant declines in almost every age group.[2] Western Europe's increase in life expectancy at birth has outpaced that in most other parts of the developed world, including the USA and Russia:[3] from 68.4 years for females and 74.7 years for males in 1970 to 75.4 years and 81.4 years, respectively, in 2000. By 2050, in rapidly ageing countries such as Italy, female life expectancy is projected to be as high as 89 years and male life expectancy as high as 84 years.[4]

The size of recent immigrant flows makes immigration a phenomenon of growing interest and controversy.[5] In 2001, the net immigration to the EU was about 1.15 million per year and it increased to 2.03 million per year in 2005.[6] Although international migration is currently the largest component of population growth in the EU, historically, migration has had a relatively modest impact on the population structure. The proportion of migrants expressed as a ratio in relation to the total population accounted for 0.34% of the total number of inhabitants in the 27 EU countries (EU-27) in 2005.[6]

Fluctuations in fertility rates exert a significant influence on population structures because declining fertility rates will have a subsequent negative effect on the size of the reproductive population in a generation's time. While the average number of children per women needed for current generations to replace themselves is 2.1, the average fertility rate of the EU-27 is currently just below 1.5.

Why is this relevant?

Longer life, of course, is an impressive testament to the rapid progress in economic, social and public health spheres in Europe. And equally, declining fertility is the consequence of increased freedom of choice regarding reproductive decisions of couples, and of women in particular.

Decreasing birth rates have already led to negative natural increases (more deaths than births) in as many as 11 of the EU-27 countries.[4] Without France (TFR 2.0) and the UK (TFR 1.84), the EU as a whole would already be experiencing more deaths than births annually.

Negative natural increases in the coming decades, however, are relatively easily offset by immigration. Immigration at the levels experienced in a number of the years early in the current century, moreover, would be sufficient to keep the EU's population from declining annually even in the mid-21st century. Given its potential future EU membership, it is noteworthy here that Turkey's natural increase of 911 000 people in 2005 was more than three times that of the entire EU-27's natural increase of 292 000. Population decline in the EU is a localised problem more than it is an EU-wide problem.

The combined effects of high post-war fertility (through the 1960s) and very low fertility since the 1970s, however, will have a significant impact on the EU's age structure in the decades to come. The proportion of the EU-27's population aged 65 years or over is projected to increase from its current 17% to 30% in 2050. Already, Europe's population pyramid is becoming increasingly inverted (see Figure 5.1). In all but six of the EU-27 countries in 2006, the number of people aged 50–64 years exceeded the number aged 0–14 years and, in four countries including the EU's largest (Germany), the number aged 65–79 years exceeded the number aged 0–14 years.[6] The major concern is whether a sufficient working-age population is available to support an increasingly older population. The increase in old-age dependency ratios is a reflection of the fact that the population structure is moving towards including an increasing proportion of older people in relation to the economically active population. While immigration can have a substantial effect on preventing or delaying population decline in Europe, it can do much less to offset population ageing.[7]

These trends portend difficult times ahead for the economies in countries with rapidly ageing populations. All other things being equal, a shrinking share of the

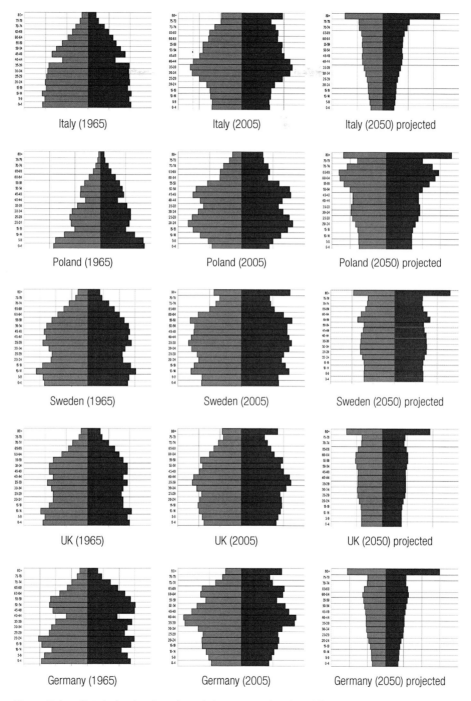

Figure 5.1   Historical and projected population structure in selected EU countries (1965, 2005 and 2050); men = light grey, women = dark grey; data from Eurostat[6]

workforce in the population implies that domestic production per capita will be lower than it otherwise would have been if the share of workers had remained stable.* At the same time, the growing proportion of elderly individuals pressures the solvency of pension and social insurance systems. As household sizes decrease, the ability to care for the elderly domestically diminishes further. Meanwhile, elderly people face growing healthcare needs and costs. Taken together, these developments could pose significant barriers to economic growth and to reaching goals on the social agenda.

Concern over these trends has sparked a debate over the most effective policies to reverse them or mitigate their impact. Not only is the affordability of European welfare systems at stake, but these unprecedented demographic trends may also have social consequences, for example for intergenerational relations. It is therefore important to understand the drivers behind these population dynamics.

This chapter focuses on one of the factors driving population change: fertility. Firstly, current trends in fertility are outlined, followed by a brief discussion of the various indicators used to measure fertility. Secondly, the determinants and drivers of fertility are explored, after which several implications of these drivers for the future are examined. Finally, the chapter concludes with some speculative remarks on possible future trends in fertility and their potential impact.

Trends in fertility

The most commonly used indicator of fertility is the TFR, also called period fertility, which for any given year is 'a measure of the number of children that a woman would have over her childbearing years if, at each age, she experienced the age-specific fertility rate of that year'.[7] TFR is often used as it is readily available, easy-to-understand information that provides an up-to-date overview of fertility at a certain point in time. TFR has changed drastically over the past four decades (Figure 5.2).

European variation in TFR is substantial. Eastern and Southern European countries have the lowest TFRs (for example, Slovakia 1.24 and Slovenia, Romania and Lithuania 1.31); higher TFRs are found in Western and Northern European countries (for example, Iceland 2.08, France 2.00 and Norway and Ireland 1.90).[8] It may therefore be fair to speak of a 'two-speed' Europe (Figure 5.3), with north-western Europe on one side (relatively slowly ageing countries) and Southern, Central and Eastern Europe on the other (relatively rapidly ageing countries). However, the period of year-after-year drops in fertility across all EU countries seems to be over: although there are still countries (for example, Germany and Romania) where fertility has continued to decrease over the past decade (Figure 5.4a), several European countries have recently recovered from their all-time lows in fertility (Figure 5.4b). In the UK, for example, the TFR has increased from 1.63 in 2001 to 1.84 in 2006. However, as will be discussed in the following sections, merely observing TFRs can be somewhat misleading because TFRs can disguise the more complex population developments involved.

---

* Some academics portray a more optimistic image of the future, arguing that harnessing the 'new economy' could offer a substitute response to ageing pressures. Increased productivity growth, due to new methods of work, would outweigh the negative growth of the workforce. This implies higher living standards, which would provide additional scope to modify pension benefit levels and contribution rates. The Organisation for Economic Co-operation and Development (OECD) has published a series of studies on the factors shaping the productivity growth process.[50]

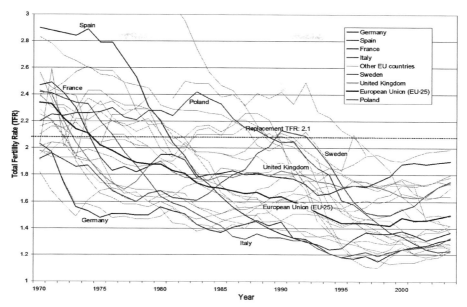

Figure 5.2   Total fertility rates in selected countries since 1970; data from Eurostat[8]

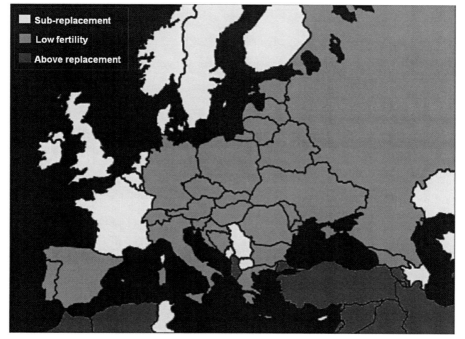

Figure 5.3   Fertility map of Europe; data from United Nations Department of Economic and Social Affairs[51]

Indicators for fertility

Distortions and misrepresentations of actual fertility trends by TFRs largely stem from
'tempo' and 'quantum' impacts on fertility.[9] Tempo effects refer to the timing of
births, which can distort TFR when women decide either to postpone or advance
childbearing. If, for the purpose of illustration, all women at year x decide to postpone
childbearing by 1 year, then the TFR for year x would be 0. Yet this would not mean

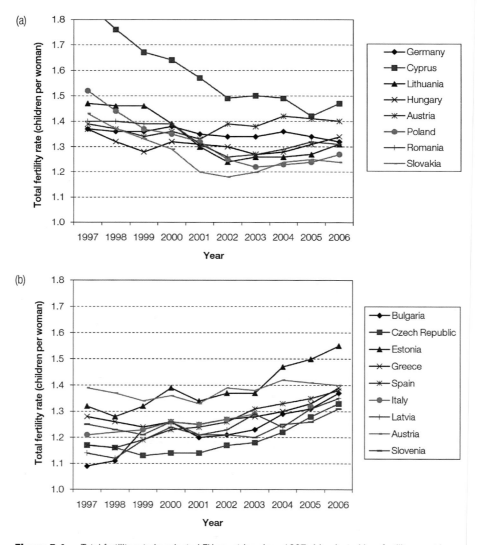

Figure 5.4 Total fertility rate in selected EU countries since 1997; (a) selected low-fertility countries
where TFR has decreased between 1997 and 2006; (b) selected low-fertility countries
where TFR has increased between 1997 and 2006; data from Eurostat[8]

that all women remain childless, it merely implies they have their children 1 year later. At year $x + 1$, TFR will be nearly double the rate of year $x - 1$. Quantum effects do imply actual variations in the average number of children women have over their reproductive lifespan, despite changes in the mean age of childbearing.

When only interested in the quantum effect of fertility, an indicator based on the total childbearing of cohorts of women can be used, by measuring the average number of births that women aged 50 years had during their reproductive years.[9] This is often referred to as the completed cohort fertility (CCF) or the completed fertility rate (CFR). The downside of CCF is, however, that it records the completed fertility of cohorts who were in the prime of their reproductive years about two or three decades previously. In other words, it is not of much help to explain what is happening today.

To sidestep this temporal obstacle, various measures have been proposed that aim to adjust the TFR for tempo effects and thus to present a more realistic figure of actual fertility.[9–11] To compare the differences between normal TFRs and adjusted TFRs, and thereby to discern the impact of tempo effects, Sobotka[12] used tempo-adjusted TFR (adjTFR), a measure proposed by Bongaarts,[9] to calculate the tempo effects for European countries. Table 5.1 provides an overview of regional TFR estimates for the period 1995–2000 and clearly indicates the possible large downturn impact of tempo effects on normal TFRs.

Table 5.1   Tempo effect and adjusted TFR in a selection of EU countries; reproduced with permission from Sobotka[12]

Country	Period	TFR	adjTFR	Tempo effect	CCF (cohort born 1960)
Austria	1995–2000	1.36	1.58	−0.22	1.7
Belgium	1995–2000	1.6	—	—	1.86
Bulgaria	1995–2000	1.2	1.48	−0.28	1.95
Czech Republic	1995–2000	1.18	1.73	−0.55	2.03
Denmark	1993–1995	1.79	2.04	−0.25	1.9
England and Wales	1995–2000	1.71	1.85	−0.14	1.97
Estonia	1996–2000	1.28	1.77	−0.49	2.03
Finland	1995–2000	1.75	1.89	−0.14	1.96
France	1999	1.79	1.96	−0.17	2.11
Germany	1995–2000	1.34	—	—	1.65
Greece	1995–1998	1.3	1.63	−0.33	1.93
Hungary	1995–1998	1.44	1.76	−0.32	2.02
Ireland	1995–2000	1.89	2.18	−0.29	2.41
Italy	1993–1996	1.21	1.64	−0.43	1.67
Latvia	1998–2000	1.17	1.55	−0.38	1.94
Lithuania	1995–1999	1.4	1.65	−0.25	1.88
Netherlands	1995–2000	1.6	1.73	−0.13	1.85
Poland	1995–2000	1.48	1.76	−0.28	2.18
Portugal	1995–2000	1.47	1.73	−0.26	1.89
Romania	1995–1999	1.31	1.52	−0.21	2.15
Slovakia	1995–2000	1.4	1.74	−0.34	2.18
Slovenia	1995–2000	1.26	1.68	−0.42	1.87
Spain	1995–1999	1.18	1.46	−0.28	1.76
Sweden	1995–2000	1.57	1.85	−0.28	2.04

adjTFR = tempo-adjusted TFR; CCF = completed cohort fertility; TFR = total fertility rate

The differences observed underline the subtleties involved in measures of fertility and emphasise the need for caution when any measure of fertility is interpreted. As Sobotka[12] noted: 'However sophisticated and complex, period measures are not a substitute for cohort fertility indicators'.

While the fertility indicators project quite a pessimistic future for Europe, it is intriguing to note that the average desired family size for the 15 EU countries before the 2004 accession wave (EU-15) still exceeds two children. Among women aged 18–34 years, the average desired number of children is 2.17.[13] A more constraint-influenced measure, expected family size; that is, the sum of the number of children that a woman already has and still plans to have, is around 0.2–0.4 less than desired family size for almost all countries. The percentages of women who give 'none' as their desired number of children are typically small, generally less than 5%. Actual childlessness, a lagging indicator as it can only be measured for women with completed fertility, is 10.6% in the EU-15.[13] However, this masks substantial intercountry differences. Ideal family size has fallen well below replacement in Austria and Germany to 1.6 in the former East Germany and to 1.7 in the former West Germany and Austria among women aged 20–34 years.[14] As many as 16.6% of women aged 18–34 years in Germany put their ideal number of children at 'none', a substantial rise from previous generations. Nonetheless, desired family size often exceeds actual (and indeed, expected) family size, prompting debate over the role of public policy in reconciling childrearing with employment and other activities.

Fertility projections

Predictions of future fertility and population size have been made under a variety of assumptions, which, if altered, can impact significantly on the projected population structure. For their population projections, the UN assumed until 1997 that fertility would eventually restabilise at replacement level. Current UN projections assume that fertility in all countries will converge at 1.85. The rationale behind an assumed recovery is that fertility decline since the 1980s can mainly be attributed to the tempo effect of parenthood delay. Assuming that couples end their postponement at some point, TFR would then catch up.

Even though some countries have experienced a slightly upward trend in fertility (for example, the UK), so far there has been little evidence for such substantial recovery of fertility rates. In fact, there is no theoretical ground for the assumption that fertility rates will converge at a particular level. Even the newly assumed stabilisation level of 1.85 might be too high in comparison with currently observed rates.[9] As a consequence, predictions of the future world population size differ under varying fertility assumptions.

Another hypothesis related to fertility trends, and particularly relevant for Europe's lowest-low fertility rates, is the possibility of the so-called 'fertility trap'. This hypothesis has been postulated by Lutz et al.[15,16] and refers to a state of very low fertility that is self-reinforcing and hence difficult to recover from. McDonald[17] has argued that such a threshold could occur at around a TFR of 1.5. Lutz et al.[15,16] have argued that this complex system of causal relations is based on a demographic, a sociological and an economic component, all of which reinforce low fertility. Demographically, low fertility can be reinforcing as a consequence of 'negative momentum' of population growth. This implies 'a force towards shrinking in the case of a history of very low fertility that has modified the population age structure to such an extent that fewer and fewer women will enter reproductive age and hence the number of births will decline, even in the hypothetical case that fertility instantly jumped to replacement level'.[16] The second sociological component is based on the concept of personal ideal family size, which is anticipated to decrease: the perceived size of the ideal family will be smaller in the future. Finally, the economic component is based upon a 'gap between personal aspirations for consumption and expected income'. Fertility is assumed to decline as relative expected income will decline 'assuming that aspirations of young adults are on an increasing trajectory while the expected income for the younger cohorts declines, partly as a consequence of population ageing induced by low fertility'.[16] A combination of these three factors could result in a tipping point where low-fertility countries would not be likely to recover quickly and thus policymakers should be aware of this hypothetical trap.

Determinants of fertility

In the paragraphs above, it was observed that fertility has been subject to substantial variations over the past few decades and assumptions about ideal family size, timing and spacing of births determine how fertility rates are projected into the future. This section discusses the many interrelated and co-dependent factors that have an influence on reproductive behaviour. Singling out factors carries the risk of oversight and oversimplification. Nevertheless, to make the various types of factor involved in the development of fertility understandable, we can distinguish three groups:

- micro-level factors at individual or family level that influence the reproductive behaviour of couples
- macro-level factors that include developments on a national or international level and that influence the reproductive behaviour of couples
- policy levers, which are efforts by governments to influence the reproductive behaviour of couples.

Micro-level factors

Micro-level factors typically relate to choices about whether to have children, when to have them and the desired number of children. Such decisions are affected by preconditions such as marriage and cohabitation and independent living situations and by the household's employment and financial situation and the costs of rearing children. Additionally, with increasing maternal age at birth, fecundity is of rapidly growing importance.

Marriage

In nearly all societies, childbearing traditionally occurs predominantly within marriage, a relationship characterised by a legally binding contract. Empirical evidence across many settings shows that the incidence of marriage responds to the same causal factors, among others, that lie behind fertility. In several Northern and Western European countries however, declining nuptiality (or marriage rate) has occurred simultaneously with increasing cohabitation rates, both as a precursor to and a substitute for marriage. In the Nordic countries and France, women aged 25–29 years are evenly split between cohabitation, marriage and single status. This has led to the phenomenon in Sweden that around 50% of children are born to unmarried parents but only 5–10% by single women.[18] The role of nuptiality as a driving force of fertility has therefore become less important in these countries.

Cohabitation and divorce

In concurrence with declining nuptiality, cohabitation rates have grown.* Untangling the complex relationships between marriage, divorce, cohabitation and fertility to uncover systematic patterns and causes is a scholarly work in progress. Public policy can affect these trends through legal and regulatory changes but it is difficult to predict how the distribution of people between the states of marriage, cohabitation and being single would respond to a tightening of divorce laws, for example. Accordingly, it is difficult to predict the effects on fertility.

Divorce rates have gone up across Europe in the past 50 years (Figure 5.5). Löfström and Westerberg[19] presented three possible effects of divorce rates on reproductive behaviour. Firstly, high divorce rates can indicate an apparent risk of becoming a lone parent and this may have a discouraging effect on fertility. Secondly, the high risk to a woman of becoming solely responsible for her household income imposes the necessity to gain a permanent position in the labour market before becoming a parent. This may delay family formation. Thirdly, women's personal negative experiences from divorces may prevent them from starting a family. In their model results, Löfström and Westerberg find that the divorce rate indeed has a negative effect on the changes in fertility.

For cohabitational unions, fertility also tends to be lower than marital fertility and cohabiting couples tend to postpone family formation longer. Hence, in countries where cohabitation is gradually substituting marriage, for example as a consequence of secularisation, fertility rates have dropped through several avenues. This fits in with the image of the 'second demographic transition' as described by Van de Kaa[20] as a regime that is characterised by a low proportion of married adults, unstable unions, high proportions of births out of wedlock and fertility rates well below replacement level.

Nevertheless, despite the predicted negative effect on fertility, these trends did not cause a steep reverse in the fertility trend in Sweden, a country with a high proportion of cohabitational unions and high divorce rates. As with the decreasing importance of marriage as driving force of family formation, cohabitation and divorce have merely imposed a timing effect on family formation.

Fecundity

The micro-level factors described above all relate to conscious decisions regarding the number or timing of children. However, not all couples who decide to have unprotected sex will immediately become pregnant. Approximately 16% of couples in the general population will not conceive within 1 year if they have regular intercourse and do not use contraception. Therefore, difficulties with natural conception are an additional factor in fertility.

Fertility and infertility are not discrete concepts; there is a grey area of reduced fertility between sterile couples on one end and fertile couples on the other. The main factor affecting the probability of getting pregnant is the period since the start of trying to become pregnant.[21] Therefore, time-to-pregnancy (TTP) estimates and cumulative probabilities of conception are used to find suitable thresholds to determine the prevalence of grades of subfertility. However, TTP is influenced by planning, use of contraceptive methods, timing of sexual activity, careseeking behaviour and past reproductive experience.[22] Probably because of different sample designs and potential selection bias, there are considerable variations between estimates of average TTP by age.[23,24]

---

* The cohabitation rate can be defined as the number of people per 1000 capita living together with someone in a consensual union when not legally married.

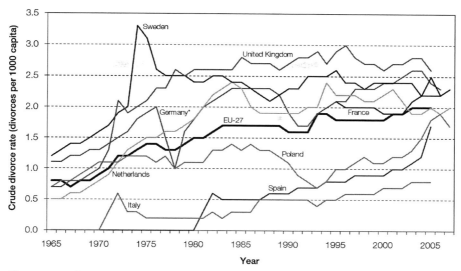

Figure 5.5   Crude divorce rates in selected EU countries and EU-27 (1965–2006); * Germany includes ex-GDR from 1991; data from Eurostat[6]

Since for every cycle there is approximately a one in four chance that a woman will become pregnant with intercourse in the fertile phase, most pregnancies (80%) will occur within the first six cycles of a couple trying. Of those who do not conceive in the first year, about half will do so in the second year.[25] Cumulative probabilities of conception decline with age of both partners. In particular, a couple's TTP increases sharply after the female age of 35 years. The inability to conceive after 1 year for older couples is often not attributable to absolute sterility but rather to reduced fecundity. Many infertile couples will conceive if they try for an additional year.

The influence of further postponement of childbirth on the TFR is likely to be limited in the short term. Estimates by Leridon and Slama[26] show that a decrease in fecundity by 15% and an increase by 2.5 years in age at first pregnancy attempt lead to a decrease in fertility by 4% and 5%, respectively. However, the persistent trend of rising female age at first childbirth indicates that decreasing fecundity may become an increasingly important factor driving fertility rates.

Macro-level factors

Macro-level trends relate to developments on a national or international level that influence the reproductive behaviour of couples. One of these could be the economic situation within a country. Economic cycles may affect the income of a household, which in turn may influence decisions on family formation. Macro-level factors can also refer to societies' collective value systems regarding female emancipation and individualisation. Macro-level effects can be seen most strikingly in the effect of World War II on childbirth (see Figure 4.1, page 34).

*Classic theories**

Halfway through the 20th century, scholars studying fertility trends observed that fertility rates tend to fall as a country's income rises and that people with high incomes tend to have lower fertility than those with low incomes. This widespread observation sparked the emergence of two new theoretical approaches during the 1960s by economists. Gary Becker and Richard Easterlin addressed the question: 'Why should children be different from nearly all the other items that people desire, where demand increases with income?'

Easterlin[27] proposed that couples' fertility responds not to their absolute level of wellbeing, but rather to the level relative to the wellbeing to which they are accustomed. The latter, he speculated, is a function of wellbeing in the households in which they grew up. To this assumption, Easterlin added the proposition that relatively small cohorts of people in a society are at an advantage in their families, in school and later in the labour market: they enjoy a higher level of wellbeing throughout. Easterlin embodied these propositions in an empirical model of relative cohort size, driven by cycles of births, accustomed wellbeing, relative wellbeing some years later and then births in the next generation. The model tracked time series data of fertility rates in the USA and some other countries fairly well.

In a very different approach to the income–fertility puzzle, Becker[28] proposed that parents' interest in children extends beyond their number to include the children's acquired characteristics, such as health and education. Parents may value this 'quality' of their children more than they do the number of children, so that increasing income induces them to substitute quality for quantity, resulting in falling fertility. Moreover, Becker emphasised that raising children is costly to parents, particularly in the opportunity cost of parental time, and most particularly in the opportunity cost of the mother's time. Hence, as labour market opportunities expand for women during the process of economic development, the cost of raising children increases. Between the incentives to invest more in fewer children and to allocate the mother's time towards market work and away from childrearing, fertility falls as income rises.

In the context of industrialised countries with good maternal and child health and nutrition, dependable government-provided old-age support, and widely available access to means of spacing and preventing births, the Becker model abstracts from the complex of intentional and unintentional factors that impinge on fertility to focus on a small number of potential causal influences. These are:

- household income
- the female partner's potential earnings in the labour market
- the degree of incompatibility of her working while caring for children
- the cost and availability of substitutes for her time in childcare
- her level of education (which influences the efficiency with which she can care for her children)
- the cost of other components of childbirth and basic childcare
- the cost of other contributors to child quality.

The theory has no unambiguous prediction for the association between household income and fertility; this depends on the child quantity–quality trade-off. Nevertheless, factors that decrease the cost of children are hypothesised to induce increased fertility.

---

* This section builds on the document *Low Fertility and Population Ageing: Causes, Consequences and Policy Options* by Grant *et al.*[7]

Influences of employment and family income

In neoclassical economic theory of fertility behaviour,[28-31] the literature assumes that the supply of female workers will grow with increasing female wages. It therefore predicts a negative relationship between the female labour market participation and the fertility rate. Numerous studies have confirmed this negative association for a wide range of countries.

In contrast to these studies, several authors have empirically studied pro-cyclical fertility. Stanfors[32] showed a positive association between fertility and family income in recent decades. Andersson[33] found that both women with a relatively low wage and women who are enrolled in education have a lower birth risk than others. He analysed the effect of a number of different economic indicators on the propensity to give birth at different birth orders in Sweden. He claimed that the increase in the number of women with such characteristics has been the main reason for the lower number of births during the 1990s.

Today, the main reason for interruption to women's employment is the birth of the first child. Part-time work has facilitated the return of women to the labour market after childbirth. The labour interruption is probably of more significance to a woman's career than her employment as such.

Influences of gender equality and education

In demographic literature some researchers argue that the process of decreasing birth rates is a result of improving gender equality and women's attempts to escape from the dependence on a male breadwinner, as evidenced by rising female employment.[34,35] Within this reasoning, female emancipation is one of the causes of declining fertility. Similar conclusions were drawn with regard to female education.

Educational status is also thought to have an impact on fertility. According to neoclassical theory,[36,37] the opportunity cost of children increases as female education rises, inducing rational individuals to reduce their demand for children. The main explanation for this is the effect that higher education has in increasing the value of women's time and their labour market opportunities.

Empirically, age of first birth is significantly higher among highly educated women than lower educated women.[38] Consequently, the increased proportion of women in higher education has contributed to a further delay of parenthood at national levels.[39] Beets *et al.*[40] have argued that if female education had not risen in the Netherlands since 1970, average female age at first birth would have been 26.5 years in 2000, instead of 29 years.

Kunzler,[41] however, has questioned whether modernisation of gender relations is to blame (or welcomed) as a cause of family decline. He argued that gender equality within the family is a prerequisite for the 'stabilisation' of the family. But also, equality between the sexes outside the family (for example in the workplace) could lead indirectly to a greater sharing of family responsibilities.[42] A study by Andersson and Duvander[43] suggested that there is at least some degree of gender equality in the way that Swedish couples deal with their family building. They found that the impacts of female and male earnings on a couple's childbearing behaviour turn out to be fairly similar.

Policy levers: efforts by governments to influence reproductive behaviour of couples

Previous sections have pointed out the impact of various macro- and micro-level factors on fertility. Many of these factors, for example those related to attitudes towards the family or gender equality, are cultural factors. If these were the most crucial determinants in childbearing behaviour then one would expect very different fertility dynamics in people from different cultural origins.[44] It appears, however, that native and foreign-born women demonstrate remarkably similar behaviour in response to recent period effects in fertility[45] and how their participation in the labour market has an impact on their childbearing behaviour.[46]

This suggests that institutional factors are important in shaping Sweden's fertility behaviour. In his book, *The Three Worlds of Welfare Capitalism*, Esping-Andersen[47] underlined the importance of a country's political and institutional characteristics in determining fertility. The questions that have intrigued many scholars in recent decades are: how important is this role, and what are the key institutional characteristics? By answering these questions, we can address how governments can implicitly or explicitly influence childbearing behaviour.

Four approaches that have a potential influence on a country's fertility rate can be distinguished:

- allowing immigrants with higher or lower fertility rates to enter the country
- influencing the use of contraceptives or the practice of abortion
- incentives to increase or decrease the desired number of children
- addressing barriers that cause a gap between desired number of children and actual number of children.

The relation between policy interventions and fertility has been the subject of lively academic debate. Scholars seem to agree that policies, such as arrangements for maternity leave and childcare and increasing cash benefits or tax exemptions for families with children, only have a limited and temporary effect on fertility. Studies from Romania and East Germany have shown an increase in fertility immediately after the introduction of these incentives but the higher fertility rates did not seem to be sustained in the long term. However, there are countries that have a sustained track record of investment in the family (for example, France) and countries that have implemented a comprehensive set of policies aimed at the improving compatibility of work and family life (for example, Sweden) that are associated with higher fertility rates.

What does this mean for the future?

Projecting the size and structure of future populations is not as difficult as predicting the weather or traffic. Historically, life expectancy in Europe shows an almost perfectly linear trend for more than a century with no sign of levelling off and, although assumptions about the future deviate slightly,[48] most statistical agencies now assume a continued increase in life expectancy. However, as with migration, predicting fertility is much harder. The United Nations (UN) assumes that global fertility will converge at 1.85, Eurostat's projections[6] assume that cohort fertility will remain constant, while Lutz's low-fertility trap hypothesis[16] argues that rates in some low-fertility countries may continue to spiral down. As visualised in Figure 5.6, the consequences of these differences for projected population structures can be substantial. The figure shows that the the UN and Eurostat projections for 2050 deviate only with regard to the population aged under 45 years, because of different fertility assumptions. The differences are larger for the very young, as the size of the cohort of their mothers deviates as well.

The macro-level factors affecting fertility outlined above tend to be more stable than micro-level factors and therefore allow for a somewhat lower degree of uncertainty

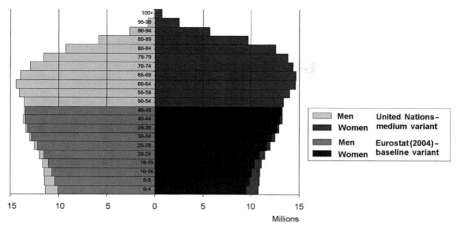

	Men	United Nations–
	Women	medium variant
	Men	Eurostat (2004) –
	Women	baseline variant

Figure 5.6   Projections of population size and structure for 2050 in EU-25 countries by Eurostat[52] and the United Nations[8]

regarding their future trends. Trends in economic development, female education levels and increasing female labour participation can be reasonably expected to follow a global trend. Therefore, according to Van de Kaa's theory[20] of demographic transition, developing economies will experience a negative correlation between economic growth and fertility. As a consequence, countries such as India and Brazil may see a considerable decrease in period fertility as female participation in the labour market increases, gender equality improves and the proportion of higher educated women grows.

What will happen in countries that have led the way in demographic transition is subject to speculation. Micro-level factors such as attitudes towards the family and perceived ideal family size will undoubtedly change, yet how (both temporal and spatial) is unclear. Furthermore, much will depend on how the drivers behind delayed parenthood – an increased proportion of women in higher education and the relative incompatibility of a career and motherhood – will develop. Will European welfare systems be generous enough to help couples combining work and family life (as in Sweden, for example) or will labour markets be flexible enough to allow for part-time work and career breaks? The question of how fertility and population will develop in the near and long-term future is inherently complex and the pursuit of a definite answer is futile. However, that should not deter us from speculation.

Over the past decade, the mean age of motherhood in Europe has increased by nearly 50 days per year on average. This would imply that, by 2050, mothers will be on average around 6 years older; in a country such as Spain, that would be at about 37 years of age. However, as fecundity decreases with age, the prevalence of couples who have difficulties conceiving can be expected to increase if these trends of postponement continue. The tempo effect of fertility will then affect the quantum effect, which will lead to further deviation between desired and completed fertility and increases in involuntary childlessness at later ages.

These trends may lead to a further increase in the demand for fertility treatment. Although the efficacy of assisted reproductive technologies currently declines steeply after the age of 35 years, advances in reproductive medicine may allow women to conceive at older ages in the future, perhaps even beyond their menopause. Although cryopreservation is currently offered mainly to women with ovarian cancer, it is already available on a commercial basis as a matter of choice for women who wish to preserve their fertility for social or professional reasons. In a special report in *Nature*,[49] scientists echoed these speculations and predicted an end to infertility in the future with the potential for any person of any age to have children by means of reproductive treatment.

If age were no longer a barrier to parenthood, it could be that couples will have more children over their lifetime but have them at later ages. A widening gap between generations would have a myriad of consequences. The structure of the population and relationships between the sexes and generations both in and outside the family will change irrevocably. Aside from demographic consequences, there will also be societal impacts, for example for the chronological order of life phases (for example, career planning and education), roles in childcare and inheritance.

Contraception has provided couples, and women in particular, with the freedom to choose when not to have children, and the mass introduction of the oral contraceptive pill had an unprecedented demographic and societal impact in the 20th century. The impact of a second reproductive revolution in the 21st century may be of similar magnitude. As low fertility, population ageing and migration are currently at the top of European political agendas, governments will continue to be challenged by demographic developments. While the contraceptive pill was controversial several decades ago, it is now a fact of life. There is little doubt that society will adapt to these developments as well.

Acknowledgement

I would to thank Joachim Krapels and Daniel Jones, research assistants at RAND Europe, for their research support.

References

1. Meadows DH, Meadows DL, Randers J, Behrens III WW. *The Limits to Growth*. New York: Universe Books; 1972.
2. Ahn N, Genova R, Herce JA, Pereira J. *Bio-Demographic Aspects of Population Ageing*. Research Report No. 1. Brussels: European Network of Economic Policy Research Institutes; 2004.
3. UNECE. *Statistical Yearbook of the Economic Commission For Europe*. Geneva: United Nations; 2003.
4. Eurostat. *In the Spotlight: Demographic Change: Challenge or Opportunity?* Luxembourg: Eurostat; 2008.
5. Spencer S. *The Challenges of Integration in Europe*. Oxford: Centre on Migration, Policy and Society; 2005.
6. Eurostat. *Population and Social Conditions Database*. Online database [www.eu.int/comm/eurostat/].
7. Grant J, Hoorens S, Sivadasan S, van het Loo M, DaVanzo J, Hale L, *et al. Low Fertility and Population Ageing: Causes, Consequences and Policy Options*. Santa Monica: RAND Corporation; 2004 [www.rand.org/publications/MG/MG206/].
8. Eurostat. *Population, Data Navigation Tree – Online Database*. Luxembourg: Eurostat; 2008 [epp.eurostat.ec.europa.eu].
9. Bongaarts J. On the quantum and tempo of fertility. *Popul Dev Rev* 1998;24:271.
10. Kohler HP, Philipov D. Variance effects in the Bongaarts–Feeney formula. *Demography* 2001;38:1–16.
11. Kohler HP, Billari EC, Ortega JA. The emergence of lowest-low fertility in Europe during the 1990s. *Popul Dev Rev* 2002;28:641–80.
12. Sobotka T. Is lowest-low fertility in Europe explained by the postponement of childbearing? *Popul Dev Rev* 2004;30:195–220.

13. European Foundation for the Improvement of Living and Working Conditions. *Fertility and Family Issues in an Enlarged Europe*. Luxembourg: Office for Official Publications of the European Communities; 2004.

14. Goldstein J, Lutz W, Testa MR. The emergence of sub-replacement family size ideals in Europe. *Popul Res Policy Rev* 2003;22:479–96.

15. Lutz W, Skirbekk V. Policies addressing the tempo effect in low-fertility countries. *Popul Dev Rev* 2005;31:699–720.

16. Lutz W, Skirbekk V, Testa MR. *The Low-Fertility Trap Hypothesis: Forces that May Lead to Further Postponement and Fewer Births in Europe*. Vienna: Vienna Institute of Demography, Austrian Academy of Sciences; 2007 [www.oeaw.ac.at/vid/download/edrp_4_05.pdf].

17. McDonald P. *An Assessment of Policies That Support Having Children From the Perspectives of Equity*. Vienna: Vienna Institute of Demography, Austrian Academy of Sciences; 2006 [www.oeaw.ac.at/vid/publications/VYPR2006/VYPR2006_McDonald_pp.213-234.pdf].

18. United Nations Economic Commission for Europe (UN/ECE). *Population in Europe and North America on the Eve of the Millennium: Dynamics and Policy Responses*. National report submitted by the Government of Sweden. Geneva and New York: UN/ECE; 1999.

19. Löfström A, Westerberg T. *Factors Behind Fertility Swings in Sweden 1965–1998*. Scandinavian Working Papers in Economics No. 582. Umeå: Umeå University; 2002 [swopec.hhs.se].

20. Van De Kaa DJ. Europe's second demographic transition, *Popul Bull* 1987;42:1–59.

21. Gnoth C, Godehardt E, Frank-Herrmann P, Friol K, Tigges J, Freundl G. Definition and prevalence of subfertility and infertility. *Hum Reprod* 2005;20:1144–7.

22. Olsen J, Juul S, Basso O. Measuring time to pregnancy: methodological issues to consider. *Hum Reprod* 1998;13:1751–6.

23. Juul S, Karmaus W, Olsen J. Regional differences in waiting time to pregnancy: pregnancy-based surveys from Denmark, France, Germany, Italy and Sweden. *Hum Reprod* 1999;14:1250–4.

24. Jensen TK, Scheike T, Keiding N, Schaumburg I, Grandjean P. Selection bias in determining the age dependence of waiting time to pregnancy. *Am J Epidemiol* 2000;152:565–72.

25. National Institute for Clinical Excellence. *Fertility: Assessment and Treatment for People with Fertility Problems*. Clinical Guideline 11. London: NICE; 2004.

26. Leridon H, Slama R. The impact of a decline in fecundity and of pregnancy postponement on final number of children and demand for assisted reproduction technology. *Hum Reprod* 2008;23:1312–19.

27. Easterlin RA. *Population, Labor Force, and Long Swings in Economic Growth*. New York: National Bureau of Economic Research; 1968.

28. Becker GS. An economic analysis of fertility. In: National Bureau Committe for Economic Research. *Demographic and Economic Changes in Developed Countries*. Princeton, NJ: National Bureau Committee for Economic Research, Princeton University Press; 1960.

29. Becker GS. *A Treatise on the Family*. Cambridge, MA: Harvard University Press; 1981.

30. Becker GS, Lewis HG. On the interaction between the quantity and quality of children. *J Polit Econ* 1973;81:279–99.

31. Butz WP, Ward MP. The emergence of countercyclical US fertility. *Am Econ Rev* 1979;45:737–60.

32. Stanfors MA. Explaining fertility variation in twentieth century Sweden. Sixth Conference of European Historical Economics Society, 9–10 September 2005, Istanbul, Turkey. [www.ata.boun.edu.tr/ehes/Istanbul Conference Papers- May 2005/Stanfors, Maria.pdf].

33. Andersson G. Childbearing trends in Sweden 1961–1997. *Eur J Popul* 1999;15:1–24.

34. Beck U, Beck-Gernsheim E. *The Normal Chaos of Love*. Cambridge: Polity Press; 1995.

35. Popenoe D. American family decline, 1960–1990: a review and appraisal. *J Marriage Fam* 1993;55:527–55.

36. Caldwell JC. Toward a restatement of demographic transition theory. *Popul Dev Rev* 1976;4:579–616.

37. Willis R. A new approach to the economic theory of fertility. *J Polit Econ* 1973;81:s14–63.

38. Gustafsson S, Kalwij A. *Education and Postponement of Maternity: Economic Analyses for Industrialized Countries*. European Studies of Population #15. Dordrecht: Springer; 2006.

39. Billari F, Philipov D. *Education and the Transition to Motherhood: A Comparative Analysis of Western Europe*. Vienna: Vienna Institute of Demography, Austrian Academy of Sciences; 2004.

40. Beets G, Dourleijn E, Liefbroer A, Henkens K. *De Timing van het Eerste Kind in Nederland en Europa.* Den Haag: Ministerie van Sociale zaken en Werkgelegenheid/Elsevier; 2000.

41. Kunzler J. Paths towards a modernization of gender relations, policies, and family building. In: Kaufmann FX, Kuijsten A, Schulze HJ, Strohmeier KP, editors. *Family Life and Family Policies in Europe: Problems and Issues in Comparative Perspective.* Oxford: Oxford University Press; 2002. p. 252–98.

42. Milivoja S. *The European Population Committee's Recent Demographic Studies and Their Relevance for Social Cohesion.* Strasbourg: Council of Europe; 2002 [www.coe.int/t/e/social_cohesion/ population/No_2_The_European_Population_Committee%E2%80%99s_Recent_Demographic_ Studies.pdf].

43. Andersson, G, Duvander A. *Second and Third Births in Sweden During the 1980s and the 1990s: the Effect of the Labour-Market Attachment of Both Partners.* Paper presented at the European Population Conference in Warsaw, August 2003.

44. Andersson G. *A Study on Policies and Practices in Selected Countries That Encourage Childbirth: The Case of Sweden.* Rostock: Max Planck Institute for Demographic Research; 2005.

45. Andersson G. Childbearing after migration: fertility patterns of foreign born women in Sweden. *Int Migr Rev* 2004;38:747–75.

46. Andersson G, Scott K. Labour-market status and first-time parenthood: the experience of immigrant women in Sweden, 1981–96. *Popul Stud (NY)* 2005;59:21–38.

47. Esping-Andersen G. *The Three Worlds of Welfare Capitalism.* Oxford: Blackwell; 1990.

48. Oeppen J, Vaupel J. Broken limits to life expectancy. *Science* 2002;296:1029–31.

49. Life after SuperBabe (editorial). *Nature* 2008;454:253.

50. Dang T, Antolin P, Oxley H. *Fiscal Implications of Ageing: Projections of Age-Related Spending.* Paris: OECD Publishing; 2001.

51. United Nations. *World Population Prospects: The 2006 Revision Population Database.* CD-ROM Edition. New York: United Nations, Department of Economic and Social Affairs, Population Division; 2007.

52. Eurostat. EUROPOP2004 – Trend Scenario, National Level. Eurostat website – Population and social conditions [epp.eurostat.ec.europa.eu].

Chapter 6
Demographics

Discussion

Gordon Smith: It was interesting that Stijn bracketed China with India and Brazil. One of the things that struck me as you were talking was the effect of the prolonged one-child-per-couple policy in China. The economic consequences of that are very dramatic. Would you really bracket China with India and Brazil, given that it had this policy for such a long time? Is there any projection of what will happen in China specifically given the liberalisation towards more children?

Stijn Hoorens: I have not studied these countries in detail but I deliberately left out China because of its one-child policy. You can see in China that there will be a massive problem with their labour force much earlier than in countries such as India precisely because of that.

Diana Mansour: Dr Botting, I understand the problems looking at birth rate, but you showed in England and Wales that there was a small increase in birth rate over the last 3–4 years (Figure 4.1, page 34). Have you any idea whether that is because women who previously delayed having children are now catching up and so we had a dip before it increased? Or is this increasing migration?

Beverley Botting: I'll answer in two parts. Given that we are seeing the increasing rates in the older ages, that goes together with the assumption that it is 'catch-up' and later births. When we look at the cohort graphs (Figure 4.4, page 37), we see, even for the younger women, that they are starting to converge. Again, it makes a suggestion of catch-up. Migrant mothers is an interesting point because what we have seen, particularly in the last couple of years, is a larger increase in births to mothers from the accession countries, and Poland particularly in the most recent data. One interesting tabulation from my research was the top ten countries mothers came from. Poland came from nowhere up into the top five, which I do not think is surprising. It is interesting because in the past overseas-born mothers were a very heterogeneous group. Particularly the mothers from India and Pakistan somewhat tended to (a) have births younger and (b) have more births. But what we are seeing now is fewer new births coming in through those mothers. We now have mothers from the accession countries who tend to have similar, or lower, fertility, albeit at slightly younger ages than UK-born mothers. At the moment that is not having a big effect but a large percentage of our births are to overseas-born mothers.

Siladitya Bhattacharya: You mentioned the age at first childbirth that we know is rising. Do you know anything about the age at last childbirth? Are women having their last child at an older age, and is this an increasing trend?

Beverley Botting: Let me first of all tell you about the problem with the quality of the data. Births are taken from birth registration data and the legislation for this was made in the 1930s. At that point, it was felt that if you had a child outside of marriage, it was an unfortunate accident. You didn't insult a woman by asking her if she had had previous unfortunate accidents! Therefore, the ability to identify firstborn children is a mixture of two measures. We are able to ask women about births within marriage and how many previous children they had. We are not allowed to do that for women who are not married. It is also a slightly complicated question because it says 'How many [children] have you had by this or any former husband?' without actually specifying whether you had to be married at that time – but that is an aside. So that's one of the main problems. By using data from the General Household Survey,[1] we have been able to make some estimates as well. So we have a mixture of knowledge and some survey-based data. Making assumptions when most births are inside marriage gives a much firmer basis for those calculations but we now have almost 50% of births occurring outside marriage – so we have got some odd assumptions there. Recently we have been able to access birth notification data where we do have better parity information. We are in the process of revising some of the extrapolations based on the information from birth notification. That was a very long background to say that (a) it's been difficult to get the data about first birth and (b) therefore the result is that we haven't done any of the late work. It is an interesting question. I hope we will be able to do it now we have the birth notification data.

Siladitya Bhattacharya: Thank you, I think. [laughter]

Beverley Botting: I am sorry – it is a statistician's answer.

Maya Unnithan: I wonder whether you would consider the flow of technologies which assist procreation from the low-fertility to high-fertility countries to blur things. You are saying that fertility in high-fertility countries will decrease over time. But what about the fact that technologies of conception are increasingly being made available to infertile people in the high-fertility contexts?

Stijn Hoorens: You are talking about assisted reproductive technologies [ART]?

Maya Unnithan: Yes.

Stijn Hoorens: The graph I showed with the two speeds (Figure 5.3, page 45) is indeed a snapshot of Europe at this very moment. I explained why it is so difficult to predict fertility. The increase in the UK has been somewhat unexpected and this may happen in other countries as well. It is happening in several other countries. I am not saying that this dichotomy is something fixed or will remain into the future. Low-fertility countries won't necessarily remain low. Regarding assisted reproductive technologies, I am uncertain what you mean.

Maya Unnithan: I was talking about infertile populations and increased access to ART in high-fertility countries such as India and China and whether such access would contribute to keeping fertility levels high.

Stijn Hoorens: It might flip the trend? No, I do not expect that. We have done some studies on the contribution of ART to national demographic statistics. We did some simulations on what would happen if, say, the UK doubled or trebled its access to ART. What would happen to fertility rates? The contribution turned out to be quite marginal, of the order of 0.2–0.4 children per woman even if access was doubled or trebled. So I do not think that at the moment, with present levels of access that ART, that it will be a significant contribution. It may be in the future if IVF is extremely cheap.

Susan Bewley: It would have to be more effective first as well?

Stijn Hoorens: Yes, exactly.

Gita Mishra: A couple of comments for Dr Botting. With regard to the age of natural menopause in the UK, the MRC National Survey of Health and Development has been following men and women born in 1946 up to now. I am part of the study group. What we have done every year, for women between the ages of 47 and 54 years, is give them a questionnaire on their menstrual patterns to get a handle on the age of natural menopause. We have a representative sample and I can say that the age of natural menopause is 51.5 years. Tomorrow, I will talk more about the studies [Chapter 17]. The other comment relates to thinking about women's reproductive health and its consequences in later life. As you mentioned, childlessness is going up. I think it is important for us to realise whether it is involuntary or voluntary childlessness – because that has a big impact on health. Is there any way the Office for National Statistics can collate such data or statistics?

Beverley Botting: No. In the past we had surveys which looked at family formation intentions. We all know that people don't necessarily always end up with exactly what their intentions were 20 years previously. The last time we looked at survey estimates, about a third were probably voluntarily childless – so they never tested their fertility, as it were. I think that there will always be some people who have chosen to remain childless and the best evidence we have is from some of the surveys.

Peter Braude: Firstly, thank you very much, both of you, for some very good facts which were very helpful in discussions. Beverley, you've made me once again ashamed to be a fertility specialist. When I look at those numbers of multiple pregnancies in the over-45s, there is no excuse. I suspect those are all women who will have received ovum donation. It is totally and absolutely avoidable. We know that the procedure's success rate is extremely high in that group [ovum recipients] and women don't need multiple embryos put back. Although when you read some of the books or look at talk shows they suggest that it is a good idea for you to want to have twins. There is a message going on out there that is the wrong way to talk. I suspect that in your 40- to 45-year-olds there was a mixed population – some are having their own babies and others were ovum donation.

Beverley Botting: Yes. That is why it is nice to start in 1988 because you see the underlying rate, in terms of what would be the natural expected rate of multiples. Really, the increase within 40- to 44-year-olds is quite small. Don't forget that the numbers are still very small in that category

Peter Braude: But they're entirely avoidable. Stijn, can I ask you one other thing about your figures? We are talking about births, and I appreciate the concern about how many of these are real children, in terms of adults surviving. Especially when you look at those figures from Africa and South America, where you say they have got higher than doubling populations; I suspect they might be even higher. We seem to be concentrating on this small place called Europe, in terms of numbers of people. We need to think about Asia, Africa and South America. Surely in the equation one has to think not just about Poles moving but the idea that there may be much larger populations migrating and moving which will change this directly. When we try to talk about Europe, it's going to be very different. There will be increasing population drops if people survive it. Again, the survival issue, because if you look at Africa particularly, what is AIDS going to do? Not just to the children that are born, but they are not going to be contributing. Some of the countries will get nowhere unless we do something about it.

Stijn Hoorens: I think that is an absolutely valid and important point. The trouble with migration is as before: demographers can run various scenarios with zero migration, current migration, double migration, sometimes higher order migration, and you can test what the consequences on population level would be. But that does not tell you the whole picture, particularly not on the social and economic level.

Peter Braude: But have we been right? Have we ever been right? [laughter] I'm not being facetious. Have we ever been right about trying to predict what would happen to population? Especially when you look at those graphs of what happened earlier to the world's population? I was brought up with the idea of the world population growing. As it is, these are horrendous numbers and a real problem. But have we ever been right in terms of what is actually happening to populations in Europe and America?

Stijn Hoorens: Regarding migration and fertility studies, the massive decline in fertility was unanticipated. The sustained low levels of fertility in Europe were unanticipated. If you go back to the literature of 15–20 years ago, most demographers expected that this was a temporal postponement effect. They thought that total fertility rates would converge back to around two children per woman. And it has not happened. You won't ever be able to predict natural disasters and political conflict.

References

1.   Office for National Statistics. *General Household Survey (GHS)* [www.ons.gov.uk/about/who-we-are/our-services/unpublished-data/social-survey-data/ghs/index.html].

Section 2

Basic science of
reproductive ageing

Chapter 7
Is ovarian ageing inexorable?

Roger Gosden and Lucinda Veeck Gosden

Establishment of the follicle reserve

In the eggs of many invertebrate animals, a specific patch of cytoplasm is predetermined for creating germ cells, but mammalian eggs have no equivalent region. Instead, germ cells emerge during a process called epigenesis under the influence of inductive factors from neighbouring cells. Their progenitors are first recognisable in the proximal epiblast of mouse blastocysts shortly after implantation when a tiny cluster of Stella-positive cells is directed to a germ cell fate by BMP4 secreted by the extraembryonic ectoderm. Prdm1 (formerly Blimp1) is a key transcription factor in germ cells that regulates cell fate by repressing the somatic cell programme expressed in neighbouring cells.[1] As germline stem cells (GSCs, also called primordial germ cells) emerge, they acquire alkaline phosphatase activity and migrate along the hind gut towards the gonadal ridge using a combination of morphogenetic movements and amoeboid motion. They express canonical genes, *Dazl*, *c-Kit* and *Vasa*, and undergo epigenetic reprogramming involving global demethylation of DNA (including imprinted genes) and histone modifications to produce a chromatin architecture resembling that of undifferentiated pluripotent stem cells.[2] The life history of human germ cells is less well known but probably similar to rodents, apart from having a much longer schedule: the time to generate follicles from GSCs is several months compared with only 1–2 weeks for rodents. Oogenesis is completed by birth in most species.

Human GSCs have a high nuclear to cytoplasmic ratio and lack notable cytoplasmic specialisation. They continue multiplying after arriving in the ovary and enter meiosis at 2–3 months of gestation, when they are regarded as oocytes. Their passage from leptotene to diplotene of prophase I takes several weeks and the chromosomes are highly conspicuous during intermediate stages (zygotene and pachytene) as the chromatin contracts and synapsis creates tetrads for genetic recombination. Entry into meiosis is unsynchronised in human ovaries and continues almost to the time of birth, when GSCs have completely disappeared. The number of germ cells peaks at 6–7 million in mid-gestation but declines to fewer than 1 million at birth.[3] A large number disappear by apoptosis in pachytene cells in which meiotic chromosome pairing errors are common.[4,5]

Nuclear maturation pauses at diplotene when chromatin becomes more diffuse. Oocytes then become associated with 'nests' of somatic cell cords growing in from the surface epithelium and perhaps connected with the rete system.[6] These nests bud to form primordial follicles consisting of a non-growing oocyte surrounded by a single layer of pregranulosa cells resting on a basement membrane, but the theca cells are still undifferentiated. Survival and development depend on granulosa cells since any naked germ cells disappear after birth and the primordial follicles are the only source of future gametes (see the section below on factors regulating the primordial-to-primary follicle transition).

Few follicles grow to Graafian sizes and no more than 400–500 follicles ovulate in a lifetime of uninterrupted menstrual cycles. Mature oocytes are arguably the rarest cells in the body and their post-ovulatory survival is brief unless they are fertilised, transforming them into founders of a virtually 'immortal' lineage. Thus, oocytes are highly specialised for fertilisation and, at the same time, capable of generating totipotent embryonic cells, a paradox seemingly explained by the dominance of RNA regulatory networks during late stages of maturation when they are transcriptionally silent until the genome becomes active during cleavage.[7]

In conclusion, oogenesis is a sequential process involving germ cell induction, migration, multiplication and genetic recombination before oocytes reach the diplotene stage and become dormant. With very few exceptions, these events occur only in fetal ovaries. Maturation of germ cells to produce fertile gametes begins at puberty, involving growth and maturation in a follicular niche, regulation by autocrine, paracrine and endocrine factors and depends on metabolic cooperativity with granulosa cells. It is challenging to mimic the complex changes occurring in the ovary in an artificial culture environment, even though it is a desirable goal for generating fertile oocytes for research and clinical treatment.

Follicle dynamics during ageing

The total number of oocytes (follicles) declines continuously after birth such that, by the time of menarche, only a quarter of a million follicles remain, or even fewer in girls prone to premature ovarian failure.[8] If the follicle store is fixed before birth, the number and rate of follicle depletion must have evolved to provide sufficiency for the prime reproductive years and to be commensurate with longevity of the species. It is not surprising, therefore, that the numbers of follicles at puberty are scaled allometrically in different species, implying that larger and longer-lived animals and humans have the largest endowments. There are few estimates of the rate at which follicles are lost across the lifespan but this factor too appears to be scaled allometrically according to body mass and longevity. Long-lived species use follicles more parsimoniously; for example, the follicle population half-life in young women is 7 years and in mice a mere 100 days.[9]

If evolution has moulded the size and dynamics of the follicle store, we can infer that genetic factors are operating but it is still enigmatic as to why such large age-specific variations exist between apparently normal individuals.[10,11] There is a ten-fold variation in follicle numbers between human ovaries of the same age and even genetically homozygous mice have three-fold differences: these are likely to have an impact corresponding to the potential length of the reproductive lifespan.[12] It might seem surprising that fecundity starts waning so early and so variably between individuals but it is consistent with a widely held evolutionary theory of ageing that posits that the force of natural selection declines with age.[13] However, explanations for the peculiarly early loss of follicles responsible for human menopause are controversial.

Once follicles have initiated development, they continue growing without pause until they either become atretic (the fate of the majority) or are selected to grow to Graafian sizes capable of ovulation. Although puberty is a major endocrine transition, there is no major change in the rate of follicle loss overall, nor indeed during pregnancy, lactation or ovarian suppression by contraceptive steroids (despite changes in antral follicles). This is unsurprising because the number of small follicles is unaffected by serum gonadotrophin levels and the follicle-stimulating hormone receptor is not expressed until after the primordial follicle stage.[14] Consequently, repeated cycles of gonadotrophin treatment are not expected to have a significant impact on ovarian ageing, as indicated in women receiving fertility treatment at the age of menopause.[15]

The rate of follicle disappearance is not, however, constant in adult women and, by the fourth decade, or slightly earlier, it accelerates more or less in parallel with the rising incidence of oocyte aneuploidy and infertility.[16] Follicles disappear more than twice as fast in the premenopausal decade, causing the timing of ovarian depletion and menopause to advance by two decades compared with calculations based on the rate being constant with age.[17] There is a similar decline in sonographically detectable antral follicles, reflecting the availability of recruitable preantral stages (Figure 7.1).

Extrapolation of the follicle decay curve indicates that about 1000 follicles remain at the median menopausal age of 51 years.[17] Whether this residue is unable to mature because of an inappropriate hormonal milieu or accumulated age changes in follicles or both is still unclear. At any rate, the close temporal correspondence between follicle depletion and the final menses strongly supports the general belief that menopause is a consequence of primary ovarian ageing, as opposed to hypothalamic–pituitary dysfunction, which is a dominating factor in small animals.[18,19] Further corroboration comes from a mathematical model that found remarkable concordance between the

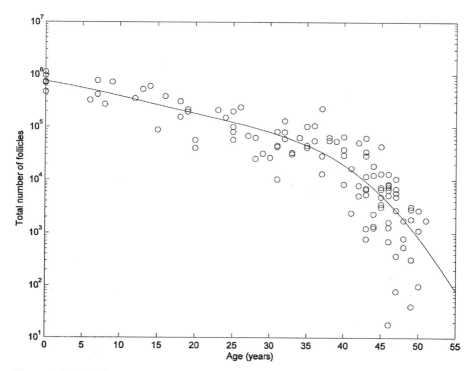

Figure 7.1 Variations with age in follicle number in human ovaries (by kind permission of Malcolm Faddy, Queensland University of Technology).

distribution of menopausal age predicted from follicle numbers and the observed distribution in a white race population.[20]

In this section, attention has been drawn to ovarian ageing as an inexorable process, which has sometimes been simplistically compared to an hourglass. The number of follicles established at birth and the subsequent rate of loss determines the time of follicle depletion and hence menopause. In the absence of follicle neoformation, menopause is an inevitable consequence of ageing and its timing quite predictable, in theory, if the total size of the follicle store could be accurately measured. Surveys have shown that menopausal age is relatively independent of lifestyle, ethnicity and reproductive history and, unlike menarcheal age,[21] there has not been a historical shift: there is rather strong evidence of genetic determination.[22,23]

Factors regulating the primordial-to-primary follicle growth transition

Primordial follicles are the basic developmental units in the ovary that remain dormant until they are recruited sequentially to become primary follicles, at which stage the oocyte enters a growth phase, the granulosa cells multiply and a zona pellucida starts to form. As expected at any developmental transition, there is a major increase in gene expression,[24] although the rate of carbohydrate metabolism is surprisingly constant.[25] This process is independent of systemic fluctuations in gonadotrophins and evidently triggered by an intrafollicular clock that probably resides in the oocyte rather than in the somatic cells.[26] The two cell types are loosely coupled in primordial follicles but after growth initiation there is increased physical and metabolic intimacy, with molecular shuttling via gap junctions between cells and across the perivitelline space.

According to Skinner,[27] the mechanism of the primordial-to-primary follicle transition has been evolutionarily conserved, as expected with a process that crucially affects fertility and the reproductive lifespan. Considering the limited number of follicles and the risks of explosive follicle growth, the mechanism might be expected to be under rigorous inhibitory control. Under conditions of organ culture, there is a spontaneous surge of follicle growth initiation, a phenomenon that has served experimental tests on the effects of potential regulatory molecules.

Using this *in vitro* model, several members of the transforming growth factor-beta (TGFβ) family have been found to play a role in regulating the follicle transition (Figure 7.2). Antimüllerian hormone (AMH) is specifically expressed by granulosa cells at secondary and later follicle stages and appears to serve as an inhibitor of recruitment from the pool of small follicles. In culture, AMH suppressed the number of newly growing follicles in human ovarian explants without affecting their survival[28] and, when the gene was deleted by a targeted mutation in mice, follicle recruitment was enhanced, causing the reserve to be prematurely depleted.[29] AMH is the only paracrine regulator known to have inhibitory effects on follicle recruitment but its physiological significance remains uncertain.

Bone morphogenetic proteins (BMPs) exert a number of effects on follicle development as well as on earlier stages of oogenesis. BMP4 secreted by theca/stroma cells promotes the primordial-to-primary follicle transition and increases oocyte survival[30] while BMP15 from the oocyte affects subsequent development. Another TGFβ molecule, GDF9, is required for granulosa cells to continue multiplying after the primary follicle stage[31] and has an inhibitory effect on Kit ligand (KL) which, in turn, interacts with the tyrosine kinase receptor for KL (c-Kit) expressed in the oocyte.[26] Mutations of either c-Kit or KL affect follicle growth at various stages[32,33] and KL in culture induces follicle growth initiation.[34]

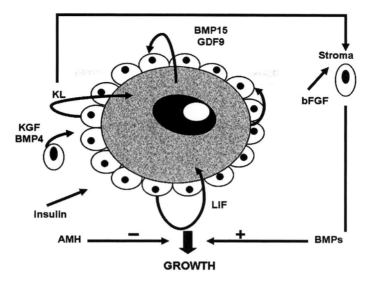

Figure 7.2 Stimulatory and inhibitory factors regulating primordial follicle activation; AMH = antimüllerian hormone, BMP4 and BMP15 = bone morphogenetic proteins, bFGF = basic fibroblast growth factor, GDF9 = growth differentiation factor 9, KGF = keratinocyte growth factor, KL = Kit ligand, LIF = leukaemia inhibiting factor

The follicle transition is also stimulated in cultured ovaries by other types of cytokines/ growth factors, including leukaemia inhibitory factor (LIF) and keratinocyte growth factor (KGF; a mesenchymally derived factor), insulin and basic fibroblast growth factor (bFGF), but neither insulin-like growth factor I (IGF-I) nor epidermal growth factor (EGF) have any effect.[27] A role has been revealed for the phosphatidylinositol-3-kinase (PI3K) signalling pathway, which is important in cell growth and migration. *Foxo3* and *Pten*, a tumour suppressor gene, are major negative regulators of PI3K that, when either are deleted in mice, trigger global activation of the follicle population soon after birth and hence lead to premature ovarian failure.[35,36] These findings are consistent with oocytes being regulators of the onset of follicle growth.

Taken together, these data suggest that the primordial-to-primary follicle transition is controlled by a number of factors, some of which are intrinsic to the oocytes while others are secreted as paracrine signals from neighbouring granulosa or even by stroma/theca cells. There does not appear to be a simple trigger but rather a balance of inhibitory and stimulatory factors that determines when each follicle starts to develop (and this may also be true for the alternative fate of apoptosis). The process is controlled spatially as well as temporally because follicles initiate growth preferentially at the cortico-medullary boundary, which indicates that changes in the local environment, or 'niche', could be crucial for follicle fate and, possibly, be amenable to pharmacological manipulation. If the inhibitory 'tone' could be enhanced, follicles might be spared from recruitment until later in life, which could be beneficial for women at risk of premature ovarian failure or those with disorders of early follicle growth. For women with normal ovaries, postponing the menopause by follicle conservation could eventually become possible, but this would not promote fertility if late-ovulated oocytes were of poor quality.

Germline stem cells in the postnatal ovary

Current concepts of ovarian ageing and the aetiology of the menopause can be traced back to a theory originally propounded by the great 19th century German anatomist Heinrich Wilhelm Goffried von Waldeyer-Hartz ('Waldeyer'). He claimed that the number of oocytes in the ovary is fixed early in life and not renewable in adulthood but, after the turn of the century, a contrary view came to the fore, namely that oocytes are continually replaced from germline stem cells. The controversy seemed to be settled by Zuckerman's seminal paper at the Laurentian Hormone Conference in 1950, at which he provided an overwhelming endorsement of Waldeyer's theory.[37] He based most of his arguments on painstaking counts of follicles in animal ovaries, the absence of early stages of meiosis after birth and results from experimental surgery, including destruction of the ovarian surface epithelium (claimed to be the source of new oocytes). His conclusions were subsequently confirmed by many independent observers and belief in a finite store of follicles became dogma until recently.

Papers published by Harvard researchers challenging the theory were therefore unexpected and reopened the old controversy in 2004. Johnson et al.[38] presented evidence that mouse follicles are renewed continuously in adulthood, a finding they attributed at first to GSCs in the ovarian surface epithelium. Their doubts were based on the old argument that the number of follicles in the ovary is insufficient to account for the entire reproductive lifespan given the high incidence of follicular atresia. They drew on new evidence found in adult mouse ovaries showing candidate GSC-like cells in the ovarian surface epithelium, expression of molecular markers of early meiosis, follicular regeneration after administering ovotoxic drugs and formation of chimaeric follicles after fusing pairs of ovaries.[38] There was insufficient stem cell activity to account for follicle replenishment but this theoretical problem seemed to be bypassed by GSC-like activity in the bone marrow, with the presumption that germ cell precursors are carried in the bloodstream to the ovaries where they replace follicles lost by atresia. Furthermore, data from bone marrow transplant studies supported their claims.[39] The cardinal observations have not been confirmed independently, however, nor have ovulable and fertile oocytes been derived from bone marrow or indeed from any other extra-ovarian source.[40–42]

Before these highly publicised studies in mice, Bukovsky's group suggested that follicle renewal occurs in adult human ovaries, based on immunohistochemical and culture methods. They inferred that oocytes and granulosa cells are generated continuously from bipotential stem cells of mesenchymal origin,[43–45] and stem cell-like cells have been described more recently in the ovarian surface epithelium.[46] These claims were contradicted in another study by the absence of molecular markers of early germ cells in adult human ovarian tissue, although they were expressed in fetuses.[47]

While the controversy has brought a welcome review of scientific dogma, the new studies have, on balance, confirmed the theory originally propounded by Waldeyer and Zuckerman. We cannot, however, dismiss the possibility of as-yet unidentified GSCs in the postnatal ovary, although, if they exist at all, they must be inactive: technology has yet to find ways of stimulating their activity. There is, however, more progress towards creating new germ cells from pluripotential stem cells. This is likely to be more rapid with male germ cells because when nuclei are haploid and epigenetically reprogrammed they can be injected to fertilise oocytes, whereas production of fertile female gametes requires maturation of a highly complex cytoplasm besides the initiation of meiosis and reprogramming of the nucleus.[48,49] After culturing mouse embryonic stem cells expressing a fluorescent reporter gene (*Oct4-GFP*) for several weeks, Hübner *et al.*[50] isolated cell aggregates resembling ovarian follicles and 'oocyte-like' cells enclosed by a membrane containing zona pellucida proteins. There were also cystic structures resembling blastocysts suspected to be derived from parthenogenetically activated oocytes. Oocyte-like cells have also been reported in another study of embryonic stem cells[51] and even from cultures of fetal pig skin.[52] The provenance and character of these structures are still poorly characterised but this progress is remarkable considering the long and complex life history of germ cells *in vivo* and the fact that specific and changing ovarian environments are poorly mimicked in culture. Thus, while the crowning achievement of producing oocytes competent for post-fertilisation development is probably still remote, these pioneering studies have at least shown this is a realistic goal.

Conclusion

The population of primordial follicles formed before birth appears to be the only source of oocytes available in adult life; hence, ovarian ageing is determined by the size of the follicle store and its rate of attrition. For the foreseeable future, however, oocytes will continue to be a limiting resource in research and assisted reproduction because of their scarcity and variable quality. Various technologies exist or are emerging for preserving oocytes, including cryopreservation and vitrification, but there is also a theoretical basis for slowing ovarian ageing by reducing primordial follicle recruitment, although possibly without a benefit for oocyte quality. Finally, the recent generation of germ cells from pluripotential stem cells in culture could be a foundation and the best long-term hope for a radical new technology to create oocytes *de novo*.

References

1. Hayashi K, de Sousa Lopes SM, Surani MA. Germ cell specification in mice. *Science* 2007;316:394–6.
2. Hajkova P, Ancelin K, Waldmann T, Lacoste N, Lange UC, Cesari F, *et al.* Chromatin dynamics during epigenetic reprogramming in the mouse germ line. *Nature* 2008;452:877–81.
3. Forabosco A, Sforza C. Establishment of ovarian reserve: a quantitative morphometric study of the developing human ovary. *Fertil Steril* 2008;88:675–83.
4. Baker T. A quantitative and cytological study of germ cells in human ovaries. *Proc Biol Sci* 963;158:417–33.
5. Speed RM. The possible role of meiotic pairing anomalies in the atresia of human fetal oocytes. *Hum Genet* 1988;78:260–6.
6. Byskov AG, Skakkebaek NE, Stafanger G, Peters H. Influence of ovarian surface epithelium and rete ovarii on follicle formation. *J Anat* 1977;123:77–86.
7. Seydoux G, Braun RE. Pathway to totipotency: lessons from germ cells. *Cell* 2006;127:891–904.
8. Goswami D, Conway GS. Premature ovarian failure. *Hum Reprod Update* 2005;11:391–410.
9. Gosden RG, Telfer E. Numbers of follicles in mammalian ovaries and their allometric relationships. *J Zool* 1987;211:169–75.
10. Block E. Quantitative morphological investigations of the follicular system in women; variations at different ages. *Acta Anat (Basel)* 1952;14:108–23.
11. Charleston JS, Hansen KR, Thyer AC, Charleston LB, Gougeon A, Siebert JR, *et al.* Estimating human ovarian non-growing follicle number: the application of modern stereology techniques to an old problem. *Hum Reprod* 2007;22:2103–10.
12. Faddy MJ, Telfer E, Gosden RG. The kinetics of preantral follicle development in ovaries of CBA/Ca mice during the first 14 weeks of life. *Cell Tissue Kinet* 1987;20:551–560.

13. Williams GC. Pleiotropy, natural selection and the evolution of senescence. *Evolution* 1957;11:398–411.

14. Oktay K, Briggs D, Gosden RG. Ontogeny of follicle-stimulating hormone receptor gene expression in isolated human ovarian follicles. *J Clin Endocrinol Metab* 1977;82:3748–51.

15. Elder K, Mathews T, Kutner E, Kim E, Espenberg D, Faddy M, *et al.* Impact of gonadotrophin stimulation for assisted reproductive technology on ovarian ageing and menopause. *Reprod Biomed Online* 2008;16:611–16.

16. te Velde ER, Pearson PL. The variability of female reproductive ageing. *Hum Reprod Update* 2002;8:141–54.

17. Faddy MJ, Gosden RG, Gougeon A, Richardson SJ, Nelson JF. Accelerated disappearance of ovarian follicles in mid-life: implications for forecasting menopause. *Hum Reprod* 1992;7:1342–6.

18. Richardson SJ, Senikas V, Nelson JF. Follicular depletion during the menopausal transition: evidence for accelerated loss and ultimate exhaustion. *J Clin Endocrinol Metab* 1987;65:1231–17.

19. Felicio LS, Nelson JF, Gosden RG, Finch CE. Restoration of ovulatory cycles by young ovarian grafts in aging mice: potentiation by long-term ovariectomy decreases with age. *Proc Natl Acad Sci U S A* 1983;80:6076–80.

20. Faddy MJ, Gosden RG. A model conforming the decline in follicle numbers to the age of menopause in women. *Hum Reprod* 1996;11:1484–6.

21. van Noord PA, Dubas JS, Dorland M, Boersma H, te Velde E. Age at natural menopause in a population-based screening cohort: the role of menarche, fecundity, and lifestyle factors. *Fertil Steril* 1997;68:95–102.

22. de Bruin JP, Bovenhuis H, van Noord PA, Pearson PL, van Arendonk JA, te Velde ER, *et al.* The role of genetic factors in age at natural menopause. *Hum Reprod* 2001;16:2014–18.

23. Murabito JM, Yang Q, Fox C, Wilson PW, Cupples LA. Heritability of age at natural menopause in the Framingham Heart Study. *J Clin Endocrinol Metab* 2005;90:3427–30.

24. Dharma SJ, Modi DN, Nandedkar TD. Gene expression profiling during early folliculogenesis in the mouse ovary. *Fertil Steril* 2008 May 24 DOI: 10.1016/j.fertnstert.2008.02.088.

25. Harris SE, Leese HJ, Gosden RG, Picton HM. Pyruvate and oxygen consumption throughout the growth and development of murine oocytes. *Mol Reprod Dev* 2009;76:231–8.

26. Matzuk MM, Burns KH, Viveiros MM, Eppig JJ. Intercellular communication in the mammalian ovary: oocytes carry the conversation. *Science* 2002;296:2178–80.

27. Skinner MK. Regulation of primordial follicle assembly and development. *Hum Reprod Update* 2005;11:461–71.

28. Carlsson IB, Scott JE, Visser JA, Ritvos O, Themmen AP, Hovatta O. Anti-Müllerian hormone inhibits initiation of growth of human primordial ovarian follicles *in vitro*. *Hum Reprod* 2006;9:2223–7.

29. Durlinger AL, Gruijters MJ, Kramer P, Karels B, Ingraham HA, Nachtigal MW, *et al.* Anti-Müllerian hormone inhibits initiation of primordial follicle growth in the mouse ovary. *Endocrinology* 2002;143:1076–84.

30. Nilsson EE, Skinner MK. Bone morphogenetic protein-4 acts as an ovarian follicle survival factor and promotes primordial follicle development. *Biol Reprod* 2003;69:1265–72.

31. Dong J, Albertini DF, Nishimori K, Kumar TR, Lu N, Matzuk MM. Growth differentiation factor-9 is required during early ovarian folliculogenesis. *Nature* 1996;383:531–5.

32. Manova K, Nocka K, Besmer P, Bachvarova RF. Gonadal expression of c-kit encoded at the W locus of the mouse. *Development* 1990;110:1057–69.

33. Huang EJ, Manova K, Packer AI, Sanchez S, Bachvarova RF, Besmer P. The murine steel panda mutation affects Kit ligand expression and growth of early ovarian follicles. *Dev Biol* 1993;157:100–9.

34. Parrott JA, Skinner MK. Kit-ligand/stem cell factor induces primordial follicle development and initiates folliculogenesis. *Endocrinology* 1999;140:4262–71.

35. Castrillon DH, Miao L, Kollipara R, Horner JW, DePinho RA. Suppression of ovarian follicle activation in mice by the transcription factor Foxo3a. *Science* 2003;301:215–18.

36. Reddy P, Liu L, Adhikari D, Jagarlamudi K, Rajareddy S, Shen Y, *et al.* Oocyte-specific deletion of *Pten* causes premature activation of the primordial follicle pool. *Science* 2008;319:611–13.

37. Zuckerman S. The number of oocytes in the mature ovary. *Rec Prog Horm Res* 1951;6:63–108.

38. Johnson J, Canning J, Kaneko T, Pru JK, Tilly JL. Germline stem cells and follicular renewal in the postnatal mammalian ovary. *Nature* 2004;428:145–50.

39. Johnson J, Bagley J, Skaznik-Wikiel M, Lee HJ, Adams GB, Niikura Y, *et al.* Oocyte generation in adult mammalian ovaries by putative germ cells in bone marrow and peripheral blood. *Cell* 2005;122:303–15.

40. Eggan K, Jurga S, Gosden R, Min IM, Wagers AJ. Ovulated oocytes in adult mice derive from non-circulating germ cells. *Nature* 2006;441:1109–14.

41. Begum S, Papaioannou VE, Gosden RG. The oocyte population is not renewed in transplanted or irradiated adult ovaries. *Hum Reprod* 2008;23:2326–30.

42. Lee HJ, Selesniemi K, Niikura Y, Niikura T, Klein R, Dombkowski DM, *et al.* Bone marrow transplantation generates immature oocytes and rescues long term fertility in a preclinical mouse model of chemotherapy-induced premature ovarian failure. *J Clin Oncol* 2007;25:3198–204.

43. Bukovsky A, Keenan JA, Caudle MR. Immunohistochemical studies of the adult human ovary: possible contribution of immune and epithelial factors to folliculogenesis. *Amer J Reprod Immunol* 1995;33:323–40.

44. Bukovsky A, Caudle MR, Svetlikova M, Upadhyaya NB. Origin of germ cells and formation of new primary follicles in adult human ovaries. *Reprod Biol Endocrinol* 2004;2:20.

45. Bukovsky A, Svetlikova M, Caudle MR. Oogenesis in cultures derived from adult human ovaries. *Reprod Biol Endocrinol* 2005;3:17.

46. Virant-Klun I, Zech N, Rozman P, Vogler A, Cvjeticanin B, Klemenc P, et al. Putative stem cells with an embryonic character isolated from the ovarian surface epithelium of women with no naturally present follicles and oocytes. *Differentiation* 2008;76:843–56.

47. Liu Y, Wu C, Lyu Q, Yang D, Albertini DF, Keefe DL, *et al.* Germline stem cells and neo-oogenesis in the adult human ovary. *Dev Biol* 2007;306:112–20.

48. Toyooka Y, Tsunekawa N, Akasu R, Noce T. Embryonic stem cells can form germ cells *in vitro*. *Proc Natl Acad Sci U S A* 2003;100:11457–62.

49. Geijsen N, Horoschak M, Kim K, Gribnau J, Eggan K, Daley GQ. Derivation of embryonic germ cells and male gametes from embryonic stem cells. *Nature* 2004;427:148–54.

50. Hübner K, Fuhrmann G, Christenson LK, Kehler J, Reinbold R, De La Fuente R, *et al.* Derivation of oocytes from mouse embryonic stem cells. *Science* 2003;300:1251–6.

51. Lacham-Kaplan O, Chy H, Trounson A. Testicular cell conditioned medium supports differentiation of embryonic stem cells into ovarian structures containing oocytes. *Stem Cells* 2006;24:266–73.

52. Dyce PW, Wen L, Li J. In vitro germline potential of stem cells derived from fetal porcine skin. *Nature Cell Biol* 2006;8:384–90.

Chapter 8

The science of ovarian ageing: how might knowledge be translated into practice?

Stephen G Hillier

Introduction

Fecundity declines as women age, owing to the continual loss of oocyte-containing follicles from their ovaries[1–3] and the simultaneous reduction in oocyte[4] and embryo quality.[5] At around 38 years of age, several years before the menstrual cycle ceases, the rate of oocyte loss increases towards total depletion of the follicular stock.[6] The associated increase in circulating follicle-stimulating hormone (FSH) reflects the accelerated follicular loss and explains several features of ovarian ageing, including shortening of the follicular phase of the menstrual cycle and increased incidence of dizygotic twinning.[7] The concomitant decrease in oocyte quality is in line with the increased incidence of miscarriages and chromosomal aberrations that occur after the age of 35 years.[8] This chapter briefly reviews key aspects of the autocrine, paracrine and endocrine control systems involved and flags the most helpful diagnostic biomarkers of ovarian ageing. The conclusion is that little or nothing can be done at the moment to slow the process. However, if the mechanisms involved can be better understood, ovarian stimulation to obtain oocytes for assisted reproductive technology procedures from older women could be conducted more efficiently and effectively on a case-by-case basis.

Why ovaries shrink with age

Newborn girls' ovaries contain a finite stock of around seven million oocytes as non-growing primordial follicles.[1] Each primordial follicle comprises an oocyte in the prophase of the first meiotic division, surrounded by an incomplete or whole layer of flattened spindle-shaped cells and separated from the surrounding ovarian stroma by a basement membrane. It is estimated to take 2–3 months for a primordial follicle to reach full maturity and ovulate. However, in a typical woman's lifespan, only 400 or so follicles ever do so.[6] The remainder initiate growth but become atretic at intermediate stages of maturity owing to programmed cell death (apoptosis).[9,10] The size of the initial oocyte stock, the rate of growth initiation and the proportion that degenerates are genetically determined variables.[11–13] Controversial experimental evidence from mice has challenged the dogma that females are incapable of *de novo* oocyte and follicle production during postnatal life.[14] The extent to which neo-oogenesis operates in women's ovaries is equivocal.[15] However, by the onset of the menopause, all functional oocytes have disappeared and the ovaries have approximately halved their weight compared with the start of the reproductive years (Hillier SG, unpublished observation).

The follicular lifespan

All ovarian follicles are doomed to degenerate through atresia unless they receive adequate trophic support from specific growth-differentiation factors or gonadotrophins at critical stages in their development. The few that ovulate will have been rescued from atresia through intrinsic (paracrine) and extrinsic (endocrine) signalling mechanisms that become fully operational during adulthood.[9] Critical checkpoints through which follicles must pass on this journey are:

1. activation, which occurs continuously from birth to senescence independently of gonadotrophic support
2. progression, requiring tonic stimulation by FSH
3. recruitment, requiring adult (intercyclic) levels of FSH stimulation
4. selection to ovulate, requiring follicular-phase levels of FSH and luteinising hormone (LH).[16]

Follicular atresia

Atresia is the natural process whereby follicles that are denied sufficient endocrine or paracrine support undergo involution through cellular apoptosis.[9,10] Development-related paracrine cues initiate follicle growth, modulate responsiveness to FSH and LH and set 'threshold' levels of gonadotrophic stimulation to ensure follicular survival (see the section below on follicular selection and dominance). Age-related increases in ovarian expression of apoptosis-related genes such as *Bcl2a1b*, *Casp1* and *Casp11* may help establish reduced responsiveness to FSH,[17] meaning that follicles in older ovaries may require more FSH to survive. Pro-apoptotic signals also modulate follicular survival. For example, theca-derived nodal, a member of the transforming growth factor-beta (TGFβ) superfamily of growth-differentiation factors, promotes granulosa cell apoptosis through downstream regulatory SMAD2 signalling and suppression of the phosphatidylinositol-3-kinase (PI3K)/Akt pathway.[18] Inactivation of the pro-apoptotic *Bax* gene in mice delays age-related ovarian failure, holding out the possibility that methods for postponing ovarian failure might eventually prove feasible in women.[19,20]

Follicular activation

Activation of follicular growth involves the transition of resting primordial follicles into growing primary follicles containing an enlarging oocyte surrounded by a single layer of pregranulosa cells.[9] A proportion of the follicular stock is always activating more-or-less continuously from birth until the menopause, by which time the oocyte stock has dissipated.[12] The process is independent of stimulation by FSH, based on its persistence in hypophysectomised rodents and animals with *Fshb* (encoding the FSHβ subunit) or *Fshr* (FSH receptor) gene knockouts.[21,22] Women with mutation-inactivated *FSHR* have primary or early-onset amenorrhoea and infertility. Their ovaries contain relatively abundant primordial and primary follicles with rare tertiary follicles, broadly consistent with arrested preantral follicular development.[23]

Paracrine communication between oocytes and surrounding somatic (granulosa) cells is the essence of follicular activation. The prototypic oogenic signal is granulosa-derived Kit ligand (KL), also known as stem cell factor (SCF), which stimulates oocyte growth and survival via the oocyte-expressed tyrosine kinase receptor for KL.[24] TGFβ-superfamily signalling is also critical to follicular activation and progression (see various reviews[25–27]). This was convincingly demonstrated by targeted gene deletion of *Gdf9*, encoding growth-differentiation factor-9 (GDF9), which prevented follicles growing beyond the two-layer granulosa cell stage and resulted in sterility in female mice.[28,29] Since GDF9 is an oocyte-specific gene product, this experiment proves that oocyte-derived GDF9 is vital to normal folliculogenesis.[26] Oocyte-derived bone morphogenetic protein-15 (BMP15; also known as GDF9b) is another candidate for involvement in follicular activation, because overexpression of *Bmp15* leads to accelerated folliculogenesis and an early onset of acyclicity in transgenic mice.[30] Ovarian phenotypes associated with primary or secondary amenorrhoea in women with *BMP15* mutations have also been reported.[31,32] Gene dosage is also a factor, because *Bmp15* mutation has been associated with both infertility (homozygotes) and superovulation (heterozygotes) in sheep.[33,34]

The molecular mechanism of follicular activation is through de-repression of oocyte growth involving the PI3K/Akt signalling pathway.[24] Transgenic experiments in mice have established that follicular activation is held in abeyance by members of the subfamily of forkhead box transcription factors (FOXO)[35] such as FOXO3a.[36] FOXO3a activity is suppressed by PI3K/Akt signalling, therefore stimulation of this pathway (via Kit, for example) leads to follicle activation.[24,37] In resting primordial follicles, PI3K/Akt signalling is naturally suppressed by the PTEN (phosphatase and tensin homologue deleted on chromosome 10) protein, which inhibits PI3K and Akt and thereby maintains FOXO3a activity. This explains why rates of follicular activation, oocyte loss and ovarian ageing are enhanced in transgenic mice bearing oocyte-specific *Foxo3a*[38,39] or *Pten*[40] gene knockouts. It remains to be determined whether these findings translate to women, in which case genetic mutations impacting PTEN–PI3K/Akt signalling could explain between-women differences in rates of oocyte loss and hence differences in timing of the onset of the menopause.[36]

Follicular progression

The primary-to-secondary follicle transition involves expansion of the oocyte, development of multiple granulosa cell layers and formation of the outer thecal cell layer. There is experimental evidence that TGFβ-superfamily signalling (TGFβ1, activin, GDF9 and antimüllerian hormone, AMH), acting via the intermediary of granulosa cell connective tissue growth factor (CTGF) formation, is responsible for the initiation of theca cell formation.[41] This stage of development is also independent of FSH support but critically dependent on paracrine signalling. Throughout folliculogenesis, granulosa cells strongly express TGFβ-superfamily genes encoding homo- or heterodimeric proteins that orchestrate the entire process of oogenesis at autocrine and paracrine levels. As shown in Figure 8.1, AMH and inhibin/activin subunits (INHBA and INHBB) predominate in primary and secondary follicles. At later stages of maturation, expression of the inhibin α subunit (INHA) increases, accounting for follicular formation of inhibin A (INHA/INHBA) or inhibin B (INHA/INHBB) (see the section below on follicular recruitment). AMH (AMH/AMH) has been shown to suppress early stages of follicular growth and onset of responsiveness to FSH *in vitro*.[42] Activins (homodimers or heterodimers of INHBA and INHBB) mainly enhance granulosa cell proliferation and promote responsiveness to FSH, although variable effects have been observed *in vitro*, possibly related to the choice of experimental model.[43,44] The efflux of AMH, activins and inhibins from immature follicles explains their presence in blood and why their measurement can offer a means of assessing ovarian reserve (see the section below on biomarkers of ovarian ageing).

Follicular progression to the point of antrum formation seems more or less automatic.[9] However, once preantral follicles reach diameters of around 200 micrometres, they increasingly require stimulation by FSH to prevent atresia.[21] Antrum formation is the morphological hallmark of FSH action, caused by fluid-filled spaces that appear between granulosa cells gradually coalescing into a single large cavity.[45] Antral (tertiary) follicles achieve moderate dimensions (around 5 mm in diameter) throughout infancy with only minimal stimulation by FSH.[46,47] However, full preovulatory growth to a diameter of 20 mm or more requires sustained stimulation by FSH at blood levels associated with ovulatory menstrual cycles. Thus, all developing antral follicles are destined to undergo atresia before puberty, whereas they are candidate preovulatory follicles in adult ovaries (see the section below on follicular recruitment).

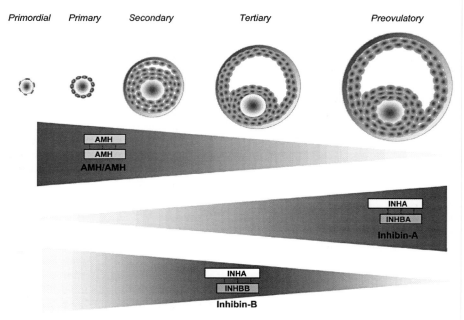

Figure 8.1 Development-related TGFβ-superfamily members provide biomarkers of ovarian ageing. The primordial to preovulatory follicular lifespan is associated with a characteristic signature of TGFβ-superfamily gene signalling. Primary preantral follicles contain granulosa cells expressing AMH (AMH/AMH), which is thought to suppress early-stage follicular growth and responsiveness to FSH. AMH protein levels in blood are proportionate to the number of follicles held in reserve. Inhibin B (INHA/INHBB) is a product of the intermediately mature follicular cohort from which the inhibin A (INHA/INHBA)-secreting preovulatory follicle is selected in ovulatory menstrual cycles. Inhibin B levels therefore reflect the number of growing follicles potentially available for preovulatory recruitment. Inhibin A is a paracrine driver of thecal androgen synthesis, which is essential for follicular estrogen synthesis and, hence, it is a biomarker of preovulatory follicular maturity

Follicular recruitment

Pituitary secretion of FSH increases at the start of each menstrual cycle, mainly owing to withdrawal of the negative feedback action of estradiol produced by the previous corpus luteum.[48] Granulosa cells in antral follicles increasingly express the inhibin α subunit, regulated by FSH.[49] Dimerisation of INHA with inhibin/activin A (INHBA) or B (INHBB) subunits produces inhibin A or inhibin B, respectively. The intercyclic FSH rise causes multiple inhibin B-secreting antral follicles with diameters of up to around 5 mm to enter preovulatory development.[50] The inhibins feed back negatively on pituitary FSH secretion to terminate the intercyclic FSH rise.[3] The evidence from ovulation induction using exogenous FSH is that each follicle within this cohort has a 'threshold' requirement for FSH below which it must be stimulated by FSH if it is to be protected from atresia and be recruited to preovulatory development.[51,52] Subtle (10–30%) differences exist between individual follicles at this stage of development with respect to the threshold amount of FSH required to initiate preovulatory development, which explains how one follicle is eventually selected to mature and ovulate (see the section below on follicular selection and dominance). Paracrine signalling via TGFβ-superfamily members is integral to the establishment of follicular thresholds for stimulation by FSH and LH that lead to follicular dominance, with activins sensitising granulosa cells to FSH and inhibins sensitising thecal cells to LH.[16,44] The reduced ovarian response to superovulation therapy with age would be consistent with a reduction in the number of antral follicles at this critically FSH-dependent stage of development.

Follicular selection and dominance

Usually only one of the several follicles that are recruited into preovulatory development via the intercyclic FSH rise survives to ovulate. This 'dominant' follicle continues to develop in the face of the subsiding mid to late follicular phase serum FSH level because, as a direct consequence of previous stimulation by FSH, its granulosa cells now express receptors for LH and therefore respond directly to LH as well as FSH.[16,53] During its final week of maturation, the preovulatory follicle increasingly secretes estradiol, driven by endocrine (LH) and paracrine (inhibin A) signalling. LH-dependent stages of oocyte and cumulus cell maturation remain critically dependent on paracrine signalling involving TGFβ-superfamily members throughout, notably GDF9 and BMP15.[54] Induction of epidermal growth factor (EGF)-like growth factors and transactivation of EGF receptor (EGFR) signalling is also integral to LH-induced ovulation.[55] As with follicular activation approximately 3 months earlier (see above), release of the preovulatory oocyte from meiotic arrest involves a molecular de-repression mechanism, this time through withdrawal or inactivation of second messenger cAMP.[56]

Genes, environment and ovarian ageing

Genetic factors influence the size of the initial oocyte endowment and subsequent rates of follicle formation, growth and atresia in mice.[13] It is also clearly established that ovarian ageing is heritable in women.[57] Of the 11 000 or so gene transcripts detected in mice, 530 undergo statistically significant expression changes with age.[58] Gene knockouts in mice associated with particularly striking examples of premature ovarian failure include zinc-finger transcription factor (*Zfx*),[59] *Oct4*,[60] *Fanca*,[61] *Foxo3a*,[38] *Foxl2*,[62] *Pten*,[36] *Dazl*,[63] *Bcl-x*,[64] *Amh*,[42] *Nobox*,[65] *Rb1* (retinoblastoma)[66] and *Ar* (androgen receptor).[67]

While it would be naïve to suppose that mouse models can faithfully reproduce the biology of human ovarian ageing, it is reasonable to suppose that the underlying regulatory mechanisms are similar.[26,68] Thus, in a review of mouse models of ovarian follicle development, Barnett et al.[69] pointed out that '*FANCL* patients exhibit POF, which is mimicked by *Fanca*[−/−] mice and *Gcd* mice.[70] The *Zfx*[−/−] mouse mimics the ovarian dysgenesis phenotype that occurs in Turner syndrome.[59,71] In addition, *Foxl2*[−/−] and *atm*[−/−] mice display ovarian failure similar to that in patients with blepharophimosis–ptosis syndrome (BPES)'.[71,72] The few candidate genes that have been unequivocally associated with fertile lifespan in women include *FMR1* (fragile X syndrome)[73,74] and *FOXL2*.[75,76] A polymorphism in *AMHR2* (AMH type II receptor) has also been associated with early onset of menopause,[77] as have missense mutations in *BMP15*.[31] However, many proposed gene associations with premature ovarian failure remain conjectural or controversial,[78] including *FSHR*,[79] *INHA*,[80,81] *ESR1* (estrogen receptor α),[82] *FOXO3A* and *FOXO1A*,[83] *BMP15*[84,85] and *GDF9*.[84,86]

Less controversial is the deleterious impact of ovotoxic environmental substances,[87] smoking[88,89] and exposure to chemotherapy or radiotherapy[90] on ovarian reserve in women. Nutrition is also potentially important, because dietary restriction initiated at weaning or during adulthood delays ovarian ageing in mice[91,92] and alters global gene expression in the ovary.[93] However, because calorie restriction suppresses ovulation, it is difficult to distinguish between direct effects of nutrition on the ovary and secondary effects due to aberrant endocrine signalling.

Biomarkers of ovarian ageing

The development-related changes in TGFβ-superfamily gene expression throughout folliculogenesis create an efflux of potential biomarkers in blood or urine that can be measured to reflect follicle number and stage of maturity. Such assays potentially provide a rational basis for the endocrine diagnosis of ovarian sufficiency, in combination with conventional markers of ovarian status (FSH and estradiol) and ultrasonographic measurements of follicle size and number.[94]

FSH and estradiol

FSH and estradiol provide classic measures of female reproductive status, based on the dynamic equilibrium that exists between pituitary FSH secretion and preovulatory follicular estrogen biosynthesis.[3,95] Menstrual cycles become irregular as the menopause approaches and ovarian estrogen production diminishes accordingly.[96] Eventually, complete estrogen withdrawal and the associated reduction in ovarian inhibin secretion combine to enhance pituitary FSH production to levels that diagnose ovarian failure.[97] The basal FSH level increases throughout reproductive life, with a major change occurring 2–7 years before the final menstrual period.[98] However, both basal FSH and its rate of increase vary considerably from woman to woman and the pulsatile nature of FSH secretion can result in an unrepresentative result being obtained if a single sample is analysed.[99] Accordingly, FSH alone is at best a crude and indirect biomarker of ovarian sufficiency.[100]

AMH

AMH is produced in relatively large amounts by the granulosa cells of small follicles in which it is proposed to retard follicular growth and suppress responsiveness to FSH.[42] Serum AMH levels reflect the size of the primordial follicle pool and number of growing follicles in mice.[101] Therefore, as a granulosa cell-specific protein, AMH is an excellent candidate biomarker of ovarian follicular reserve.[102] Absolute relationships between AMH formation/function and follicular development in women have not been clearly established.[103,104] However, serum AMH level is suggested to provide a 'quantitative' index of the transition of resting primordial follicles to growing follicles and hence the imminence of menopause. Clinical data have confirmed that blood AMH levels provide a realistic estimate of biological age,[105] with a critical fall in the level becoming evident 5 years before the menopause.[94]

Inhibins

Development-related gene expression of activin and inhibin subunits occurs throughout the follicular lifespan, from activation to ovulation.[26,27] The clinical application of two-site immunoassays capable of distinguishing inhibin A and inhibin B has allowed clarification of the roles played by these proteins as regulators of reproductive function and as biomarkers of ovarian ageing.[106] Basal inhibin A and inhibin B levels each decline in advance of the menopause, reflecting the attrition of small antral and preovulatory follicles, respectively.[107] Typically, the serum inhibin B level falls before that of inhibin A.[108] This is because inhibin B is produced by the granulosa cells of follicles in the vanishing cohort of intermediately mature follicles from which preovulatory (that is, inhibin A-secreting) follicles are sporadically recruited when menstrual cycles succeed.[109,110] Gradual withdrawal of negative feedback suppression of pituitary FSH secretion by inhibin B can explain the age-related increase in basal FSH level[96,106] and the accelerated FSH rise that portends ovarian failure.[98,111]

Conclusion

Once activated, all human ovarian follicles are potentially capable of ovulating if they receive adequate trophic stimulation at critical stages of development. However, the number of follicles initially present, their rates of activation, progression and ovulation, and their susceptibility to atresia will vary from woman to woman. Thus, while one woman aged 35 years might retain sufficient oocytes in her ovaries to continue ovulating for a decade or more, another of the same age may have become completely barren.

Ovarian and pituitary factors that orchestrate progressive stages of follicular growth and atresia can be measured in blood to monitor ovarian reserve (that is, potential fecundity). Analytes of choice currently include AMH and inhibin B, in conjunction with the principal endocrine driver of folliculogenesis, FSH. The clinical application of assays for AMH and inhibins has helped clarify the roles of these substances in ovarian physiology and suggest a unified paracrine and endocrine mechanism to explain age-related ovarian failure. Our current understanding is thus that circulating levels of AMH and inhibin B in the blood decline with age owing to the irreversible loss of immature follicles at stages of development that characteristically secrete these substances. The progressive loss of inhibin B negative feedback on pituitary FSH secretion explains the secondary increase in blood FSH level that heralds the menopause. The rise in FSH in turn speeds up the final stages of follicular depletion by advancing the growth and differentiation of granulosa cells in residual immature follicles containing oocytes that have not completed their gonadotrophin-independent growth phase. These follicles are probably driven into atresia through discordant granulosa–oocyte paracrine signalling. Eventually, the cyclic selection of preovulatory follicles also fails, as reflected in the late perimenopausal decline in blood estradiol and inhibin A levels. As FSH rises, the process is amplified until menstrual cycles cease.

Unquestionably, human homologues of the numerous mouse genes that regulate ovarian ageing operate in women. Their future verification and evaluation in gene association studies can be expected to define genotypes that will benefit from elective clinical intervention in advance of follicular depletion and premature ovarian failure. Some of these genotypes may be amenable to targeted therapy to delay onset of the premature ovarian failure phenotype. It seems unlikely that any single successful approach to ovarian stimulation for fertility treatment in older women (or younger women with 'older' ovaries) will emerge in the near future, given the genetic and environmental complexities involved. Patient history, antral follicular count and ovarian volume assessed by vaginal ultrasonography and biomarkers of follicular reserve will continue to point the way to optimal treatment. Each woman's treatment should be personalised (by type, dose and duration of ovarian stimulation) to coax preovulatory maturation from the diminishing residual follicular cohort in her ovaries. However, this cannot compensate for the age-related attrition in oocyte and embryo 'quality', over which neither the gynaecologist nor reproductive endocrinologist currently has control.

References

1. Baker TG. Oogenesis and ovarian development. In: Balin H, Glasser SR, editors. *Reproductive Biology*. Amsterdam: Excerpta Medica; 1972. p. 398–437.
2. Broekmans FJ, Faddy MJ, Scheffer G, te Velde ER. Antral follicle counts are related to age at natural fertility loss and age at menopause. *Menopause* 2004;11:607–14.
3. Burger HG, Hale GE, Dennerstein L, Robertson DM. Cycle and hormone changes during perimenopause: the key role of ovarian function. *Menopause* 2008;15:603–12.
4. Navot D, Bergh PA, Williams MA, Garrisi GJ, Guzman I, Sandler B, et al. L. Poor oocyte quality rather than implantation failure as a cause of age-related decline in female fertility. *Lancet* 1991;337:1375–7.
5. Ziebe S, Loft A, Petersen JH, Andersen AG, Lindenberg S, Petersen K, Andersen AN. Embryo quality and developmental potential is compromised by age. *Acta Obstet Gynecol Scand* 2001;80:169–74.
6. Gougeon A, Ecochard R, Thalabard JC. Age-related changes of the population of human ovarian follicles: increase in the disappearance rate of non-growing and early-growing follicles in aging women. *Biol Reprod* 1994;50:653–63.
7. Beemsterboer SN, Homburg R, Gorter NA, Schats R, Hompes PG, Lambalk CB. The paradox of declining fertility but increasing twinning rates with advancing maternal age. *Hum Reprod* 2006;21:1531–2.
8. te Velde ER, Scheffer GJ, Dorland M, Broekmans FJ, Fauser BC. Developmental and endocrine aspects of normal ovarian aging. *Mol Cell Endocrinol* 1998;145:67–73.
9. Craig J, Orisaka M, Wang H, Orisaka S, Thompson W, Zhu C, et al. Gonadotropin and intra-ovarian signals regulating follicle development and atresia: the delicate balance between life and death. *Front Biosci* 2007;12:3628–39.
10. Krysko DV, Diez-Fraile A, Criel G, Svistunov AA, Vandenabeele P, D'Herde K. Life and death of female gametes during oogenesis and folliculogenesis. *Apoptosis* 2008;13:1065–87.
11. Faddy MJ, Gosden RG, Edwards RG. Ovarian follicle dynamics in mice: a comparative study of three inbred strains and an F1 hybrid. *J Endocrinol* 1983;96:23–33.
12. Faddy MJ, Gosden RG. A model conforming the decline in follicle numbers to the age of menopause in women. *Hum Reprod* 1996;11:1484–6.
13. Canning J, Takai Y, Tilly JL. Evidence for genetic modifiers of ovarian follicular endowment and development from studies of five inbred mouse strains. *Endocrinology* 2003;144:9–12.

14. Johnson J, Canning J, Kaneko T, Pru JK, Tilly JL. Germline stem cells and follicular renewal in the postnatal mammalian ovary. *Nature* 2004;428:145–50.

15. Tilly JL, Johnson J. Recent arguments against germ cell renewal in the adult human ovary: is an absence of marker gene expression really acceptable evidence of an absence of oogenesis? *Cell Cycle* 2007;6:879–83.

16. Hillier SG. Current concepts of the roles of follicle stimulating hormone and luteinizing hormone in folliculogenesis. *Hum Reprod* 1994;9:188–91.

17. Sharov AA, Falco G, Piao Y, Poosala S, Becker KG, Zonderman AB, et al. Effects of aging and calorie restriction on the global gene expression profiles of mouse testis and ovary. *BMC Biol* 2008;6:24.

18. Wang H, Jiang JY, Zhu C, Peng C, Tsang BK. Role and regulation of nodal/activin receptor-like kinase 7 signaling pathway in the control of ovarian follicular atresia. *Mol Endocrinol* 2006;20:2469–82.

19. Perez GI, Robles R, Knudson CM, Flaws JA, Korsmeyer SJ, Tilly JL. Prolongation of ovarian lifespan into advanced chronological age by Bax-deficiency. *Nat Genet* 1999;21:200–3.

20. Perez GI, Jurisicova A, Wise L, Lipina T, Kanisek M, Bechard A, et al. Absence of the proapoptotic Bax protein extends fertility and alleviates age-related health complications in female mice. *Proc Natl Acad Sci U S A* 2007;104:5229–34.

21. Hirshfield AN. Comparison of granulosa cell proliferation in small follicles of hypophysectomized, prepubertal, and mature rats. *Biol Reprod* 1985;32:979–87.

22. Layman LC, McDonough PG. Mutations of follicle stimulating hormone-beta and its receptor in human and mouse: genotype/phenotype. *Mol Cell Endocrinol* 2000;161:9–17.

23. Tapanainen JS, Vaskivuo T, Aittomaki K, Huhtaniemi IT. Inactivating FSH receptor mutations and gonadal dysfunction. *Mol Cell Endocrinol* 1998;145:129–35.

24. Liu K. Stem cell factor (SCF)-Kit mediated phosphatidylinositol 3 (PI3) kinase signaling during mammalian oocyte growth and early follicular development. *Front Biosci* 2006;11:126–35.

25. Eppig JJ, Chesnel F, Hirao Y, O'Brien MJ, Pendola FL, Watanabe S, et al. Oocyte control of granulosa cell development: how and why. *Hum Reprod* 1997;12(Suppl):127–32.

26. Chang H, Brown CW, Matzuk MM. Genetic analysis of the mammalian transforming growth factor-beta superfamily. *Endocr Rev* 2002;23:787–823.

27. Matzuk MM, Burns KH, Viveiros MM, Eppig JJ. Intercellular communication in the mammalian ovary: oocytes carry the conversation. *Science* 2002;296:2178–80.

28. Dong J, Albertini DF, Nishimori K, Kumar TR, Lu N, Matzuk MM. Growth differentiation factor-9 is required during early ovarian folliculogenesis. *Nature* 1996;383:531–5.

29. Carabatsos MJ, Elvin J, Matzuk MM, Albertini DF. Characterization of oocyte and follicle development in growth differentiation factor-9-deficient mice. *Dev Biol* 1998;204:373–84.

30. McMahon HE, Hashimoto O, Mellon PL, Shimasaki S. Oocyte-specific overexpression of mouse bone morphogenetic protein-15 leads to accelerated folliculogenesis and an early onset of acyclicity in transgenic mice. *Endocrinology* 2008;149:2807–15.

31. Dixit H, Rao LK, Padmalatha VV, Kanakavalli M, Deenadayal M, Gupta N, et al. Missense mutations in the BMP15 gene are associated with ovarian failure. *Hum Genet* 2006;119:408–15.

32. Laissue P, Vinci G, Veitia RA, Fellous M. Recent advances in the study of genes involved in non-syndromic premature ovarian failure. *Mol Cell Endocrinol* 2008;282:101–11.

33. Galloway SM, McNatty KP, Cambridge LM, Laitinen MP, Juengel JL, Jokiranta TS, et al. Mutations in an oocyte-derived growth factor gene (BMP15) cause increased ovulation rate and infertility in a dosage-sensitive manner. *Nat Genet* 2000;25:279–83.

34. McNatty KP, Galloway SM, Wilson T, Smith P, Hudson NL, O'Connell A, et al. Physiological effects of major genes affecting ovulation rate in sheep. *Genet Sel Evol* 2005;37 Suppl 1:S25–38.

35. Arden KC. FOXO animal models reveal a variety of diverse roles for FOXO transcription factors. *Oncogene* 2008;27:2345–50.

36. John GB, Gallardo TD, Shirley LJ, Castrillon DH. Foxo3 is a PI3K-dependent molecular switch controlling the initiation of oocyte growth. *Dev Biol* 2008;321:197–204.

37. Thomas FH, Ismail RS, Jiang JY, Vanderhyden BC. Kit ligand 2 promotes murine oocyte growth *in vitro*. *Biol Reprod* 2008;7:167–75.

38. Castrillon DH, Miao L, Kollipara R, Horner JW, DePinho RA. Suppression of ovarian follicle activation in mice by the transcription factor Foxo3a. *Science* 2003:215–18.

39. Liu L, Rajareddy S, Reddy P, Du C, Jagarlamudi K, Shen Y, *et al.* Infertility caused by retardation of follicular development in mice with oocyte-specific expression of Foxo3a. *Development* 2007;134:199–209.

40. Reddy P, Liu L, Adhikari D, Jagarlamudi K, Rajareddy S, Shen Y, *et al.* Oocyte-specific deletion of Pten causes premature activation of the primordial follicle pool. *Science* 2008;319:611–13.

41. Harlow CR, Davidson L, Burns KH, Yan C, Matzuk MM, Hillier SG. FSH and TGF-beta superfamily members regulate granulosa cell connective tissue growth factor gene expression *in vitro* and *in vivo*. *Endocrinology* 2002;143:3316–25.

42. Visser JA, Themmen AP. Anti-Müllerian hormone and folliculogenesis. *Mol Cell Endocrinol* 2005;234:81–6.

43. Knight PG, Glister C. TGF-beta superfamily members and ovarian follicle development. *Reproduction* 2006;132:191–206.

44. Hillier SG, Miró F. Inhibin, activin, and follistatin. Potential roles in ovarian physiology. *Ann N Y Acad Sci* 1993;687:29–38.

45. Mitchell LM, Kennedy CR, Hartshorne GM. Effects of varying gonadotrophin dose and timing on antrum formation and ovulation efficiency of mouse follicles *in vitro*. *Hum Reprod* 2002;17:1181–8.

46. Peters H, Byskov AG, Grinsted J. Follicular growth in fetal and prepubertal ovaries of humans and other primates. *Clin Endocrinol Metab* 1978;7:469–85.

47. Zhang K, Pollack S, Ghods A, Dicken C, Isaac B, Adel G, *et al.* Onset of ovulation after menarche in girls: a longitudinal study. *J Clin Endocrinol Metab* 2008;93:1186–94.

48. le Nestour E, Marraoui J, Lahlou N, Roger M, de Ziegler D, Bouchard P. Role of estradiol in the rise in follicle-stimulating hormone levels during the luteal-follicular transition. *J Clin Endocrinol Metab* 1993;77:439–42.

49. Burkart AD, Mukherjee A, Mayo KE. Mechanism of repression of the inhibin alpha-subunit gene by inducible 3′,5′-cyclic adenosine monophosphate early repressor. *Mol Endocrinol* 2006;20:584–97.

50. Laven JS, Fauser BC. Inhibins and adult ovarian function. *Mol Cell Endocrinol* 2004;225:37–44.

51. Brown JB. Pituitary control of ovarian function – concepts derived from gonadotrophin therapy. *Aust N Z J Obstet Gynaecol* 1978;18:46–54.

52. Schipper I, Hop WC, Fauser BC. The follicle-stimulating hormone (FSH) threshold/window concept examined by different interventions with exogenous FSH during the follicular phase of the normal menstrual cycle: duration, rather than magnitude, of FSH increase affects follicle development. *J Clin Endocrinol Metab* 1998;83:1292–8.

53. Zeleznik AJ, Hillier SG. The role of gonadotropins in the selection of the preovulatory follicle. *Clin Obstet Gynecol* 1984;27:927–40.

54. Russell DL, Robker RL. Molecular mechanisms of ovulation: co-ordination through the cumulus complex. *Hum Reprod Update* 2007;13:289–312.

55. Panigone S, Hsieh M, Fu M, Persani L, Conti M. Luteinizing hormone signaling in preovulatory follicles involves early activation of the epidermal growth factor receptor pathway. *Mol Endocrinol* 2008:924–36.

56. Vaccari S, Horner K, Mehlmann LM, Conti M. Generation of mouse oocytes defective in cAMP synthesis and degradation: endogenous cyclic AMP is essential for meiotic arrest. *Dev Biol* 2008;316:124–34.

57. van Asselt KM, Kok HS, Pearson PL, Dubas JS, Peeters PH, Te Velde ER, *et al.* Heritability of menopausal age in mothers and daughters. *Fertil Steril* 2004;82:1348–51.

58. Hamatani T, Falco G, Carter MG, Akutsu H, Stagg CA, Sharov AA, *et al.* Age-associated alteration of gene expression patterns in mouse oocytes. *Hum Mol Genet* 2004;13:2263–78.

59. Luoh SW, Bain PA, Polakiewicz RD, Goodheart ML, Gardner H, Jaenisch R, *et al.* Zfx mutation results in small animal size and reduced germ cell number in male and female mice. *Development* 1997;124:2275–84.

60. Kehler J, Tolkunova E, Koschorz B, Pesce M, Gentile L, Boiani M, *et al.* Oct4 is required for primordial germ cell survival. *EMBO Rep* 2004;5:1078–83.

61. Koomen M, Cheng NC, van de Vrugt HJ, Godthelp BC, van der Valk MA, Oostra AB, et al. Reduced fertility and hypersensitivity to mitomycin C characterize Fancg/Xrcc9 null mice. *Hum Mol Genet* 2002;11;273–81.
62. Uda M, Ottolenghi C, Crisponi L, Garcia JE, Deiana M, Kimber W, et al. Foxl2 disruption causes mouse ovarian failure by pervasive blockage of follicle development. *Hum Mol Genet* 2004;13:1171–81.
63. Ruggiu M, Speed R, Taggart M, McKay SJ, Kilanowski F, Saunders P, et al. The mouse Dazla gene encodes a cytoplasmic protein essential for gametogenesis. *Nature* 1997;389:73–7.
64. Rucker EB III, Dierisseau P, Wagner KU, Garrett L, Wynshaw-Boris A, Flaws JA, et al. Bcl-x and bax regulate mouse primordial germ cell survival and apoptosis during embryogenesis. *Mol Endocrinol* 2000;14:1038–52.
65. Rajkovic A, Panga SA, Ballow D, Suzumori N, Matzuk MM. NOBOX deficiency disrupts early folliculogenesis and oocyte-specific gene expression. *Science* 2004;305:1157–9.
66. Andreu-Vieyra C, Chen R, Matzuk MM. Conditional deletion of the retinoblastoma (Rb) gene in ovarian granulosa cells leads to premature ovarian failure. *Mol Endocrinol* 2008;22:2141–61.
67. Kimura S, Matsumoto T, Matsuyama R, Shiina H, Sato T, Takeyama K, et al. Androgen receptor function in folliculogenesis and its clinical implication in premature ovarian failure. *Trends Endocrinol Metab* 2007;18:183–9.
68. Suzumori N, Pangas SA, Rajkovic A. Candidate genes for premature ovarian failure. *Curr Med Chem* 2007;14:353–7.
69. Barnett KR, Schilling C, Greenfeld CR, Tomic D, Flaws JA. Ovarian follicle development and transgenic mouse models. *Hum Reprod Update* 2006;12:537–55.
70. Agoulnik AI, Lu B, Zhu Q, Truong C, Ty MT, Arango N, et al. A novel gene, Pog, is necessary for primordial germ cell proliferation in the mouse and underlies the germ cell deficient mutation, gcd. *Hum Mol Genet* 2002;11:3047–53.
71. Christin-Maitre S, Vasseur C, Portnoï MF, Bouchard P. Genes and premature ovarian failure. *Mol Cell Endocrinol* 1998;145:75–80.
72. Di Giacomo M, Barchi M, Baudat F, Edelmann W, Keeney S, Jasin M. Distinct DNA-damage-dependent and -independent responses drive the loss of oocytes in recombination-defective mouse mutants. *Proc Natl Acad Sci U S A* 2005;102:737–42.
73. Welt CK, Smith PC, Taylor AE. Evidence of early ovarian aging in fragile X premutation carriers. *J Clin Endocrinol Metab* 2004;89:4569–74.
74. Gleicher N, Weghofer A, Barad DH. A pilot study of premature ovarian senescence: I. Correlation of triple CGG repeats on the FMR1 gene to ovarian reserve parameters FSH and anti-Müllerian hormone. *Fertil Steril* 2008 Apr 1 DOI: 10.1016/j.fertnstert.2008.01.098.
75. Harris SE, Chand AL, Winship IM, Gersak K, Aittomäki K, Shelling AN. Identification of novel mutations in FOXL2 associated with premature ovarian failure. *Mol Hum Reprod* 2002;8:729–33.
76. Uhlenhaut NH, Treier M. Foxl2 function in ovarian development. *Mol Genet Metab* 2006;88:225–34.
77. Kevenaar ME, Themmen AP, Rivadeneira F, Uitterlinden AG, Laven JS, van Schoor NM, et al. A polymorphism in the AMH type II receptor gene is associated with age at menopause in interaction with parity. *Hum Reprod* 2007;22:2382–8.
78. Kok HS, van Asselt KM, van der Schouw YT, Peeters PH, Wijmenga C. Genetic studies to identify genes underlying menopausal age. *Hum Reprod Update* 2005;11:483–93.
79. Zerbetto I, Gromoll J, Luisi S, Reis FM, Nieschlag E, Simoni M, et al. Follicle-stimulating hormone receptor and DAZL gene polymorphisms do not affect the age of menopause. *Fertil Steril* 2008;90:2264–8.
80. Sundblad V, Chiauzzi VA, Andreone L, Campo S, Charreau EH, Dain L. Controversial role of inhibin alpha-subunit gene in the aetiology of premature ovarian failure. *Hum Reprod* 2006;21:1154–60.
81. Harris SE, Chand AL, Winship IM, Gersak K, Nishi Y, Yanase T, et al. INHA promoter polymorphisms are associated with premature ovarian failure. *Mol Hum Reprod* 2005;11:779–84.
82. Bretherick KL, Hanna CW, Currie LM, Fluker MR, Hammond GL, Robinson WP. Estrogen receptor alpha gene polymorphisms are associated with idiopathic premature ovarian failure. *Fertil Steril* 2008;89:318–24.

83. Watkins WJ, Umbers AJ, Woad KJ, Harris SE, Winship IM, Gersak K, *et al*. Mutational screening of FOXO3A and FOXO1A in women with premature ovarian failure. *Fertil Steril* 2006;86:1518–21.

84. Chand AL, Ponnampalam AP, Harris SE, Winship IM, Shelling AN. Mutational analysis of *BMP15* and *GDF9* as candidate genes for premature ovarian failure. *Fertil Steril* 2006;86:1009–12.

85. Zhang P, Shi YH, Wang LC, Chen ZJ. Sequence variants in exons of the *BMP-15* gene in Chinese patients with premature ovarian failure. *Acta Obstet Gynecol Scand* 2007;86:585–9.

86. Kovanci E, Rohozinski J, Simpson JL, Heard MJ, Bishop CE, Carson SA. Growth differentiating factor-9 mutations may be associated with premature ovarian failure. *Fertil Steril* 2007;87:143–6.

87. Hoyer PB. Reproductive toxicology: current and future directions. *Biochem Pharmacol* 2001;62:1557–64.

88. Freour T, Masson D, Mirallie S, Jean M, Bach K, Dejoie T, *et al*. Active smoking compromises IVF outcome and affects ovarian reserve. *Reprod Biomed Online* 2008;16:96–102.

89. van Asselt KM, Kok HS, van Der Schouw YT, Grobbee DE, te Velde ER, Pearson PL, Peeters PH. Current smoking at menopause rather than duration determines the onset of natural menopause. *Epidemiology* 2004;15:634–9.

90. Anderson RA, Themmen AP, Al-Qahtani A, Groome NP, Cameron DA. The effects of chemotherapy and long-term gonadotrophin suppression on the ovarian reserve in premenopausal women with breast cancer. *Hum Reprod* 2006;21:2583–92. .

91. Nelson JF, Gosden RG, Felicio LS. Effect of dietary restriction on estrous cyclicity and follicular reserves in aging C57BL/6J mice. *Biol Reprod* 1985;32:515–22.

92. Selesniemi K, Lee HJ, Tilly JL. Moderate caloric restriction initiated in rodents during adulthood sustains function of the female reproductive axis into advanced chronological age. *Aging Cell* 2008;7:622–9.

93 Sharov AA, Falco G, Piao Y, Poosala S, Becker KG, Zonderman AB, *et al*. Effects of aging and calorie restriction on the global gene expression profiles of mouse testis and ovary. *BMC Biol* 2008;6:24.

94. Sowers MR, Eyvazzadeh AD, McConnell D, Yosef M, Jannausch ML, Zhang D, *et al*. Anti-mullerian hormone and inhibin B in the definition of ovarian aging and the menopause transition. *J Clin Endocrinol Metab* 2008;93:3478–83.

95. Klein NA, Soules MR. Endocrine changes of the perimenopause. *Clin Obstet Gynecol* 1998;41:912–20.

96. Broekmans FJ, Knauff EA, te Velde ER, Macklon NS, Fauser BC. Female reproductive ageing: current knowledge and future trends. *Trends Endocrinol Metab* 2007;18:58–65.

97. Muttukrishna S, Sharma S, Barlow DH, Ledger W, Groome N, Sathananda M. Serum inhibins, estradiol, progesterone and FSH in surgical menopause: a demonstration of ovarian pituitary feedback loop in women. *Hum Reprod* 2002;17:2535–9.

98. Sowers MR, Zheng H, McConnell D, Nan B, Harlow S, Randolph JF Jr. Follicle stimulating hormone and its rate of change in defining menopause transition stages. *J Clin Endocrinol Metab* 2008;93:3958–64.

99 Ferrell RJ, O'Connor KA, Holman DJ, Brindle E, Miller RC, Rodriguez G, *et al*. Monitoring reproductive aging in a 5-year prospective study: aggregate and individual changes in luteinizing hormone and follicle-stimulating hormone with age. *Menopause* 2007;14:29–37.

100. Henrich JB, Hughes JP, Kaufman SC, Brody DJ, Curtin LR. Limitations of follicle-stimulating hormone in assessing menopause status: findings from the National Health and Nutrition Examination Survey (NHANES 1999–2000). *Menopause* 2006;13:171–7.

101. Kevenaar ME, Meerasahib MF, Kramer P, van de Lang-Born BM, de Jong FH, Groome NP, *et al*. Serum anti-mullerian hormone levels reflect the size of the primordial follicle pool in mice. *Endocrinology* 2006 ;147:3228–34.

102 Teixeira J, Maheswaran S, Donahoe PK. Mullerian inhibiting substance: an instructive developmental hormone with diagnostic and possible therapeutic applications. *Endocr Rev* 2001;22:657–74.

103. Rice S, Ojha K, Whitehead S, Mason H. Stage-specific expression of androgen receptor, follicle-stimulating hormone receptor, and anti-Müllerian hormone type II receptor in single, isolated, human preantral follicles: relevance to polycystic ovaries. *J Clin Endocrinol Metab* 2007;92:1034–40.

104. Yding Andersen C, Rosendahl M, Byskov AG. Concentration of anti-Müllerian hormone and inhibin-B in relation to steroids and age in follicular fluid from small antral human follicles. *J Clin Endocrinol Metab* 2008;93:2344–9.

105. van Disseldorp J, Faddy MJ, Themmen AP, de Jong FH, Peeters PH, van der Schouw YT, *et al*. Relationship of serum antimüllerian hormone concentration to age at menopause. *J Clin Endocrinol Metab* 2008;93:2129–34.

106. Tsigkou A, Luisi S, Reis FM, Petraglia F. Inhibins as diagnostic markers in human reproduction. *Adv Clin Chem* 2008;45:1–29.

107. Burger HG, Dudley EC, Hopper JL, Groome N, Guthrie JR, Green A, *et al*. Prospectively measured levels of serum follicle-stimulating hormone, estradiol, and the dimeric inhibins during the menopausal transition in a population-based cohort of women. *J Clin Endocrinol Metab* 1999;84:4025–30.

108. Burger HG, Cahir N, Robertson DM, Groome NP, Dudley E, Green A, *et al*. Serum inhibins A and B fall differentially as FSH rises in perimenopausal women. *Clin Endocrinol (Oxf)* 1998;48:809–13. Erratum in: *Clin Endocrinol (Oxf)* 1998;49:550.

109. Welt CK, Adams JM, Sluss PM, Hall JE. Inhibin A and inhibin B responses to gonadotropin withdrawal depends on stage of follicle development. *J Clin Endocrinol Metab* 1999;84:2163–9.

110. Welt CK, McNicholl DJ, Taylor AE, Hall JE. Female reproductive aging is marked by decreased secretion of dimeric inhibin. *J Clin Endocrinol Metab* 1999;84:105–11.

111. McTavish KJ, Jimenez M, Walters KA, Spaliviero J, Groome NP, Themmen AP, *et al*. Rising follicle-stimulating hormone levels with age accelerate female reproductive failure. *Endocrinology* 2007;148:4432–9.

Chapter 9
Basic science: eggs and ovaries

Discussion

William Ledger: Thank you both for your really interesting talks. Can I start the discussion? You have both shown us ways in which ovarian ageing can be accelerated. The question that women ask is how can they slow it down? Are you aware of anything that we, as clinicians, can advise women to do to defer the day when they lose fertility, apart from 'don't have chemotherapy and don't smoke cigarettes'?

Roger Gosden: I do not know of any genetic condition in humans which seems to be associated with a long-time rescue of primordial follicles. Sixty seems to be pretty close to the limit, maybe very exceptionally beyond that. But if that is the case, that we do not know of any women, say at 70 or 80, who have had any follicles left, that suggests to me the regulation of this process was probably polygenic. That provides greater challenges for any means for slowing down follicle usage. Because in theory we have all of the stocks. We can of course freeze eggs or ovarian tissue, but we want to do it pharmacologically. It is theoretically possible but we do not know all the targets. Steve summarised these targets and there may be more than one target. I wonder whether Steve agrees with me? My impression is that all things have a major inhibitory regulatory load. We see a lot of that in the ovary anyway. That makes sense because the danger for human biology is that you have explosive growth of all these follicles.

Stephen Hillier: Yes. We obviously both think this is important because we both showed the same FOXO3A and PTEN data. The central role that signalling pathway plays in cell growth throughout the body is indisputable, which actually limits what we might be able achieve in an oocyte. But there are molecules that suppress the destruction of FOXO. In theory, they could be developed in pharmaceuticals. PTEN is the obvious one. Another aspect is some fascinating data in mice that suggest that nutrition has a major impact on the rate at which oocytes are lost from the ovary.[1,2] Certainly you can prolong reproductive lifespan and functional lifespan of the ovary by calorie restriction.

William Ledger: There's a possibility that there's a message there! That might be encouraging for patients.

Dimitrios Nikolaou: Thank you very much for that fascinating talk. Dr Hillier's point, that treatment should be individualised and based on the biological and not the chronological age, I think is correct. I think, however, that it needs to be clarified because it has a risk of misleading people. If you think about treatment for fertility …

Stephen Hillier: Sorry, I was thinking very specifically of ovarian stimulation to harvest oocytes for ART procedures in the context of poor responders or older women who respond less effectively to blunderbuss therapies.

Dimitrios Nikolaou: We will have a chance to talk about this more tomorrow [Chapter 22 but I think we have all been following the wrong lead for years by understanding ovarian or biological age as almost exclusively quantitative: how many eggs have you got in the ovary? The hourglass concept. When it appears, with the exception of some very extreme cases, that if you take the bulk of women who come to us who ovulate on their own, almost the only thing that matters in terms of live birth is how old women are, their chronological age, because that is very strongly associated with oocyte quality. In my view, this is the single most important question to look at biologically – how do we assess egg quality and can we improve egg quality?[3]

Roger Gosden: I do not know the answer. I don't think we can answer that.

William Ledger: We will leave that as a question for tomorrow then.

Diana Mansour: A question I am often asked, and have to advise about, is when a woman says 'I've been on the pill for so long. Will that protect me and will I preserve the number of follicles?' I say 'No, that doesn't happen'. Can you explain why it isn't protective?

Stephen Hillier: I wanted to ask Roger about the whole concept of clock genes. Real clock genes operating in oocytes that intrinsically regulate the rate at which the follicles start to grow and become atretic regardless of the secondary influence of whether or not you have one ovary, or two ovaries, or high FSH [follicle-stimulating hormone], or you have had five rounds of superovulation therapy or you have been on the pill for 20 years. Don't forget that most of those things have a negative impact on ovarian cancer. That to me implies that there are direct beneficial effects of not having lots of FSH around for a long period of time, although there are other ways of explaining that. It also implies to me that there are targets responding during that period. The bottom line is that there are no animal experiments, nor do I think there are any human clinical paradigms, which suggest that you can slow down the overall process of attrition simply by removing the endocrine stimulus to more advanced stages of growth.

Roger Gosden: Yes. Some very old data show that hypophysectomy would also not count over generic general age. It is the endocrinological view they are inactive and it doesn't seem to change that clock. At some point a long time ago we looked at the expression of the FSH receptor in human follicles and a very small number do not express the receptor. So, they are non-responsive to cyclical changes and gonadotrophin changes. All those very baseline changes come to act on small follicles to start them growing, are independent from the changes in the cycle. So we wouldn't expect the contraceptive pill to affect the best eggs ageing, as animal models prove. Presumably, it's the quality of eggs as well as the quantity.

Stephen Hillier: Why haven't people looked closely at clock genes in mammalian oocytes?

Roger Gosden: We have data about Per-3 in a few papers. They are expressed, but nobody's really followed this through, not to my knowledge.

William Ledger: There's a recommendation …

Anna Kenyon: How do you feel this has a role in terms of optimising your ovulation induction regimens for women who may have limited ovarian function? And, speaking as an obstetrician, can I ask you to horizon gaze about other implications? Perhaps women will be seeking these kinds of tests in the future so they can plan their lives, or, in the case of delaying childrearing, because 'I would like you to predict the time my eggs are going to remain useful'. From an obstetric point of view, the biological age is very important for outcome. I wonder whether you could suggest any other possible uses of this technology if these tests would become available in the future in terms of predicting rather than actually being in this situation?

Roger Gosden: Do you agree that antimüllerian hormone [AMH] is the best test that we have at the moment?

Stephen Hillier: I can see that all these guys here make a living out of evidence-based medicine so I couldn't possibly comment. [laughter] In theory, if the assay is refined appropriately, the AMH inhibins and the activins ought to be. There is a very sound rational basis for hypothesising they will be very robust molecules. It is more than just the endocrine markers. Although we may not understand for many, many years, in a post-genomic, post-HapMap world, it will be possible to develop algorithms that phenotype certain patients. Some will have certain propensities and requirements for more LH [luteinising hormone] than FSH, or a longer period of something else, or whatever. I have absolutely no doubt about that whatsoever. From my own experience of ovulation and ovarian stimulation therapy, even going right back to when I worked for Robert Winston, we used to monitor individual women and adjust low-dose stimulation to their particular requirements. It was not evidence-based, but it worked (sometimes).

Siladitya Bhattacharya: One of the problems of these tests is obviously that they need a good diagnostic test. Which are the good screening tests that anticipate what might happen in 5 or 10 years?

Roger Gosden: Malcolm Faddy has published work in the *Journal of Clinical Endocrinology and Metabolism* with Frank Broekmans on AMH earlier this year.[4] I discussed this with Malcolm, who is a mathematician now based in Australia. He said we can't be sure how predictive this is. If you look at groups of women in a cohort analysis you find trends and that will look very good. If we take a blood sample from a woman at, say, age 30, can we predict whether she is going to have menopause at age 40, 45 or 55? On the basis of what we know at the moment, he said we cannot. He was also concerned that it would take a very long time before we know this, if at all, because we need to do a prospective study. I do not know whether anyone is going to do that study.

Siladitya Bhattacharya: Especially if we had a subgroup of women with polycystic ovaries, where interpreting AMH would be very difficult.

Stephen Hillier: Yes. To come back to your point that it is basically a question of clinical chemistry. Every analyte that you measure, or ask for in the laboratory, has a normal range. There are wide ranges and narrow ranges, good tests and bad tests – and that is for something like insulin or FSH. But then when you pull together all the variables and clusters and say 'What does it say about what is going to happen in 5 years' time?', that is a tough ask.

Peter Braude: We measure AMH and other things that are surrogate markers for the mother's follicles. Wouldn't counting the follicles be much easier? If you count the follicles, you know what is going to happen. I'm not saying you can predict but you can say what's happening now.

Steve Hiller: That sounds a rather old-fashioned gynaecological point of view …

Peter Braude: That is a fact. It's exactly what is happening to each woman.

Stephen Hillier: I do not think we can measure those very small follicles. Well, we cannot. We can hardly see them under a microscope.

Peter Braude: But if you want to know how they will respond, it is the small ones that you will see. Whether you can actually see …

Stephen Hillier: Well, no, I am sorry. I disagree. You want to see what a woman's reproductive potential is in 10 years' time. She needs to know about those little ones that you cannot see at the moment.

Peter Braude: Neither of you commented on that massive loss of follicles that occurs at about 8 months *in utero*. You both interrogated data from 1975. I do not know of any data subsequent to that, but what you are talking about is a log loss of follicles or oocytes. If there were going to be any strategy that is going to change the likelihood, or the possibility, of either the number of follicles or extending menopause, if that is what you wanted to achieve, it would be something directed at that. Do we know anything about that mechanism? It strikes me that that is quite important. It is also interesting when you look at PCOS [polycystic ovary syndrome]. The women have bucketloads of follicles all the time and quite late in reproductive age. Although they aren't always good eggs, they seem to have the propensity to produce large numbers of follicles even with the slightest amount of gonadotrophin.

Roger Gosden: That is certainly unknown. In PCOS we see a larger proportion of growing ones. You'd think that they would run out earlier, but they don't apparently. We do not really know the dynamics. Something that's speeded up at one stage may slow down a later stage, or there may be differences in the death rate. Regarding the question about prenatal oocytes. Clearly, if we could increase the number of follicles that survive then potentially we could extend reproductive lifespan as an alternative to slowing down the rate of recruitment. But there is a scaling relationship in nature between mouse and humans. We fit on that scale, or allometric curve, in terms of the numbers of eggs, at a comparable developmental stage with puberty in other animals. Biologists arrange this scale according to body weight actually, not longevity. So, if we had a larger store, then potentially they would last longer. The mechanisms for the wastage are hardly investigated, but we do believe that it is an apoptosis process. People speculate about whether some of these are abnormal and it is a way of removing them. I doubt whether it is all due to removing aneuploidies but we do not know because we cannot test those that are dying. By definition we can't prove whether they are abnormal. My guess is that it is part of a population regulating process and there may be ways of rescuing those follicles. Maybe if we had the opportunity to take a biopsy of the ovary, we might be able to rescue some of those. There are even a few just before birth in the preterm infant. They could be stored and then oogonia transplanted back onto the ovary later on – we could only do the experiments in animals to answer the question, but it is interesting to speculate about it.

William Ledger: Fetal surgery for restoring ooyctes is a little bit beyond even this group for 2008! [laughter]. Could we take one more question?

Donna Dickenson: The commercial sale of oocytes and ova has been allowed in the USA for 20 years. We are getting this massive phenomenon in Europe as well. We are now in the position, or we could be, to know the evidence. Do you know any studies that are going on in terms of numbers? For example, in one US study,[5] up to 70 oocytes have been extracted from one woman and similar numbers have been taken in clinics in Cyprus and Spain. We have pretty good evidence about the numbers there. The whole thing was premised, in the USA at least, on the idea that oocytes were an infinitely renewable tissue, which we've just heard isn't true. Solly Zuckerman's hypothesis,[6] which you believe is correct, is not the case. If there is a threshold of 1000 follicles which triggers menopause, do you think that there is any effect from repeated ovarian hyperstimulation, not for the woman's own benefit, but for the provision of very large numbers of eggs on a commercial basis?

Roger Gosden: That has been an interesting question for a long time. Helen Picton and I have done studies on animals which suggested that long-term stimulation does not deplete the ovary prematurely and with Kay Elder at Bourn Hall Clinic who published just a few months ago in *Reproductive Biomedicine Online* a study based on Bourn Hall Clinic patients going back a long way.[7] We followed up those women that we could find from the early days of IVF to find out when they had menopause. It was not a perfect study but there was no relationship between menopausal age and the amount of therapy they received – and some of them had a huge number of treatment cycles in those days. So, we think this is pretty reassuring and they are not going to end up with an earlier menopause no matter how many cycles of a treatment, provided there is no excessive trauma to the ovary from egg collection.

Stephen Hillier: The only thing to add is that in no way justifies repeated hyperstimulation as a strategy. There are a few worries, as you would appreciate, as to what other impact there is, apart from the ethics.

William Ledger: Thank you very much everyone.

References

1. Nelson JF, Gosden RG, Felicio LS. Effect of dietary restriction on estrous cyclicity and follicular reserves in aging C57BL/6J mice. *Biol Reprod* 1985;32:515–22.
2. Selesniemi K, Lee HJ, Tilly JL. Moderate caloric restriction initiated in rodents during adulthood sustains function of the female reproductive axis into advanced chronological age. *Aging Cell* 2008;7:622–9.
3. Nikolaou D. How old are your eggs? *Curr Opin Obstet Gynecol* 2008;20:540–4.
4. van Disseldorp J, Faddy MJ, Themmen AP, de Jong FH, Peeters PH, van der Schouw YT, *et al*. Relationship of serum antimüllerian hormone concentration to age at menopause. *J Clin Endocrinol Metab* 2008;93:2129–34.
5. Jacobs A, Dwyer J, Lee PH. Seventy ova. *Hastings Cent Rep* 2001;31:12; discussion 12–14.
6. Zuckerman S. The number of oocytes in the mature ovary. *Rec Prog Horm Res* 1951;6:63–108.
7. Elder K, Mathews T, Kutner E, Kim E, Espenberg D, Faddy M, *et al*. Impact of gonadotrophin stimulation for assisted reproductive technology on ovarian ageing and menopause. *Reprod Biomed Online* 2008;16:611–16.

Chapter 10
Male reproductive ageing

Herman Tournaye

Introduction

While the adverse effects of maternal age on reproduction are well documented and evident, reproductive effects related to advanced paternal age are less well defined. According to the Office for National Statistics,[1] in 1971 the mean age of a father at birth was 27.2 years but by 1999 this had risen to 30.1 years and by 2004 it had risen to 32 years. In the UK in 2004, more than 75 000 babies, that is, more than one in ten of all born, were born to fathers aged 40 years or over and 6489 children were born to fathers aged 50 years or over. In recent years, male reproductive ageing has come into view, mainly in the lay press. However, few well-designed studies have been conducted on this subject and major textbooks on andrology only cover the endocrine aspects of male ageing but not its reproductive effects.

Studies referring to 'testicular reserve' in men focus on the endocrine function, that is, androgen production. With ageing, testicular androgen output declines. This condition has been named andropause, partial androgen deficiency in the ageing male and testosterone deficiency syndrome, among others, but it is now currently referred to as late-onset hypogonadism.[2] Late-onset hypogonadism is defined as a clinical and biochemical syndrome associated with a deficiency in testosterone because of advanced age and is marked by a progressive development of osteoporosis, mood disorders and metabolic changes.

Ageing and exocrine testicular function

In contrast to the vast body of studies on the endocrine function of the testis, few well-designed studies exist concerning its exocrine function, that is, the output of gametes, and those studies that are available suffer from many flaws in design and methodology. Longitudinal studies do not exist and data for men aged 50 years or over are hardly reported. Many studies do not properly control for confounding factors such as abstinence period, lifestyle, exposure to gonadotoxins and male accessory gland infection (the prevalence of chronic prostatitis is known to increase with age).

From a histological viewpoint, changes with ageing have been reported. Holstein[3] described testicular histology in men aged 65–93 years. Apart from a reduction in numbers of Leydig cells, he observed disturbances in spermatogonial stem cell renewal and meiosis. However, these changes were minimal and were observed in relatively small areas distributed diffusely throughout the testis. Furthermore, these observations showed high inter-individual differences. Another study[4] comparing 36 older men (aged 61–102 years) with ten young controls (aged 29–40 years) showed a gradual decrease in Sertoli cell numbers, in spermatogonia, spermatocytes and spermatozoa. These histological changes also showed a great inter-individual variability. Only half of the older men exhibited completion of spermatogenesis. The rest showed varying degrees of maturation arrest, mainly before meiosis, and four showed a Sertoli cell-only pattern. Men with arrested spermatogenesis had a marked thickening of the basal membrane (over 10 micrometres).

Studies on sperm output in men that have controlled for abstinence period have reported consistent observations except for density. These studies have compared semen and sperm parameters with reference groups of young men (mostly aged around 20 years). All studies showed a reduction in semen volume varying from −0.5% to −1% per year. The majority of these studies showed a decrease in sperm motility and morphology from −0.2% to −0.7% and −0.2% to −0.9% per year, respectively. For density, however, changes ranging from −2.5% to +0.7% per year have been reported.[5]

Summary

Age-related changes in sperm output develop gradually without any evidence of sudden onset. All of the observed changes are within the limits of 'normality' as currently proposed by the World Health Organization.[6]

Ageing and fecundity

Effect of paternal age on fecundity

Female fecundity starts to decline after 30 years of age and is greatly reduced after age 40 years. The effect of male age on fecundity remains controversial and few studies show a similar trend in men. Many confounding factors exist that may explain the variations among different reports, including lack of proper correction for female age, decrease in coital frequency, increase in erectile dysfunction and use of medication.

The Avon Longitudinal Study of Parents and their Children (ALSPAC)[7] has studied the effect of paternal age on fecundity by analysing the likelihood of conception within 12 months of starting to try for pregnancy. After adjusting for female partner's age, body mass index (BMI), smoking habits, level of education, duration of cohabitation, alcohol consumption and use of contraception, this study showed lower odds ratios with advancing paternal age. Compared with men aged under 25 years (the reference group), the odds ratio for achieving conception within 12 months for men aged 30–34 years was 0.62 (95% CI 0.40–0.98), 0.50 (95% CI 0.31–0.81) for men aged 35–39 years and 0.51 (95% CI 0.31–0.86) for those aged 40 years or over. This study has an important shortcoming: the age at conception rather than the age at the onset of attempting to achieve a pregnancy was studied.

Another well-controlled observational antenatal clinic study[8] studied the time to pregnancy (TTP) from the onset of attempting conception in 2112 couples. A subgroup of 638 men impregnated a partner aged under 25 years. After adjusting for coital frequency, BMI, parity, menstrual pattern and menarche, living standard and lifestyle, TTP in men aged 25–30 years was 6.2 months (95% CI 4.3–8.0 months) while in men aged 40 years or over TTP was 23.2 months (95% CI 14.5–31.9 months) (Figure 10.1).

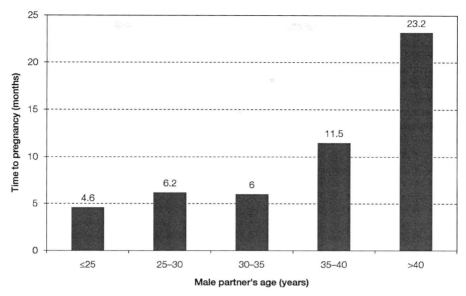

Figure 10.1 Time to pregnancy for women aged under 25 years with men at various ages (at onset of attempting conception) after adjusting for confounding factors; data from Hassan and Killick[8]

A shortcoming of both antenatal clinic studies is that they may potentially underestimate the effect of parental age because only couples who eventually conceived were included and subfertile couples may thus be under-represented.

In a study by Dunson et al.,[9] the day-specific probability for conception was studied. After adjusting for coital frequency, this prospective study showed that the probability of clinical pregnancy after intercourse on the most fertile day of the menstrual cycle in women aged 35–39 years decreased from 29% to 18% when their partners were 5 years older. In women aged under 35 years, this paternal age effect was absent.

A retrospective European multicentre study[10] also reported a paternal age effect becoming significant with increasing female age. Couples were randomly selected from census registries for an interview regarding their reproductive history. Both a 'delay' in conception (no conception after 12 months of regular sexual intercourse without using birth control methods) and 'difficulty' in having a baby (similar as 'delay' but also including getting pregnant without a live birth) were taken as fertility indicators. In women aged under 30 years, there was no paternal age effect; however, matched to a male partner aged 40 years or over, 'difficulty' was reported as being twice as high in women aged 30–34 years (OR 2.0; 95% CI 1.1–3.5) and 4.6 times higher in women aged 35–39 years (OR 4.6; 95% CI 2.8–7.5) compared with women aged under 30 years having a partner aged under 40 years. The latter category also showed a significant delay compared with the reference group (OR 3.0; 95% CI 1.8–4.9).

In another prospective study by Dunson et al.,[11] the impact of the cervical mucus quality on fecundity was studied. After adjusting for intercourse timing and female age, their data showed that a paternal age effect became evident in men aged 35 years or over when a poor mucus score was present on the day of intercourse but was absent when fertile-type mucus was present.

Summary

From the above studies, we may conclude that male age has an adverse effect on fertility, with fecundity starting to decline after 40 years of age. However, this adverse effect of paternal age is less pronounced than that of the female age. Preliminary data show that there is a synergistic effect between maternal and paternal age that contributes to reduced fertility.

Effect of paternal age on assisted reproduction outcomes

Few studies have addressed the effect of male age on the outcome of assisted reproduction. A retrospective study[12] reported a decline in pregnancy rate and an increased miscarriage rate after intrauterine insemination with advancing paternal age. Although more than 17 000 intrauterine insemination cycles were analysed, this study did not properly control for confounding factors including maternal age and hence the conclusions remain debatable.

Controlling for confounding factors is also difficult with treatments involving assisted reproductive technologies (ART). Oocyte donation studies can properly control for a maternal age effect. The few studies available in the literature (all retrospective in design) could not indicate any significant effect of paternal age on fertilisation rates or on pregnancy rates.[13,14] A retrospective study reported an influence of paternal age on the outcome of an oocyte donation programme but without providing direct evidence.[15]

A major shortcoming of all these studies is their lack of control for other possible confounding factors, for example the number of oocytes inseminated and hence ovarian reserve.

A few retrospective non-oocyte donation studies investigated the effect of paternal age on intracytoplasmic sperm injection (ICSI) outcome. These studies reported no effect on pregnancy rates but some effect on fertilisation after ICSI: a somewhat lower two pronuclear (2PN) fertilisation rate in men aged 50 years or over[16] and a slightly higher prevalence of 3PN fertilisation with increasing age of the male partner.[17]

A large retrospective *in vitro* fertilisation (IVF) study[18] based on the French national registry on IVF outcomes (FIVNAT) data investigated the paternal age effect after adjusting for female age. These data showed a synergistic effect of maternal and paternal age both contributing to failure to conceive after IVF (ICSI was excluded from this analysis). Compared with a reference group of women aged under 30 years having male partners aged under 30 years, women aged 35–37 years had double the risk of not conceiving when their partners were aged 40 years, but not if their partners were aged under 40 years. The older the women were, the more significant the paternal age effect became at earlier ages. For example, women aged 38–40 years had three times more risk of not conceiving after IVF when associated with partners aged 35–39 years (OR 3.05; 95% CI 1.44–6.48) than the reference group of women aged under 30 years associated with partners aged under 30 years. A similar synergistic age effect on IVF and ICSI has been observed in the German ART registry.[5]

Summary

Overall, studies on paternal age effects on IVF and ICSI outcomes are inconsistent in their findings. Paternal age seems to have some impact when the female partner is also older, when ovarian reserve may be compromised.

Ageing and pregnancy loss and obstetric outcome

Effect of paternal age on the risk of miscarriage

In addition to their lower chance of becoming pregnant as women age, they also have a higher chance of losing their pregnancy. The effect of ageing of the male partner on the risk for miscarriage has been studied extensively, although many studies are retrospective, span long observational periods and fail to control properly for maternal age effects, or have small sample sizes.

A large case–control study[19] of almost 14 000 pregnancies found paternal age to be a significant risk factor for miscarriage. With a paternal age of 25–29 years as a reference, women with partners aged 35 years or over had nearly a doubling in miscarriage rate when adjusting for maternal age, parity, previous miscarriages, maternal tobacco use and diabetes.

A retrospective French study[20] reported an increased risk for miscarriage associated with paternal age but only with increasing maternal age and when the male partner was aged 40 years or over.

Two large prospective cohort studies have also shown a small paternal age effect. A Californian study[21] showed an adjusted hazard ratio of miscarriage of 1.27 (95% CI 1.00–1.61) with a stronger association for first-trimester pregnancy loss. A study from Denmark[22] that controlled properly for a variety of potential confounding factors found that when the father was aged 50 years or over, the hazard ratio for late fetal death (20 weeks or more of gestation) was 3.94 (95% CI 1.12–13.8) compared with fathers aged 25–29 years (the reference group). This increased risk was independent of maternal age and was not confounded by diabetes, alcohol and coffee consumption, parity, maternal and paternal smoking, maternal and paternal occupational status or previous miscarriages. However, for early fetal death (less than 20 weeks of gestation) and for all paternal ages under 50 years, no significant paternal age effect was observed, with adjusted hazard ratios close to one. In contrast to the French study,[20] these two well-controlled studies found no interaction between maternal and paternal age and attributed the finding in the French study to a residual confounding maternal age.

Summary

Paternal age is associated with a slight increase in risk of miscarriage. This risk is not comparable to that associated with maternal ageing. An adverse association between maternal and paternal age is currently not supported by unequivocal evidence.

Effect of paternal age on birth outcomes

Most studies report no association between adverse birth outcomes and paternal age. In those studies that do find an association, this is probably attributable to poor control for confounding factors such as race, multiple birth, tobacco and alcohol exposure, and prenatal care status. A well-controlled retrospective cohort study[23] of 2 614 966 liveborn singletons investigated the independent effect of paternal age on adverse birth outcomes. Compared with infants born to fathers aged 20–29 years, infants fathered by teenagers (aged under 20 years) had an increased risk of preterm birth, low birth weight, small-for-gestational-age births, low Apgar score, neonatal mortality and post-neonatal mortality. However, a paternal age of 40 years or over was not associated with such risks.

Summary

Based on well-controlled large population-based studies, it may be concluded that advanced paternal age is not an independent risk factor for adverse birth outcomes.

Ageing and genetic anomalies

Effect of paternal age on genetic disorders

Women aged 35 years or over are at greater risk of delivering a child with a genetic disorder such as Down syndrome. On a purely hypothetical basis, an increased genetic risk related to paternal age is to be expected: while it takes about 24 cell divisions to produce a metaphase II oocyte, the number of divisions to produce spermatozoa increases with paternal age and it has been estimated that, by the age of 50 years, about 800 divisions precede production of spermatozoa. In the 1950s, Penrose[24] postulated that a DNA 'copy error' may occur at each replication, causing a transcription error later, and that these errors accumulate with advancing paternal age.

Eight infrequent genetic disorders caused by single-gene defects are exclusively paternal in origin and are known to show a strong paternal age effect. Among them is achondroplasia, a disease caused by a mutation in the fibroblast growth factor receptor 3 (*FGFR3*) gene.[25] Interestingly, while an increase in mutation rate for the *FGFR3* gene has been observed in DNA extracted from testicular spermatogenetic cells,[26] this increase was not observed in ejaculated spermatozoa[26] or observed to a lower extent than expected from the age-dependent increase in this disease.[27–28] This surprising finding has been attributed to a positive selection of mutated sperm for fertilisation. A few other genetic diseases were shown to have a weak association with advanced paternal age.[25]

For all genetic diseases with a paternal age effect, different mutagenic mechanisms are at work and there is disagreement over how these mutations increase with ageing of the father. Findings from recent studies do not support the long-lived 'copy error' hypothesis. It has also been questioned whether these genetic errors are due to age itself or are caused by changes in lifestyle or mutagenic exposure with advancing age or even cohort selection.[28]

Summary

A paternal age effect cannot be neglected in these genetic diseases and, although their prevalence is low, candidate fathers aged 40 years or over should be informed about this age effect. In view of the above observations, an age limit for sperm donors is justified. The RCOG recommends the British Andrology Society guideline of limiting the age of sperm donors to 40 years.[29]

Effect of paternal age on DNA damage to spermatozoa

DNA damage is another cause of genetic errors in spermatozoa. Although many confounding factors are present and often difficult to control for, studies have shown that paternal age is an independent factor in increasing DNA damage to spermatozoa.[28,30,31] The DNA fragmentation index was shown to increase gradually and, compared with men aged 20 years, men aged 60 years show a doubling of the DNA fragmentation rate, while men aged 80 years show a five-fold increase. Men aged 60 years or over show DNA fragmentation rates of over 30%, the threshold value associated with decreased fecundity.[28]

In most studies examining aneuploidy on spermatozoa, including trisomies and sex-chromosome disomies, no paternal age effect has been observed.[5] Also, a study on testicular biopsies[4] failed to show an increase in aneuploidy even at advanced paternal ages. Studies on newborns are more difficult to interpret because of many confounding factors apart from maternal age and their conclusions are less in agreement.[5] There exists controversy on the paternal age effect for trisomy 21. A large Norwegian study[32] showed that, after adjusting for maternal age, the effect of paternal age was weak. Another study[33] demonstrated a slight but significant paternal age effect in women aged 35 years or over.

Summary

Based on current data, advanced paternal age of itself is not an indication for performing prenatal diagnosis.

Birth defects and health consequences in children of older fathers

Effect of paternal age on birth defects

Paternal ageing has also been associated with diseases of more complex genetic predisposition, such as congenital heart defects, cleft lip and/or palate, neural tube defects, craniosynostosis, retinoblastoma, neurofibromatosis and neurological diseases. However, controversy exists concerning the influence of paternal age on these disorders. Many studies do not properly control for confounding factors, report on small case series, suffer from selection bias or have missing data on paternal demographic characteristics.[34] Archer *et al.*[35] have shown that in studies of paternal age and birth defect risk, the completeness of data may influence the validity of the findings. This study also failed to demonstrate any association between paternal age and a selection of the most prevalent birth defects. Yang *et al.*[36] found a weak association between paternal age and several selected birth defects: heart defects, tracheo-oesophageal atresia, musculoskeletal/integumental anomalies and chromosomal anomalies. Men aged 50 years or over had 1.15 times more risk for these birth defects than men aged 25–29 years (the reference group) (adjusted OR 1.15; 95% CI 1.06–1.24).

Summary

Given the weak association, paternal age appears to play only a small role in the aetiology of birth defects.

Effect of paternal age on cancer and neurodevelopmental disorders

Few studies demonstrate a link between paternal age and the risk of developing cancer, for example prostate cancer, brain cancer, leukemia and breast cancer. But again, associations are weak and data are prone to bias and confounding factors.

Finally, a number of researchers have examined the effect of paternal age on neurodevelopmental disorders such as Alzheimer's disease, autism and schizophrenia. A study of autism[37] found an association between paternal age and the prevalence of autism. After adjusting for the age of the mother and socio-economic factors, children of men who were aged 40 years or over when they became a father were 5.75 times as likely to have autism as those whose fathers were aged under 30 years. However, this study has been criticised because it lacks information about autistic traits in the parents. Fathers who themselves have autism or mild social deficits are likely to marry and have children at a later age than other men and their children inherit factors putting them at high risk of developing the condition themselves.

A study on schizophrenia,[38] using a registry of 87 907 births in Jerusalem between 1964 and 1976, found that the risk of this disorder was doubled among children of fathers in their late 40s when compared with children of fathers aged under 25 years and that this risk increased almost three times in children born to fathers aged 50 years or over. No association between paternal age and related nonaffective psychoses was observed. The study controlled for the age of the mother and other confounding factors (sex, ethnicity, education and duration of marriage) but it did not include information on family psychiatric history, which is an important confounder. Both a Swedish[39] and a Danish study[40] corroborated these observations. Fathers aged 44 years or over had a 2.8 times greater risk of having a child with schizophrenia compared with fathers aged 20–24 years (the reference group).[39] In the Danish cohort, using the same age group as a reference, the risk of schizophrenia doubled in daughters of fathers aged 50–54 years and in sons of fathers aged 55 years or over. It tripled in daughters of fathers aged 55 years or over.[40]

Another study[41] controlled for schizoid family traits and demonstrated again an association between paternal age and schizophrenia in fathers without a family history.

In another study using Israeli data,[42] an association between paternal age and lower scores on nonverbal (performance) intelligence quotient tests was observed. For Alzheimer's disease, data are less conclusive. The paternal age effect on these neurodevelopmental disorders is assumed to result from *de novo* mutations or abnormal methylation of paternally imprinted genes; however, direct evidence supporting this hypothesis is currently lacking.

Another study[43] addressed the adverse health consequences of advanced paternal age by examining the mortality rates in children. After adjusting for maternal age, the mortality rate ratio in children was 1.77 (95% CI 1.28–2.45) in fathers aged 45–49 years and 1.59 (95% CI 1.03–2.46) in fathers aged 50 years or over compared with children of fathers aged 25–29 years. Apart from mortality because of congenital disorders, surprisingly, the researchers found an association between paternal age and death caused by injury and poisoning, indicating the importance for controlling for social and behavioural confounding factors.

Summary

Although many of the reported adverse health outcomes discussed above are controversial because of methodological shortcomings of registry-based cohort studies, some of them, for example schizophrenia, have been replicated in a number of studies and therefore their potential impact should be discussed with candidate fathers who want to procreate at an older age. However, as socio-economic factors are known to be important determinants for health and longevity, the potential socio-economic advantages for offspring born to older fathers should not be neglected.

Conclusion

In comparison with maternal age, the impact of paternal age on fertility is less, although synergies may exist. Paternal ageing does not affect the risk of miscarriage and increased paternal age on its own is not an indication for prenatal diagnosis since the absolute risk for genetic anomalies in offspring is low. Because some infrequent single-gene defects are associated with increased paternal age, an age limit for sperm donors is justified. There is no clear association between adverse health outcome and paternal age but longitudinal studies are needed.

References

1   Office for National Statistics [www.statistics.gov.uk].

2   Nieschlag E, Swerdloff R, Behre HM, Gooren LJ, Kaufman JM, Legros JJ, et al. Investigation, treatment, and monitoring of late-onset hypogonadism in males: ISA, ISSAM, and EAU recommendations. J Androl 2006;27:135–7.

3   Holstein AF. Morphological evidence for the involution of spermatogenesis during senescence. In: Holstein AF, editor. Reproductive Biology and Medicine. Berlin: Diesbach; 1989. p. 66–77.

4   Dakouane M, Bicchieray L, Bergere M, Albert M, Vialard F, Selva J. A histomorphometric and cytogenetic study of testis from men 29–102 years old. Fertil Steril 2005;83:923–8.

5   Kühnert B, Nieschlag E. Reproductive functions of the ageing male. Hum Reprod Update 2004;10:327–39.

6   World Health Organization. Laboratory Manual for the Examination of Human Semen and Semen–Cervical Mucus Interaction. Cambridge: Cambridge University Press; 1992.

7   Ford WCL, North K, Taylor H, Farrow A, Hull MGR, Golding J. Increasing paternal age is associated with delayed conception in a large population of fertile couples: evidence for declining fecundity in older men. Hum Reprod 2000;15:1703–8.

8   Hassan MA, Killick SR. Effect of male age on fertility: evidence for the decline in male fertility with increasing age. Fertil Steril 2003;79(Suppl 3):1520–7.

9   Dunson DB, Colombo B, Baird D. Changes with age in the level and duration of fertility in the menstrual cycle. Hum Reprod 2002;17:1399–403.

10 de la Rochebrochard E, Thonneau P. Paternal age ≥40 years: an important risk factor for infertility. Am J Obstet Gynecol 2003;189:901–15.

11 Dunson DB, Bigelow JL, Colombo B. Reduced fertilization rates in older men when cervical mucus is suboptimal. Obstet Gynecol 2005;105:788–93.

12 Belloc S, Cohen-Bacrie P, Benkhalifa M, Cohen-Bacrie M, De Mouzon J, Hazout A, et al. Effect of maternal and paternal age on pregnancy and miscarriage rates after intrauterine insemination. Reprod Biomed Online 2008;17:392–7.

13 Gallardo E, Simón C, Levy M, Guanes PP, Remohí J, Pellicer A. Effect of age on sperm fertility potential: oocyte donation as a model. Fertil Steril 1996;66:260–4.

14 Paulson RJ, Milligan RC, Sokol RZ. The lack of influence of age on male fertility. Am J Obstet Gynecol 2001;184:818–22.

15 Girsh E, Katz N, Genkin L, Girtler O, Bocker J, Bezdin S, et al. Male age influences oocyte-donor program results. J Assist Reprod Genet 2008;25:137–43.

16 Aboulghar M, Mansour R, Al-Inany H, Abou-Setta AM, Aboulghar M, Mourad L, et al. Paternal age and outcome of intracytoplasmic sperm injection. Reprod Biomed Online 2007;14:588–92.

17 Spandorfer SD, Avrech OM, Colombero LT, Palermo GD, Rosenwaks Z. Effect of parental age on fertilization and pregnancy characteristics in couples treated by intracytoplasmic sperm injection. Hum Reprod 1998;13:334–8.

18 de La Rochebrochard E, de Mouzon J, Thépot F, Thonneau P. Fathers over 40 and increased failure to conceive: the lessons of in vitro fertilization in France. Fertil Steril 2006;85:1420–4.

19 Kleinhaus K, Perrin M, Friedlander Y, Paltiel O, Malaspina D, Harlap S. Paternal age and spontaneous abortion. Obstet Gynecol 2006;108:369–77.

20 de la Rochebrochard E, Thonneau P. Paternal age and maternal age are risk factors for miscarriage; results of a multicentre European study. Hum Reprod 2002;17:1649–56.

21 Slama R, Bouyer J, Windham G, Fenster L, Werwatz A, Swan SH. Influence of paternal age on the risk of spontaneous abortion. Am J Epidemiol 2005;161:816–23.

22   Nybo Andersen AM, Hansen KD, Andersen PK, Davey Smith G. Advanced paternal age and risk of fetal death: a cohort study. *Am J Epidemiol* 2004;160:1214–22.

23   Chen XK, Wen SW, Krewski D, Fleming N, Yang Q, Walker MC. Paternal age and adverse birth outcomes: teenager or 40+, who is at risk? *Hum Reprod* 2008;23:1290–6.

24   Penrose LS. Parental age and mutation. *Lancet* 1955;269:312–13.

25   Glaser RL, Jabs EW. Dear old dad. *Sci Aging Knowledge Environ* 2004;2004:re1.

26   Dakouane GM, Serazin V, Le Sciellour CR, Albert M, Selva J, Giudicelli Y. Increased achondroplasia mutation frequency with advanced age and evidence for G1138A mosaicism in human testis biopsies. *Fertil Steril* 2008;89:1651–6.

27   Tiemann-Boege I, Navidi W, Grewal R, Cohn D, Eskenazi B, Wyrobek AJ, *et al.* The observed human sperm mutation frequency cannot explain the achondroplasia paternal age effect. *Proc Natl Acad Sci U S A* 2002;99:14952–7.

28   Wyrobek AJ, Eskenazi B, Young S, Arnheim N, Tiemann-Boege I, Jabs EW, *et al.* Advancing age has differential effects on DNA damage, chromatin integrity, gene mutations, and aneuploidies in sperm. *Proc Natl Acad Sci U S A* 2006;103:9601–6.

29   British Andrology Society. British Andrology Society guidelines for the screening of semen donors for donor insemination. *Hum Reprod* 1999;14:1823–6.

30   Singh NP, Muller CH, Berger RE. Effects of age on DNA double-strand breaks and apoptosis in human sperm. *Fertil Steril* 2003;80:1420–30.

31   Schmid TE, Eskenazi B, Baumgartner A, Marchetti F, Young S, Weldon R, *et al.* The effects of male age on sperm DNA damage in healthy non-smokers. *Hum Reprod* 2007;22:180–7.

32   Kazaura MR, Lie RT. Down's syndrome and paternal age in Norway. *Paediatr Perinat Epidemiol* 2002;16:314–19.

33   Fisch H, Hyun G, Golden R, Hensle TW, Olsson CA, Liberson GL. The influence of paternal age on Down syndrome. *J Urol* 2003;169:2275–8.

34   Kirby RS. Vital statistics: a poor source of data for investigating the association between paternal age and birth defects. *Hum Reprod* 2007;22:3265–7.

35   Archer NP, Langlois PH, Suarez L, Brender J, Shanmugam R. Association of paternal age with prevalence of selected birth defects. *Birth Defects Res (Part A)* 2007;79:27–34.

36   Yang Q, Wen SW, Leader A, Chen XK, Lipson J, Walker M. Paternal age and birth defects: how strong is the association? *Hum Reprod* 2007;22:696–701.

37   Reichenberg A, Gross R, Weiser M, Bresnahan M, Silverman J, Harlap S, *et al.* Advancing paternal age and autism. *Arch Gen Psychiatry* 2006;63:1026–32.

38   Malaspina D, Harlap S, Fennig S, Heiman D, Nahon D, Feldman D, Susser ES. Advancing paternal age and the risk of schizophrenia. *Arch Gen Psychiatry* 2001;58:361–7.

39   Dalman C, Allebeck P. Paternal age and schizophrenia: further support for an association. *Am J Psychiatry* 2002;159:1591–2.

40   Byrne M, Agerbo E, Ewald H, Eaton WW, Mortensen PB. Parental age and risk of schizophrenia: a case–control study. *Arch Gen Psychiatry* 2003;60:673–8.

41   Sipos A, Rasmussen F, Harrison G, Tynelius P, Lewis G, Leon DA, *et al.* Paternal age and schizophrenia: a population based cohort study. *BMJ* 2004;329:1070–3.

42   Malaspina D, Reichenberg A, Weiser M, Fennig S, Davidson M, Harlap S, *et al.* Paternal age and intelligence: implications for age-related genomic changes in male germ cells. *Psychiatr Genet* 2005;15:117–25.

43   Zhu JL, Vestergaard M, Madsen KM, Olsen J. Paternal age and mortality in children. *Eur J Epidemiol* 2008;23:443–7.

Chapter 11
The science of the ageing uterus and placenta
Gordon CS Smith

Introduction

The scientific study of ageing of the uterus and placenta is clinically relevant because of the associations between advanced maternal age and outcome of pregnancy. The details of these associations are addressed in other sections of this book. However, some clinical observations are also included in this chapter to demonstrate parallels between the scientific observations and the clinical outcomes that are thought to be related. The subject is addressed in terms of the ageing myometrium, decidua and placenta. The key clinical parallels are the association between advanced age and the risks of both complicated childbirth and antepartum stillbirth. The association with complicated childbirth is paralleled with the evidence that ageing adversely affects the myometrium. The association with stillbirth will be paralleled with evidence that ageing affects formation and development of the placenta, from implantation onwards. Some of the evidence relating to ageing and implantation may also be relevant to ageing and fecundity, but this is not discussed in detail.

Molecular and cellular aspects of ageing

The scientific literature on the mechanisms of ageing is vast and I make no attempt to summarise it here. However, I will briefly discuss two biological mechanisms that are thought to be important in ageing, namely telomere length and failure of autophagy.

Telomere length and ageing

Telomeres are lengths of repetitive sequences of non-coding DNA that are found at the end of chromosomes and are capped with binding proteins. In the human neonate, average telomere length is 15–20 kb and average telomere length shortens over the lifetime of an individual. When a critical threshold of telomere length is reached, it is thought that this triggers cell senescence. This leads to a live cell (hence the process is distinct from apoptosis) that is unable to undergo further cell divisions. Moreover, the altered pattern of protein expression changes the phenotype of the cell. The progressive change of cells within a tissue towards senescence is thought to be part of the basis for the visible effects of ageing. The factors controlling cell senescence are illustrated in Figure 11.1.

The relationship between telomere length and cell senescence is thought to have the role of limiting the number of divisions that a cell can undergo. With each cell division, there is the potential for mutations that predispose to cancer. Stochastically, the more divisions that a cell undergoes, the more likely it is that it will accumulate a combination of mutations that will lead to cancer. Telomere length can be increased by the enzyme telomerase. However, in healthy cells, this enzyme is only found in embryonic tissues, male germline cells and stem cells. Telomerase is also found in cancer cells and is thought to be part of the basis for their property of indefinite cell division. Interestingly, telomere length does not appear to be involved in ageing in some other mammals, such as mice and rabbits. Hence, other pathways can be involved in these processes. The subject is reviewed in depth elsewhere.[1]

Autophagy and ageing

Telomere length appears to be a mediator of ageing in cells that undergo repeated cell divisions. However, cells that do not undergo repeated cell divisions, such as cardiomyocytes and neurons, also age and other mechanisms exist. When aged cells of this type are examined ultrastructurally, there are a number of observations characteristic of ageing, specifically the presence of autofluorescent particles and abnormal organelles, in particular mitochondria. Lysosomes are the primary intracellular organelle involved in autophagy. The autofluorescent particles seen in aged tissues represent lysosomes that have accumulated lipofuscin, a complex high-molecular-weight polymer, the exact composition of which varies according to the cell type. Lipofuscin is formed in the process of lysosomal degradation and accumulates within the lysosome. The quantity of lipofuscin is increased in situations where

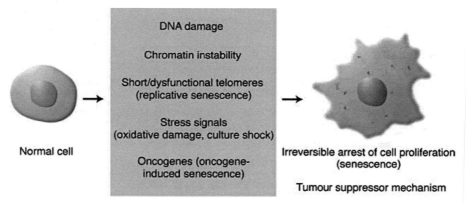

Figure 11.1 Mechanisms of senescence. In addition to progressive telomere shortening leading to irreversible growth arrest, other pathways include DNA damage, chromatin instability, overexpression of oncoproteins and a variety of stress signals (including oxidative damage). While morphologically the cells appear similar (but with a greatly enlarged size), only replicative senescence shows shortened telomeres. The other mechanisms occur with normal-length telomeres. However, all of these mechanisms may contribute to a potent tumour suppressor pathway, initially limiting the growth of potentially malignant cells. Reproduced with permission from Shay and Wright[1]

autophagy is increased and in the presence of increased concentrations of reactive oxygen species (ROS), in particular hydrogen peroxide (due either to increased ROS production or decreased scavenging). Failure of autophagy of abnormal intracellular organelles is another feature of ageing in post-mitotic cells. The major organelle involved is the mitochondrion and this is manifested by the accumulation of abnormal mitochondria exhibiting a variety of ultrastructural abnormalities. The vulnerability of these organelles is thought to be due to the poor capacity for repair of mitochondrial DNA and their increased exposure to endogenous ROS. Autophagy and ageing are also reviewed in depth elsewhere.[2]

Studying the effects of ageing on the uterus and placenta

Scientific study of the effect of ageing on the uterus can be directed towards either animal studies or the study of human clinical material. The approach to animal studies is clearly much more straightforward, as ageing is under the control of the experimenter and its effects can be isolated. The approach to studying the effects of ageing in women is much more complex. Many of the key issues relate to pregnancy and childbirth and the factors that determine the age that a woman chooses to start a family are clearly highly complex. It is inevitable that many major maternal characteristics, such as smoking status, educational achievement and socio-economic status, will differ systematically in relation to maternal age. Moreover, many of a woman's physical characteristics and medical comorbidities will vary with age, for example body mass index, the presence of diabetes and connective tissue disorders. Finally, parity is a major determinant of pregnancy outcome and performance. Effects of age must be separated from parity, with which age will be correlated in most populations. Hence, the characterisation of some biological property of the uterus or placenta in relation to the age of the mother requires a standardised population (for example, primiparous women in labour at term) plus detailed information on other maternal characteristics. Moreover, the analytical approach used will tend to have to involve procedures to account for confounding by the associated features. This necessitates the use of complex statistical tools to handle multivariate assessment of associations. However, basic scientists, being founded in the experimental paradigm, often lack skills in such methods and, indeed, there is a tendency in the biological sciences to be somewhat distrustful of complex statistical modelling. Genuine progress in the future in translational studies to address ageing will require researchers to possess knowledge of all three of clinical obstetrics, basic science and biostatistics.

Ageing and the myometrium

Clarifying the clinical evidence

Previous studies have demonstrated that the risk of caesarean delivery increases with advancing maternal age. However, it is currently unclear whether the association reflects a biological effect of advanced age[3,4] or is a consequence of physician and maternal preference.[5,6] Resolving the question of whether a true epidemiological association exists is clearly crucial before studying the science. Clinically, there are variable definitions of age threshold that mark a woman as being at increased risk of complications. However, in practice, age is not regarded as an issue among women aged under 30 years. Hence, the presence of any association between age and outcome up to 30 years of age is unlikely to be explained by an effect of age on medical decision making. Another aspect of addressing this question is the indication for caesarean section. In cases where the mother or physician has concerns, a decision is often made for a planned caesarean section. Hence, if one were looking for biological determinants of caesarean section, such as poor progress in labour, the analysis should focus on women in otherwise uncomplicated labour at term and also determine whether similar associations were observed for other markers of dysfunctional labour, such as

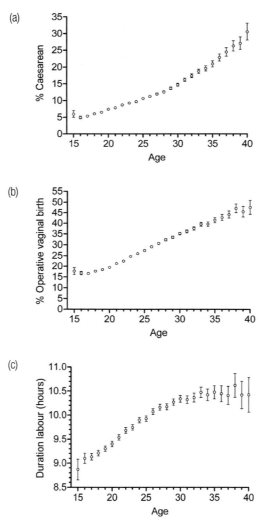

Figure 11.2 Maternal age and the outcome of labour: (a) proportion of women being delivered by emergency intrapartum caesarean section in relation to age of mother ($n = 583847$); bars are binomial 95% confidence intervals; (b) proportion of nulliparous women who required operative vaginal delivery in relation to maternal age among the 518787 women delivered by a means other than emergency caesarean section; bars are binomial 95% CIs; (c) mean duration of spontaneous labour in relation to maternal age ($n = 409703$); bars are 95% CIs of the mean; reproduced from Smith et al.[9]

operative vaginal delivery. Hence, if there is a true association between maternal age and the risk of caesarean section, one would expect to see this across the whole of the age range and to see a similar association with operative vaginal birth. We have addressed this by studying over 500 000 first births of women in labour at term with a singleton infant in a cephalic presentation. This demonstrated a linear relationship between the age of the mother across the age range of 16–30 years and the risk of caesarean delivery, operative vaginal birth and long duration of labour (Figure 11.2). This suggested that there is a true biological effect of age and that, when studying the biological effects of ageing on the myometrium, age should be treated as a continuum.

Basic scientific studies of ageing and myometrial structure and function

I have been unable to find any animal studies addressing the effects of ageing on myometrial function. However, two studies of human myometrium have demonstrated evidence of failure of autophagy in tissue from older women. Gosden *et al.* (1978)[7] examined nonpregnant human myometrium obtained at the time of hysterectomy and demonstrated the presence of cytoplasmic lipofuscin inclusions in uterine smooth muscle cells from older women (across the age range 15–45 years). These inclusions were approximately 1 micrometre in diameter and demonstrated autofluorescence. Analysis of specimens in relation to age demonstrated no cases with a high concentration of these particles in four women aged 25 years or less and high concentrations in nine of 11 women aged 36 years or over ($P = 0.01$ by Fisher's exact test, not reported in the paper). The functional significance of lipofuscin was not studied. A second study that addressed myometrial ultrastructure in relation to ageing was published in Russian in 1983.[8] These authors examined lower uterine segment samples obtained at the time of caesarean section and reported dissociation of myofilaments, mitochondrial destruction and abnormal appearances of the endoplasmic reticulum in association with age. However, there was no apparent control group and no attempt at quantitative analysis. We have performed preliminary studies on myometrium also obtained from the lower uterine segment at the time of caesarean section and were able to see similar ultrastructural features in samples from a woman aged 40 years (Figure 11.3).

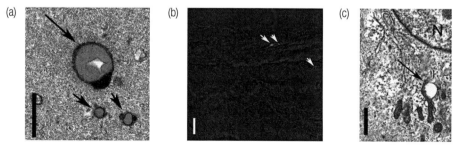

Figure 11.3 Electron and confocal microscopy of human lower uterine segment myometrium from a woman aged 40 years: (a) transmission electron microscopy demonstrating one large and two smaller lipofuscin granules (arrows) within a myometrial cell (bar = 1 micrometre); (b) confocal microscopy of frozen section of myometrium demonstrating autofluorescence of lipofuscin particles (bar = 10 micrometres); (c) transmission electron microscopy demonstrating a vacuolated mitochondrion (arrow) and normal mitochondria, adjacent to the nucleus (N) (bar = 1 micrometre); micrographs courtesy of Cordeaux Y, Charnock-Jones DS, Burton GB and Smith GC (unpublished data)

We have also completed a study of the function of human myometrium in relation to maternal age.[9] Myometrial biopsies were obtained from 62 non-labouring women undergoing routine elective caesarean section at 38–40 weeks and were studied using a standard organ-bath system. Spontaneous contractile activity was quantified by integrating the area under the tension curve: the ratio of the area under the curve before and during exposure to 50 mmol/l potassium was calculated and log-transformed to normalise the distribution. This value was termed the 'contraction unit' (see Figure 11.4a). Spontaneous contractions were also assessed for coupling: the presence of two or more distinct peaks before the return to baseline (examples in Figure 11.4), which is associated with dysfunctional labour *in vivo*.[10] Both assessments were made blind to the mother's age.

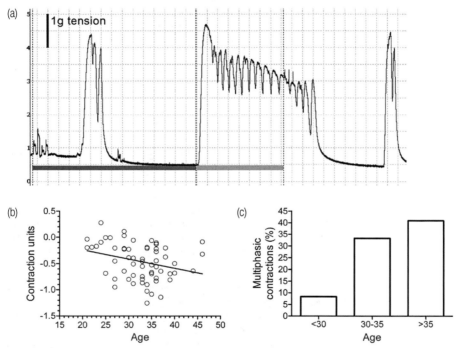

Figure 11.4 Myometrial contractility in relation to maternal age. (a) Trace of isometric tension from myometrial strip obtained from a 40-year-old woman being delivered by planned ceasarean section. The dark grey line represents the 15 minutes before addition of potassium, and the light grey line 7 minutes in the presence of 50 mmol/l of potassium. The area under the curve is the space between the tension trace and the baseline, indicated by the dark and light grey lines. The $\log_{10}$ of the ratio of these two areas is the contraction unit. The spontaneous contraction before the addition of potassium and the contraction following potassium being washed out are both multiphasic. (b) Mean spontaneous contractile activity (quantified as contraction units) of isolated strips of myometrium obtained from women ($n = 62$) at the time of planned caesarean section in relation to the age of the donor; regression line: $y = 0.1078 - 0.0174 \times$ age (95% CI for slope −0.0326 to −0.0022). (c) Proportion of spontaneous contractions that were multiphasic in relation to maternal age ($n = 62$, 181 samples). Reproduced from Smith *et al.*[9]

Spontaneous contraction of isolated myometrial strips declined with advancing age (Figure 11.4b).[9] Regression modelling demonstrated a significant negative association between spontaneous activity and maternal age, with a coefficient of -0.086 for a 5-year increase in age (95% CI -0.161 to -0.012, $P = 0.02$). The other maternal characteristics associated with the degree of spontaneous contraction were previous vaginal births and week of gestation (both factors were positively associated). However, the association between maternal age and the spontaneous contractility was virtually unaffected by adjustment for these and other maternal characteristics. The probability of spontaneous contractions being coupled increased with advancing maternal age (Figure 11.4c). A 5-year increase in age was associated with 93% increase in the odds of coupling (95% CI 41–163%; $P < 0.001$). This was also virtually unaltered by adjusting for maternal characteristics.

Understanding why ageing might impair myometrial function

Both the clinical and scientific data indicated a decline in myometrial function with advancing age across the whole range of maternal age. For example, the associations between age and obstetric outcome were all strikingly linear across the maternal age range of 20–29 years. I have advanced a hypothesis that the association may be explained by hormonal effects on the uterus.[9] Women who delay childbirth using the combined oral contraceptive pill, barrier methods, non-hormonal intrauterine devices or sexual abstinence (which collectively constitute the majority of women) will have repetitive cyclical stimulation by estrogens and progestogens. Myometrium expresses both estrogen and progesterone receptors and these hormones have profound effects on myometrial growth, metabolism and contractility (see review[11]). Hence, I have hypothesised that the adverse effect of advancing maternal age on myometrial contractility may be a consequence of this prolonged cyclical stimulation of the myometrium by estrogen and progesterone.[9]

This hypothesis is falsifiable, as it predicts that early menarche would be independently predictive of the risk of dysfunctional labour. Moreover, the hypothesis makes three predictions about any relationship between age at menarche and the risk of obstetric complications. Firstly, a given year increase in the age at menarche would be expected to have the same protective effect on the risk of intervention as the same decease in maternal age at the time of birth. Secondly, the association between age at menarche and the risk of intervention should be independent of other maternal characteristics associated with age at menarche, such as height and obesity. Finally, it is hypothesised that the true underlying association that mediates both the association with maternal age and any association with the age at menarche is an effect of the gynaecological age of the women, that is, the interval from menarche to first birth. Hence, the hypothesis would predict that the association would also disappear when adjusted for that interval.

The hypothesis has recently been tested using data from the Avon Longitudinal Study of Parents and their Children (ALSPAC) cohort, a multicentre prospective cohort study of women attending for prenatal care in south-west England in 1990–92. This analysis, currently only available in abstract form,[12] reported the relationship between age at menarche and the risk of operative delivery (a composite of caesarean section, forceps delivery or vacuum extraction) among 3739 primiparae recruited to the study who experienced labour at term with a singleton liveborn infant in a cephalic presentation. When adjusted for height, body mass index, marital status, smoking status, induction of labour, week of gestation at delivery and birthweight percentile, the odds ratio for operative delivery associated with a 5-year increase in age at menarche (OR 0.71; 95% CI 0.54–0.92; $P = 0.01$) was very similar to the odds ratio for a 5-year decrease in age at delivery (OR 0.72; 95% CI 0.66–0.79; $P < 0.001$). There was no association between age at menarche and the risk of operative delivery following adjustment for the interval between menarche and the first birth (adjusted OR 0.99; 95% CI 0.78–1.25; $P = 0.91$). Hence, these further clinical observations are consistent with a biological model that predicts that prolonged prepregnancy stimulation of the uterus by the female sex hormones has a harmful effect on the myometrium. This in turn raises the possibility that the effect of delaying childbirth on the outcome of labour varies according to the method of contraception used, which could be of clinical and public health relevance. With the 'physiological' model of human reproduction, operating at the time when humans were evolving, menarche would be soon followed by pregnancy and pregnancies would be interspersed with prolonged periods of breastfeeding. Hence, exposure to changing levels of sex hormones would generally occur quite gradually, except in the immediate period following childbirth. In contrast, modern women experiencing a physiological menstrual cycle and women using the combined pill have a pattern of hormonal exposure characterised by relatively rapid fluctuations in the levels of estrogens and progestogens. This pattern will result in rapid, cyclical fluctuations in the expression levels of sex-hormone responsive genes in the uterus. If this is the key determinant of age-related deterioration in uterine function, then it is possible that hormonal contraceptive methods that do not involve rapid changes in sex hormone levels, such as long-acting progestogens, may preserve uterine function better than barrier methods or the combined pill. Hence, understanding the biological basis of the relationship between maternal age and uterine function may allow identification of contraceptive strategies that better preserve uterine function among women wishing to delay childbirth.

Ageing and the decidua

A number of studies have addressed the effect of ageing in the decidua. The context of these studies is often factors controlling implantation, particularly that failure of implantation may lead to apparent infertility. Clinical applications of such studies include understanding fecundity and the factors that determine the success of assisted reproductive technologies. However, there is a body of work indicating that placental dysfunction, the basis of many complications during late pregnancy, may be explained by suboptimal formation of the placenta in very early pregnancy. This subject is reviewed in detail elsewhere.[13] Hence, understanding the effects of ageing on the earliest stages of pregnancy may also ultimately reveal mechanisms that lead to the increased risk of stillbirth among older women.

Informative studies in women are limited for the reasons elaborated above, namely that assessment of the effect of age is difficult to separate from other maternal associations. For example, expression of lectin, as determined by semi-quantitative immunohistochemistry, did not differ among nonpregnant women in the mid-luteal phase of the menstrual cycle, comparing those aged under 30 years with those aged 40 years or over. However, there was no information on, or adjustment for, other maternal characteristics, such as smoking, body mass index and parity.[14] Studies have, however, been conducted in a range of rodent species, where the effect of age can be studied more effectively in isolation. Some studies addressed implantation directly. For example, implantation appeared to be delayed in aged golden hamsters compared with young animals when studied using electron microscopy. However, overall rates of failure of implantation did not appear to differ according to the age of the animals.[15] Other studies have used experimental manipulations in one uterine horn to simulate some aspects of implantation and compared the appearances with the contralateral horn. Induction of experimental hyperaemia in one uterine horn stimulated vascular development and growth of the myometrium and stroma in young hamsters (3–5 months) but not older animals (13–15 months).[16] In ovariectomised rats treated with ovarian hormones, unilateral sesame oil was used as a deciduagenic stimulus, injected into one horn but not the other, and the responses of the injected and control horn were compared in relation to the age of the animal. Rats aged 2 years showed no response whereas rats aged 4–10 months demonstrated a response to the stimulus. A number of microscopic differences were also noted, namely more lysosomes and fewer luminal microvilli in epithelial cells of older animals. In the stromal cells, more lipofuscin deposits were also observed, as seen in the myometrium of older women, and the cellular composition of the stroma also varied.[17] In aged mice, those that had undergone ovariectomy at 2 months had a greater decidual response compared with controls. However, the controls had not had sham operations at 2 months and the experiment was weak.[18] In ovariectomised mice, the effect of estrogen and progesterone to stimulate uterine growth was similar in young (4 months) and aged (10 months) animals. However, the decidual response to a standardised stimulus was reduced in the older animals.[19]

Collectively, these studies indicate that there is evidence that decidualisation and implantation may be adversely affected by maternal age. However, high-quality studies in women are required to clarify the clinical importance of any such effects.

Ageing and the placenta

Stillbirth is one of the most common major complications of pregnancy, affecting approximately one in 200 potentially viable pregnancies. It is the major cause of perinatal death and is the endpoint of a number of pathophysiological pathways of variable clarity. However, assessment of the evidence suggests that the majority of stillbirths are manifestations of underlying placental dysfunction.[20] Advanced maternal age is one of the most consistent associations with stillbirth.[21,22] One aspect of this literature that is worth clarifying is that ageing of the placenta often refers to the structure and function of the placenta in relation to gestational age. Hence, some studies will refer to the aged placenta and make no reference to maternal age but rather focus on the placenta of women who deliver post-dates. A detailed discussion of this is clearly outside the scope of this review, but the subject is reviewed elsewhere.[23]

As in the case of studies of ageing in the decidua, such evidence as could be found in relation to ageing and the placenta generally failed to control for associated maternal characteristics. The placentas of healthy older women who had a normal pregnancy outcome exhibited reduced levels of apoptosis and increased levels of proliferation in trophoblast cells of the placenta. It was speculated that increased trophoblast activity was compensating for 'the disadvantages of age-related hypofunction'. The effect was seen as a continuum across the range of ages. However, the study included minimal information on the other characteristics of the cohort and, in particular, it is not clear whether all the women were of the same parity.[24] A panel of enzymes involved in metabolism, including those of the cytochrome P450 family, were studied in first-trimester termination of pregnancy specimens.[25] It was found that cytochrome P450 1A (CYP1A) activity was lower with advancing maternal age but was increased among women who smoked. The authors commented: 'there was no significant difference in the ages of the women who smoked compared with non-smokers in our study ($P = 0.12$) which rules out the potential confounding effect of younger women being more likely to smoke and thus skewing the data in relation to maternal age and smoking'. However, a P value of 0.12 suggests a trend towards statistical significance. Moreover, the study only had ten non-smokers and 17 smokers and the borderline P value may simply indicate insufficient power to show the effect. The appropriate approach would have been a regression model with the enzyme activity as the dependent variable and age and cigarette use as predictors. This illustrates the point raised at the beginning of this chapter about the analysis of translational research studies that use an observational design.

There were fewer available studies on maternal age and the placenta in animals. However, one study compared young rats (3–5 months) with old rats (9–12 months) and observed that the placental weight was greater in the last quarter of pregnancy in the older animals (40–70%). This was despite the fact that there was no significant difference in the weights of the pups. Hence, the fetal-to-placental weight ratio was decreased in the older animals. However, the older animals were multiparous and the younger animals nulliparous, hence the comparison failed to isolate the effect of age from parity. The authors speculated that hypertrophy of the placenta was required to maintain fetal growth in the face of less favourable maternal physiology.[26] Quantitative analysis of macrophages was performed in young nulliparous mice, older nulliparous mice and older multiparous mice. Consistent with the better outcome in multiparous animals, the number of placental macrophages was increased in the older multiparous mice. In contrast, the number of macrophages was decreased in older nulliparous mice compared with young nulliparous animals.[27] There is also evidence in thoroughbred mares that ageing is associated with impaired placentation. Microplacentome development in the placenta of an aged mare exhibited reduced 'extent and intimacy' of the border for fetomaternal exchange, which was in turn postulated to result in impaired fetal growth.[28] However, very significant differences exist in the formation and structure of the human placenta compared with these animal species. Given that stillbirth is the major single cause of perinatal death and that advanced maternal age is one of the most prevalent risk factors for this outcome, high-quality translational studies on the effect of maternal age on placentation are required.

Conclusion

The present state of the literature strongly indicates direct biological effects of ageing on the uterus and the placenta. A combination of biological epidemiology and smooth muscle studies indicates a mechanistic basis for the effect of ageing on performance during labour, namely that prolonged prepregnancy stimulation of the uterus by estrogens and progestogens may adversely affect its function. Further studies are required to clarify the molecular mechanism of these effects and whether different approaches to hormonal contraception may be protective in relation to the myometrium. There is a paucity of high-quality biological studies that address the mechanisms by which delaying childbirth increases the risk of antepartum stillbirth and there is an urgent need for translational studies in this area. The approach to such studies will require excellence in both basic sciences and in the design of clinical observational research.

References

1. Shay JW, Wright WE. Hallmarks of telomeres in ageing research. *J Pathol* 2007;211:114–23.

2. Terman A, Gustafsson B, Brunk UT. Autophagy, organelles and ageing. *J Pathol* 2007;211:134–43.

3. Main DM, Main EK, Moore DH. The relationship between maternal age and uterine dysfunction: a continuous effect throughout reproductive life. *Am J Obstet Gynecol* 2000;182:1312–20.

4. Adashek JA, Peaceman AM, Lopez-Zeno JA, Minogue JP, Socol ML. Factors contributing to the increased cesarean birth rate in older parturient women. *Am J Obstet Gynecol* 1993;169:936–40.

5. Gareen IF, Morgenstern H, Greenland S, Gifford DS. Explaining the association of maternal age with Cesarean delivery for nulliparous and parous women. *J Clin Epidemiol* 2003;56:1100–10.

6. Bell JS, Campbell DM, Graham WJ, Penney GC, Ryan M, Hall MH. Do obstetric complications explain high caesarean section rates among women over 30? A retrospective analysis. *BMJ* 2001;322:894–5.

7. Gosden RG, Hawkins HK, Gosden CA. Autofluorescent particles of human uterine muscle cells. *Am J Pathol* 1978;91:155–74.

8. Drampian GK, Okoev GG, Allaverdian AG. [Ultrastructural characteristics of the myometrium in the lower segment of the uterus in elderly primigravidas]. *Akush Ginekol (Mosk)* 1983;8:18–21.

9. Smith GC, Cordeaux Y, White IR, Pasupathy D, Missfelder-Lobos H, Pell JP, *et al*. The effect of delaying childbirth on primary cesarean section rates. *PLoS Med* 2008;5:e144.

10. Ferreira CJ, Odendaal HJ. Does coupling of uterine contractions reflect uterine dysfunction? *S Afr Med J* 1994;84:20–3.

11. Hertelendy F, Zakar T. Regulation of myometrial smooth muscle functions. *Curr Pharm Des* 2004;10:2499–517.

12. Smith GCS. Age at menarche and the risk of operative first delivery. *Am J Obstet Gynecol* 2009;SMFM Abstract number 375.

13. Smith GC. First trimester origins of fetal growth impairment. *Semin Perinatol* 2004;28:41–50.

14. Noci I, Gheri G, Bryk SG, Sgambati E, Moncini D, Paglierani M, *et al*. Aging of the human endometrium: peri-implantation phase endometrium does not show any age-dependent variation in lectin binding. *Eur J Obstet Gynecol Reprod Biol* 1996;64:11–21.

15. Parkening TA. An ultrastructural comparison of implantation in young and senescent golden hamsters. *Anat Embryol (Berl)* 1975;147:293–307.

16. Sorger T, Soderwall A. The aging uterus and the role of edema in endometrial function. *Biol Reprod* 1981;24:1135–44.

17. Craig SS. Effect of age upon uterine response to deciduagenic stimulus. *Acta Anat (Basel)* 1981;110:146–58.

18. Goodrick GJ, Nelson JF. The decidual cell response in aging C57BL/6J mice is potentiated by long-term ovariectomy and chronic food restriction. *J Gerontol* 1989;44:B67–71.

19. Holinka CF, Finch CE. Age-related changes in the decidual response of the C57BL/6J mouse uterus. *Biol Reprod* 1977;16:385–93.

20. Smith GC, Fretts RC. Stillbirth. *Lancet* 2007;370:1715–25.

21. Fretts RC, Schmittdiel J, Mclean FH, Usher RH, Goldman MB. Increased maternal age and the risk of fetal death. *N Engl J Med* 1995;333:953–7.

22. Huang L, Sauve R, Birkett N, Fergusson D, van Walraven C. Maternal age and risk of stillbirth: a systematic review. *CMAJ* 2008;178:165–72.

23. Fox H. Aging of the placenta. *Arch Dis Child Fetal Neonatal Ed* 1997;77:F171–5.

24. Yamada Z, Kitagawa M, Takemura T, Hirokawa K. Effect of maternal age on incidences of apoptotic and proliferative cells in trophoblasts of full-term human placenta. *Mol Hum Reprod* 2001;7:1179–85.

25. Collier AC, Tingle MD, Paxton JW, Mitchell MD, Keelan JA. Metabolizing enzyme localization and activities in the first trimester human placenta: the effect of maternal and gestational age, smoking and alcohol consumption. *Hum Reprod* 2002;17:2564–72.

26. Rahima A, Bruce NW. Fetal and placental growth in young, primiparous and old, multiparous rats. *Exp Gerontol* 1987;22:257–61.

27.   Lagadari M, Blois S, Margni R, Miranda S. Analysis of macrophage presence in murine placenta: influence of age and parity status. *Am J Reprod Immunol* 2004;51:49–55.

28.   Abd-Elnaeim MM, Leiser R, Wilsher S, Allen WR. Structural and haemovascular aspects of placental growth throughout gestation in young and aged mares. *Placenta* 2006;27:1103–13.

Chapter 12
Basic science: sperm and placenta

Discussion

William Ledger: Thank you both for excellent talks. That was fascinating. Gordon, could you just speculate on whether the cervix might be similarly affected as the uterus? Do we have any new information on that?

Gordon Smith: Cervical tissue is obviously much harder to get. It's relatively straightforward to obtain lower uterine segment at caesarean section. You can obtain cervical biopsies but it is tricky to do so.

Mandish Dhanjal: Did you look at the effect on women of the oral contraceptive pill?

Gordon Smith: We don't have that information. We only have basic information on contraception and not such that we could do an informative analysis on it. That is certainly intriguing. If we think again about the evolutionary idea, you would have gradual increases in estrogen and progesterone during pregnancy and then suppression of both during breastfeeding. It does raise a possibility that maybe something in the cyclical nature of both the ovarian cycle and combined oral contraception in stimulating the uterus, withdrawing, stimulating the uterus, withdrawing, could lead to an adverse effect. Hence, it is not clear that the combined pill would be all that different from the spontaneous ovarian cycle. The intriguing thing is that long-acting progestogens may have a pattern of stimulation that is closer to the physiological, and may have less of an effect. You can really only tell in animal studies, where you can study manipulations of the hormonal environment directly.

Roger Gosden: One animal study which we carried out many years ago that probably has not been noticed because it was published as an abstract by the Physiological Society was directly to address the question about the long history of exposure to ovarian steroids.[1] This experiment was carried out in the mouse and it involved embryo transfer to standardise the quality of the eggs or embryos. The animals were divided into various groups and controls and the main treatment group was long-term ovariectomised mice. After many months, the animals were tested for fertility by embryo transfer compared with various controls. The background to this was that rodents have very dramatic uterine ageing. This is more important than the quality of the eggs. The uterine capacity goes down, so if you transfer eggs from young animals into old recipients they never take. But in this experiment, the removing of the ovaries, and the long-term ovariectomy state, potentiated fertility dramatically.

Gordon Smith: That is one of the things I wanted to do, and I have submitted unsuccessful grant applications to study this. The hypothesis would also make a prediction: if you take a rat or mouse and age it, there will be a difference between those in whom you suppressed the hypophyseal–pituitary axis and not. The way we proposed to do this was with long-acting GnRH [gonadotrophin-releasing hormone] analogue. You'd look at the effect of, say, 6 months with or without an estrus cycle, on the aged animal – but the grant-giving body resisted the temptation so I haven't an answer.

Alastair Sutcliffe: Thank you for your eloquent hypothesis. How is that different from the known patterns of striated muscle that gradually reduces its strength over years?

Gordon Smith: This is where it's important to look at the epidemiological data. What you see is the same proportional change going from 16 to 21 as you see going from 36 to 41. The epidemiological association doesn't have the characteristics of a deterioration with age because you can actually see the variation over that period of time. With the hypothesis, if it really was just a general age-related deterioration, you wouldn't predict there would be an independent effect of menarche which was lost when we adjusted for the interval between menarche and first birth. So, it is two-fold.

William Ledger: Does it happen in athletes who train?

Gordon Smith: I would predict it would. I would need 3000 athletes to test that.

William Ledger: Next thing the newspapers will try to get us to 'exercise your uterus' or something. [laughter]

Gordon Smith: Maybe it's exercised too much …

Dimitrios Nikolaou: There are many possible obstetric outcomes but I guess some are more important than others. For example, cephalopelvic disproportion is important, but not as important as intrauterine growth restriction or stillbirth. You said that depends on placentation.

Gordon Smith: Yes. One of the things that I would really emphasise with this is that if you are going to study age you have to isolate it from maternal comorbidities and other general characteristics. You can only do that in an animal study or if you use a very sophisticated biostatical approach. Reviewing the literature on the placenta for my chapter I could not identify any human study that made any attempt to isolate the effect of age statistically. There was not much to the animal studies in the placenta as well. We are doing a large-scale prospective cohort study in a first pregnancy where we are taking serial serum samples, collecting the placenta at birth and all the demographic data and medical data you require to address this. But looking at the literature, I was unable to find a human study that made a serious attempt to isolate age. The most obvious confounder is parity. It is so obvious that parity is going to tend to vary with age and virtually everything about pregnancy varies according to parity. It is difficult to interpret some of the published studies when authors do not take into account whether it's a first or subsequent pregnancy.

Gordon Smith: There are data about pre-eclampsia and eclampsia which show increased risks at the extremes of age.

Stephen Hillier: I wondered whether there were any endocrine data in relation to age and parturition. I'm thinking particularly about factors such as relaxin and these various peri-paracrine growth factors, etc., that could be adjusted to age. If you imagine that, it would still be consistent with your hypothesis but it would not necessarily be a direct effect of estrogens or progesterones on the uterus but secondary effects that might kick in at the time of parturition.

Gordon Smith: The literature is really, really sparse. What I presented today is pretty much everything I could find in relation to myometrium. I think animal studies are where you could really begin to pick this apart. It is very difficult to do in observational human studies.

Stephen Hillier: Of course. I just wanted to know whether the data were there.

Mandish Dhanjal: Are there any data on the way the older mother's myometrium responds to Syntocinon® [oxytocin] in a primigravid woman compared with a younger one?

Gordon Smith: Yes. The clinical data are that older women tended to need longer courses of Syntocinon and greater total doses compared with younger women if they were having labour augmented.

Maya Unnithan: And has that been looked at in the human *in vitro*?

Gordon Smith: No. Again, what we wanted to do is a systematic description of myometrial contractility in relation to the age of the mother. I want to characterise this dose response *in vitro*.

Roger Gosden: Herman, I am very grateful to you for putting together all this information about the ageing male. I have underestimated the importance. Do you think that testicular ageing can be accounted for largely by vascular ageing? I've looked at a few microscope sections of ageing human testes and there are a couple of very obvious phenomena. One is that the tubules seem to fail as a unit rather than seeing proportionate decreases in each. I would like you to confirm that. Secondly, we see quite a lot of fibrosis going on. I wondered whether stenosis of the testicular artery or reduced perfusion of other regions within the testis could explain the phenomenon?

Herman Tournaye: You are probably right. In fact, there are few studies available, the older one from Holstein.[2] They all describe large individual changes but also, within one testis, there are always patchy areas where you see that there are fewer spermatogonia, but there are other areas where sperm production is perfect. That is in my view a hypothesis but there is, as far as I know, no proof that could implicate vascular changes.

Roger Gosden: Would it be too difficult to do Doppler ultrasound studies in relation to this matter?

Herman Tournaye: Yes. What you are talking about is probably in the microvascularisation.

Susan Bewley: Herman, you made a chance remark at the beginning about how this is suddenly a topic of interest in the media. From your work and knowledge on male reproductive ageing, is it really new that we are getting anxious about older men? Is it to do with our general anxieties about life and health – that as we get healthier we worry more? Is it something to do with the discourse about women ageing? Or maybe our worries about pollution and falling sperm counts? Have you any thoughts about why it is a new anxiety?

Herman Tournaye: Someone else might comment much better than me. There is a trend of more older fathers now. It is a trend everywhere and I think it is in the statistics of the UK. So that's one thing, there are more candidate fathers up to old age, although, on the other hand, I think it is indeed because of the female ageing. If you look at what has happened really in the scientific world, in the last few years, there are some studies. That number tremendously increased. So, for me there is a big disproportion between the interest 2 years ago that scientists put into the area and that of the layman just assuming overnight. I think it is catchy, it is trendy also …

Susan Bewley: Do you think we want to be as anxious about male reproductive ageing as female reproductive ageing?

Herman Tournaye: I don't think we should, you know. I think you need to inform patients about the risks. Clearly, the risks are completely different with what's happening in the female with ageing. Keep everything in proportion – that is my feeling.

Peter Braude: Maybe it's disaffected men on a second family who are picking out younger women and so now they've got to think about new children and that's when they begin to worry about ageing?

Gordon Smith: It is intriguing that two FGF [fibroblast growth factor] sub-types are associated with these mutations. Is there some aspect of the effectiveness of sperm that is controlled by FGF and by knocking out the receptor you preferentially increase the likelihood of the sperm fertilising the egg. It made me think there must be something about FGF that controls sperm function. So is there any evidence for that?

Herman Tournaye: At least the more recent molecular studies[3] today show that Penrose's copy-error hypothesis[4] does not explain this properly.

Gordon Smith: And does the sperm make FGF? Or is there any reason the sperm respond? [silence]

William Ledger: Even among this group we have lacunae in knowledge. [laughter] Does anyone else want to ask a question or make a comment?

Maya Unnithan: You didn't seem to mention hormonal changes or did I miss it?

Herman Tournaye: I didn't want to mention it because you have many societies now covering this issue. I mean, for many years the pharmaceutical companies did not have a good drug to sell. Now, for about the past 7–10 years they have good drugs to sell and they are looking for markets. So the endocrine function in the ageing male: there are books, there are meetings, there are societies, whatever you want, and then it is clear that every man's testosterone output is going down gradually but nobody knows exactly when it's too low. There are no reference values. You can be very young and have the same value as somebody who is very old but feel very well. So, let us say that it is clear that the endocrine function is going down with ageing; it was called andropause but there is no sudden stop as in menopause. So now the terminology used is late-onset hypogonadism, but again it is a natural phenomenon. They call it a disease. There is a lot of marketing in that.

William Ledger: Right. We'll end on that non-controversial note! [laughter].

References

1.   Felicio LS, Finch CE, Gosden RG, Nelson JF. Effects of long-term ovariectomy on the potential for oestrous cyclicity and pregnancy disclosed by ovarian grafts in ageing mice. *J Physiol* 1984;346:122P.

2.   Holstein AF. Morphological evidence for the involution of spermatogenesis during senescence. In: Holstein AF, editor. *Reproductive Biology and Medicine*. Berlin: Diesbach; 1989. p. 66–77.

3.   Tiemann-Boege I, Navidi W, Grewal R, Cohn D, Eskenazi B, Wyrobek AJ, *et al*. The observed human sperm mutation frequency cannot explain the achondroplasia paternal age effect. *Proc Natl Acad Sci USA* 2002;99:14952–7.

4.   Penrose LS. Parental age and mutation. *Lancet* 1955;269:312–13.

Section 3

Pregnancy: the ageing
mother and medical
needs

Chapter 13

The effect of age on obstetric (maternal and fetal) outcomes

Anna Kenyon and Susan Bewley

Introduction

Numerous studies have reported multiple adverse outcomes associated with childbearing at an advanced maternal age. The clinical importance (as opposed to the statistical significance) of the outcomes reported in these studies is variously concluded, with a few suggesting no increased risk.[1-6] This may be accounted for by subtle differences in study design and data collection. When considering adverse obstetric outcome with respect to maternal age, a cautionary note is therefore advised when reviewing research.

Study designs and pitfalls

Population size is an important consideration. Adverse outcomes, particularly stillbirth, occur infrequently. Only 10–20% of mothers in most populations are aged 35 years or over, 2–4% are 40 years or over[1,7-10] and 0.005% are 50 years or over.[11] Large sample sizes are therefore required to determine an effect of age on outcome. Maternal parity also influences obstetric outcome. Primiparity is reported to be most frequent in those aged 20–29 years, with a trough at 40–49 years and then a modest increase at 50 years or over.[12] In the UK, maternal age at the birth of the first child is steadily increasing (Figure 13.1).[13,14] Any study of a population of older mothers is therefore likely to include an ever-increasing proportion of primiparous women. Great (or grand) multiparity is also more frequently seen among older mothers in some studies:[9] 16% of those aged 40–49 years were grand multiparae compared with 7.0% at 30–39 years and 2.6% at 20–29 years.[12] Those entering their first pregnancy at age 40 years have different risks to those of the same age entering their second or further pregnancies and their outcome must be reviewed with this in mind.

Pregnancies in older mothers are more likely to be as a result of assisted reproductive technologies (ART). Women who conceive via ART (*in vitro* fertilisation [IVF] or ovulation induction) have a higher risk of pregnancy-induced hypertension, gestational diabetes, preterm birth and caesarean section. Even in those studies where mothers have been age and parity matched for singleton[14-17] and multiple pregnancies,[18-20] these outcomes are still statistically significant.[14]

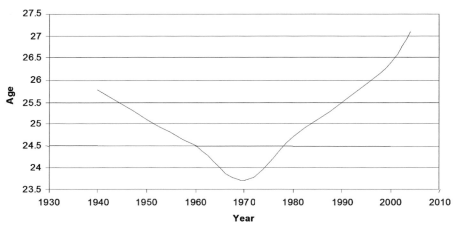

Figure 13.1 Average maternal age at birth of the first child in the UK, 1940–2004; data from Birth Statistics 2004 (Office for National Statistics); reproduced with permission from Nwandison and Bewley[14]

When reviewing studies regarding outcome, consideration must also be given to plurality. Multiple pregnancy is associated with adverse outcome at all ages. Multiple pregnancies occur more frequently in women of advancing age both spontaneously (dizygotic twinning) and as a result of multiple embryo transfer. As the length of the follicular phase, and thus the overall menstrual cycle, shortens with advancing age, a slight increase in follicle-stimulating hormone (FSH) levels during selection of the dominant follicle occurs. This results in the release of two ova in some cycles.[14] Overall, multiple pregnancy rates that have been reported include 2.7% for mothers aged 20–29 years,[12] 1.4% at 20–34 years,[21] 4.1% at 30–39 years,[12] 2.2% at 35–39 years,[21] 2.6% at 40 years or over,[21] 5% at 40–49 years[12] and 37% at 50 years or over.[12] Not all studies describe the proportion of multiple pregnancies arising as a result of ART and, indeed, this may not be known if women do not disclose ART (and especially ovum donation) to their obstetric caregivers. Studies that report obstetric outcome in older mothers must take account of the larger number of multiple pregnancies and the effect of this on the frequency of adverse outcome events observed.

Few studies are prospective. The largest studies, in excess of a million women,[7,11,12,22,23] are all retrospective and derived from national data registries. The largest prospective study, of 36 056 women, only had 1364 women (4%) aged 40 years or over.[1] This limits the social and biological variables that can be recorded[24] and that may have independently affected the outcomes observed. For example, older mothers are more likely to attend early for antenatal care[8] and to be married, of a higher socio-economic group, multiparous and white,[1,9,12,21] which are groups where obstetric outcome might be expected to be better. They are also more likely to deliver in the private sector where intervention rates may be higher.[25] Thus, if anything, we might hypothesise that the particular effect of age on outcome might be attenuated downwards, but exaggerated for intervention rates.

Not all studies include those pregnancies ending prematurely, such as those with chromosomal or lethal congenital abnormalities, the prevalence of which rises with age.[26] Fetal loss and stillbirth are similarly variously defined. Those statistics for determining absolute pregnancy success rates per pregnancy embarked upon (prepregnancy counselling) do not guide practice for women and doctors seeking age-specific risk associated with continuing pregnancies (in antenatal clinics), nor guide practice regarding surveillance or interventions to protect against those losses occurring late.

The control groups used for comparison (for example, age 20–29, 30–39, over 45, or 40 years or more) also vary widely. As age is likely to represent a continuum of risk,[1,26] this is likely to be relevant in terms of the degree of effect observed. Older mothers often have children with older fathers and very few studies correct for this.[27]

Lastly, it should be borne in mind that a statistically significant increase in risk does not necessarily equate with a clinically significant increase in risk. Cleary-Goldman et al.,[1] in a large prospective investigation of singleton pregnancies, advocated that in such large studies where statistical significance is reached ($P < 0.05$) as a result of the large sample size, a higher level of risk should be demanded to ensure that any observed differences in outcome equate with a clinically meaningful difference. This is particularly important when retrospectively trawling through multiple outcomes seeking an association. Cleary-Goldman et al. suggested that an adjusted odds ratio (AOR) of greater than 2.0 and $P < 0.05$ would represent a clinically meaningful difference while acknowledging that an OR less than 2.0 and $P < 0.05$ would be a statistically significant difference.[1] Not all studies apply such robust criteria and this may explain the differing conclusions drawn.

Obstetric outcome

The risk of fetal loss according to maternal age at conception follows a J-shaped curve, with a steep increase after the age of 35 years (Figure 13.2).[7,21,26] Nybo Andersen et al.[26] reported that approximately 20% of all wanted pregnancies in women aged 35 years will result in fetal loss (defined as stillbirths, miscarriages or ectopic pregnancies), rising to 54.5% at age 42 years. The risk of miscarriage is even more alarming: a woman aged 35–39 years has a risk of miscarriage of 24.6%, rising to 51% at 40–44 years and 93.4%

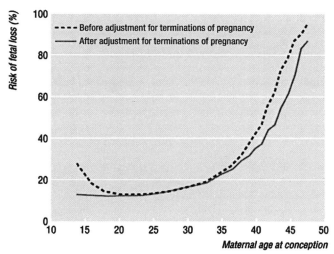

Figure 13.2   Risk of fetal loss from miscarriage, ectopic pregnancy and stillbirth according to maternal age at conception; reproduced with permission from Nybo Andersen et al.[26]

at 45 years or over.[26] This study only explored those women reaching hospital and not miscarriages at home. A further increase in risk of fetal loss for women aged 35 years was observed if terminations of pregnancy (for all causes) were also considered. This study could not, however, account for use of ART, multiple pregnancies or ovum donation, all of which are factors known to be associated with a poorer obstetric outcome.[7]

The association of age and miscarriage is widely agreed but that of adverse obstetric outcome later is less clear. In their prospective study of 36 056 singleton pregnancies, Cleary-Goldman et al.[1] agreed a rise in miscarriage rates (OR 2.0 and OR 2.4 at age 35 years or over and at age 40 years or over, respectively) and chromosomal abnormalities (OR 4.0 and OR 9.9 at age 35 years or over and at age 40 years or over, respectively) in older mothers. However, when the effects of race, parity, body mass index, education, marital status, smoking, pre-existing medical conditions, previous adverse obstetric outcome and use of ART were controlled for, the authors showed that there was no statistically significant association between age 35 years or over and other outcomes such as threatened miscarriage, pre-eclampsia, gestational hypertension, preterm labour and operative vaginal delivery. Maternal age of 40 years or over was an independent risk factor for gestational diabetes (AOR 2.4), placenta praevia (AOR 2.8), placental abruption (AOR 2.3), caesarean section (AOR 2.0) and perinatal mortality (AOR 2.2).[1] Interestingly, this study did not show advancing age to be associated with hypertensive complications despite confirming that chronic hypertension was more common among older women. The authors suggested this was as a result of controlling for covariates associated with gestational hypertension and pre-eclampsia such as history of medical conditions and use of ART.[1]

Hoffman[7] looked only at singleton pregnancies in a multiethnic population and compared women aged 35–39 years (13 902) and aged 40 years or over (3953) with those aged under 35 years. The author noted a higher percentage of maternal complications including chronic hypertension, diabetes, gestational diabetes and pre-eclampsia in women aged 35 years or over. However, after correcting for race, parity, chronic hypertension, pre-eclampsia, diabetes, gestational diabetes and gestational age at delivery, the risk of having an infant of low birth weight was increased for mothers aged 40 years or over (birth weight less than 2500 g AOR 1.4; 95% CI 1.24–1.58, and birth weight less than 1500 g OR 1.5; 95% CI 1.17–1.93). The odds ratio for preterm birth (before 28 weeks) was also increased in women aged 40 years or over compared with those aged under 35 years (AOR 1.27; 95% CI 1.06–1.53).[7]

Salihu et al.,[12] in a large retrospective US study of 12 066 854 pregnancies, found that women aged 30 years or over with a singleton pregnancy had higher risks of all morbidity and mortality indices compared with women aged 20–29 years (Figure 13.3). Risks of pre-eclampsia, eclampsia, placental abruption and placenta praevia also all showed an increasing linear trend with age. Among multiple births, the relative risk for adverse fetal outcomes were still higher among older mothers but the magnitude of these differences was less (Figure 13.4) (note different scale of y-axis).[12]

Others have confirmed the increased incidence of placenta praevia in older mothers: AOR 10.5; 95% CI 5.4–20 in nulliparous, and AOR 2.7; 95% CI 1.8–3.6 in multiparous women aged 40 years or over compared with those aged 20–29 years.[9] The absolute number of women aged 40 years or over was small in this study and represented only 0.25% of nulliparous and 0.13% of multiparous women.

Parity

Older mothers are more likely to be nulliparous. Gilbert et al.[9] retrospectively studied 24 032 pregnant women over a 2-year delivery period, of which 2772 (20%) were

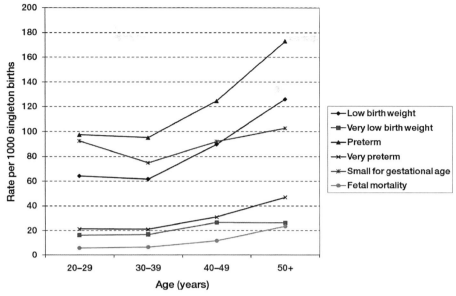

Figure 13.3   Crude rates for fetal morbidity and mortality among singletons by maternal age in the USA, 1997–99; data from Salihu *et al.*[12]

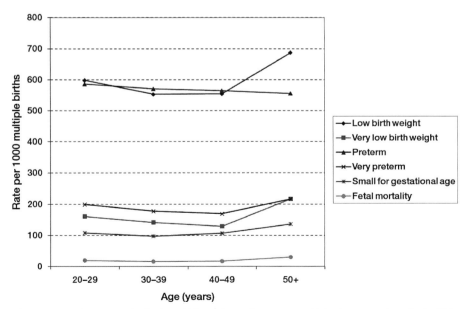

Figure 13.4   Crude rates for fetal morbidity and mortality among multiples by maternal age in the USA, 1997–99; data from Salihu *et al.*[12]

both nulliparas and aged 40 years or over. These women were compared both with multiparous women aged 40 years or over and with those aged 20–29 years (the control group).[9] No comment was made regarding plurality but Figure 13.5 shows the risks of birth asphyxia, fetal growth restriction and malpresentation. The risks all increased with age but also with nulliparity.

Plurality

Even without consideration of maternal age, multiple pregnancies have increased rates of obstetric complications (pre-eclampsia, gestational diabetes, postpartum haemorrhage, stillbirth and caesarean section).[12,22] Luke and Brown[22] considered the effect of plurality and age on pregnancy outcome and corrected for race, smoking status, maternal education and trimester of prenatal care in women without diabetes or chronic hypertension. The authors demonstrated that multiple pregnancies were associated with increased risks of pregnancy-induced hypertension (AOR 2.45; 95% CI 2.42–2.48 for twins, and AOR 3.04; 2.86–3.22 for triplets) and delivery before 29 weeks (AOR 8.10; 95% CI 7.97–8.24 for twins, and AOR 33.89; 95% CI 32.21–35.66 for triplets, compared with singletons). Within the same plurality, increasing maternal age was associated with reported significantly higher risks of pregnancy-induced hypertension and excessive bleeding (including placental abruption, placenta praevia, and excessive bleeding during labour and delivery) (Table 13.1). However, for twins and triplets there was a lower risk for tocolysis and infant mortality with rising age.[22] The magnitude of the reported increased risks are, however, small. None of the outcomes was associated with an AOR of greater than 2.0, which Cleary-Goldman *et al.*[1] have recommended as being a clinically meaningful increase in risk.[1]

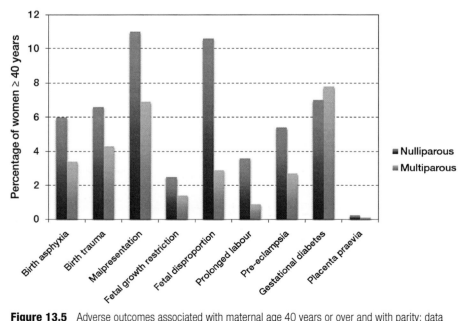

Figure 13.5 Adverse outcomes associated with maternal age 40 years or over and with parity; data from Gilbert *et al.*[9]

Table 13.1 Complications of pregnancy and delivery by maternal age and plurality in women without diabetes or chronic hypertension; adjusted for maternal race, parity and smoking status and compared with women aged 20–29 years; reproduced with permission from Luke and Brown[22]

	Age (years)	Singletons AOR (95%CI)	Twins AOR (95%CI)	Triplets AOR (95%CI)
Pregnancy-induced hypertension	30–34	0.99 (0.99–1.00)	1.01[a] (0.97–1.04)	1.15[a] (0.99–1.35)
	35–39	1.17 (1.16–1.18)	1.08[b] (1.03–1.12)	1.11[a] (0.93–1.33)
	40 or over	1.50 (1.47–1.52)	1.49 (1.39–1.60)	1.52[c] (1.16–1.98)
Delivery before 29 weeks of gestation	30–34	1.08 (1.06–1.09)	0.88 (0.84–0.92)	0.69 (0.58–0.82)
	35–39	1.32 (1.29–1.34)	0.83 (0.78–0.88)	0.58 (0.47–0.71)
	40 or over	1.55 (1.50–1.60)	0.72 (0.65–0.81)	0.52 (0.37–0.75)
Excessive bleeding	30–34	1.16 (1.15–1.17)	1.15 (1.08–1.23)	0.96 (0.68–1.36)
	35–39	1.42 (1.40–1.42)	1.32 (1.23–1.41)	1.13 (0.78–1.65)
	40 or over	1.76 (1.72–1.80)	1.75 (1.57–1.96)	1.06 (0.59–1.88)

AOR = adjusted odds ratio

Excessive bleeding included placental abruption, placenta praevia and excessive bleeding during labour and delivery

All results were significant at $P < 0.001$ except [a] not significant, [b] 0.001, [c] 0.002

Plurality and ovum donation

Porreco et al.[5] attempted to address the specific effect of ovum donation on pregnancy outcome in older mothers while also considering plurality. Women aged 45 years or over were recruited and matched for parity and plurality with a woman aged under 36 years. Forty-eight percent of the pregnancies were multiple. Thirty-nine of 50 women aged 45 years or over (78%) conceived by ovum donation and IVF. One-third of the women in the control group also conceived after ART. Pre-eclampsia was significantly more prevalent among the women aged 45 years or over (OR 2.67; 95% CI 1.04–6.82) even though 22% of those in the control group developed pre-eclampsia. One of 11 women (9%) aged 45 years or over conceiving spontaneously developed pre-eclampsia compared with 20/39 (51%) conceiving with ART and donor eggs (P 0.016).[5] There were no other differences in diabetes, chronic hypertension, tocolysis, fetal growth restriction, gestational age at delivery or birth weight.[5] Henne et al.[28] reported an increase in preterm labour, pre-eclampsia and protracted labour in women conceiving after ovum donation, after having corrected for parity.

Stillbirth

Stillbirths affect one in 200 pregnancies.[29] The degree of risk that advanced maternal age poses has been investigated in several studies (Table 13.2). The studies varied in terms of the reference population but increased rates of stillbirth were reported consistently.

Wyatt et al.[30] examined fetal loss (miscarriage or intrauterine fetal death) at 15 weeks of gestation or more in a large cohort of women (264 653) but excluded those with fetal chromosomal or structural abnormalities, insulin-dependent diabetes or multiple pregnancies. An age-specific risk of fetal loss after these corrections was then calculated. Age 35 years or over was associated with an OR of 2.4 (compared with the 27-year-old women who had the lowest risk of loss (that is, the reference age with OR of 1), rising to OR 5.2 at age 40 years and OR 6.4 at age 43 years.[30]

Table 13.2   Studies reporting risks of stillbirth by maternal age

Reference	Stillbirth definition	Study population	Population age in years (n)	Comparator age (years)	Risk (95% CI)			
					35–40 years	≥40 years	≥45 years	≥50 years
Donoso and Carvajal (2008)[11]	Fetal death	2 817 959	≥50 (217)	20–34				OR 3.7 (1.2–10.5)
Hoffman et al. (2007)[7] [a]	Fetal death	126 402	≥40 (3953)	<40		AOR 2.28 at 40–41 weeks, AOR 2.93 at 28–31 weeks (1.76–4.92)		
Luke and Brown (2007)[22]	Infant death (unspecified)	22 991 306	≥ 40 (4 982 612 singletons)			AOR 1.44[b] (1.38–1.50)		
Jacobsson et al. (2004)[23]	Intrauterine fetal death after 28 weeks	1 566 313	40–44 (31 662), >45 (1205)	20–29		AOR 2.1 (1.8–2.4) for 40–44 years	AOR 3.8 (2.2–6.4)	
Salihu et al. (2003)[12]	Loss after 20 weeks	12 066 854	40–49 (3 982 062), >50 (539)	20–29		AOR 1.94 (1.67–2.26) singletons at 40–49 years, AOR 0.72 (0.43–1.2) multiples at 40–49 years		AOR 2.20 (1.01–4.75) singletons, AOR 1.6 (0.4–3.0) multiples
Gilbert et al. (1999)[9]	Infant death	1 160 000	≥40 (24 032)	20–29		AOR 1.2 (0.8–1.8) nulliparous, AOR 1.5 (1.3–1.8) multiparous		
Jolly et al. (2000)[8]	Stillbirth	385 120	35–40 (41 327), >40 (7331)	18–34	OR 1.41 (1.17–1.70)	OR 1.83 (1.29–2.61)		
Reddy et al. (2006)[10]	Stillbirth	5 458 735	35–39 (545 873), >40 (109 174)	<35	RR 1.54 (1.38–1.72)	RR 2.54 (2.14–3.03)		
Bateman and Simpson (2006)[21]	Stillbirth	5 874 203	35–39 (650 723), ≥40 (130 857)	20–34	OR 1.28 (1.24–1.32)	OR 1.72 (1.63–1.81)		

AOR = adjusted odds ratio; OR = odds ratio

[a] Adjusted for ethnic group, parity, hypertension, pre-eclampsia, gestational diabetes

[b] Adjusted for race/parity

Reddy et al.[10] assessed the relationship between maternal age and risk of stillbirth defined as death at 20 weeks of gestation or more. Among 5 458 735 pregnancies, 10% of mothers were aged 35–39 years and 2.2% were aged 40 years or over. For singleton pregnancies excluding congenital anomalies, the risk of stillbirth at 37–41 weeks of gestation for women aged 35–39 years was one in 382 and for women aged 40 years or over it was one in 267 continuing pregnancies. Compared with women aged under 35 years, the relative risk of stillbirth was 1.32 (95% CI 1.22–1.43) for women aged 35–39 years and 1.88 (95% CI 1.64–2.16) for women aged 40 years or over at 37–41 weeks of gestation (Figure 13.6). The effect of maternal age persisted despite accounting for medical disease, parity, race and ethnicity.[10]

The risk appears to occur in a continuum with rising age,[21,26] The largest increase in risk for women aged 35 years or over may start at 39 weeks of gestation and peak at 41 weeks. Extremes of gestation are associated with the highest weekly risk of stillbirth (more than 41 weeks followed by 20–23 weeks) and women aged 40 years or over appear to have the largest risk.[10]

Nybo Andersen et al.,[26] defining stillbirth as loss of a child beyond gestational age 28 weeks, reported a risk of stillbirth in the general population (63 472 women) to be 4.3 per 1000. As they had shown for other variables (termination of pregnancy, miscarriage and ectopic pregnancy), the curve was J-shaped but less of an effect of age was noted than for miscarriages and ectopic pregnancies. Nulliparous women had a slightly higher risk compared with multiparous women.[26] Hoffman et al.,[7] in a retrospective review of 126 402 singleton pregnancies in the USA, of which 3.3% of women were aged 40 years or over, reported that the odds ratio for a woman aged 40 years or over suffering a stillbirth at 40–41 weeks was 2.28 (95% CI 1.82–4.40) compared with women aged under 35 years at the same gestation.[7]

Fretts and Duru[31] suggested that the risk of stillbirth in women aged 40 years or over may be as high as one in 116 pregnancies at more than 37 weeks of gestation.[30] This increased risk was still observed when corrections were made for coexisting medical

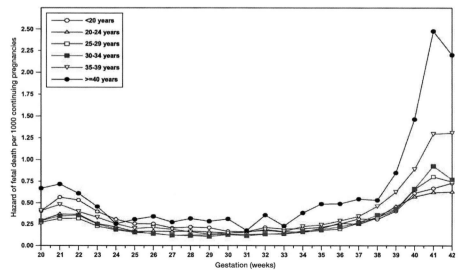

Figure 13.6 Hazard (risk) of stillbirth for singleton births without congenital anomalies by gestational age in the USA, 2001–2002; reproduced with permission from Reddy et al.[10]

conditions, which are not only more common in women of advanced age but are also independently associated with stillbirth (pre-eclampsia, gestational diabetes and multiple pregnancies).[7,32,33] Fretts et al.[32] reported that, even when recognised coexisting conditions that contribute to fetal death were controlled for, women aged 35 years or over had a risk of fetal death twice as high as that among their younger counterparts.

Placental abruption and umbilical cord complications appear to rise with increasing age.[21] Cleary-Goldman et al.[1] suggested that for singleton pregnancies in women aged over 40 years the risk of abruption is OR 2.3. Other important maternal risk factors such as nulliparity and obesity[29] are also seen to rise in women of advanced maternal age.[13,14,33] However, the most significant contribution to the increased risk of stillbirth in women of advanced age is the increased risk of unexplained fetal death (OR 2.2; 95% CI 1.3–3.8).[21]

It could be argued that women aged 20 years should not be compared with those aged 40 years delivering at the same time but rather with women aged 40 years 20 years later, as there may be a temporal benefit for women from improved overall outcomes in obstetric populations over the intervening two decades. Older mothers have benefited from the reduction in stillbirth in general populations over time and this has been confirmed by Fretts et al.[32] Between the years 1960 and 1993, stillbirth rates declined overall and, in women aged 35 years or over, the rate of stillbirths per 1000 births decreased from 16.5 in 1960 to 5.8 in 1990–93. The absolute risk of stillbirth has greatly reduced. However, the higher relative risk for older women persists and exactly what clinicians should do to reduce this is not clear.[24,34]

Labour

Human physical performance peaks at age 25 years but more women are now entering pregnancy beyond this age.[35] A Dublin group employing 'active management of labour' in all nulliparous women attending their unit in spontaneous labour undertook an analysis of outcome with respect to age. In a population where 1091 of 10 737 women were aged 35 years or over, the need for oxytocin and the incidence of prolonged labour, instrumental delivery, intrapartum caesarean section and intrapartum caesarean section because of dystocia all increased with increasing maternal age. The proportion of oxytocin-augmented labours resulting in caesarean section rose from 2.8% for women aged under 20 years to 3.5% at 20–24 years, 4.9% at 25–29 years, 5.5% at 30–34 years and 7.4% in those aged 35 years or over.[35] The observed differences were not accounted for by differences in birth weight, epidural use or gestational age.[35] Heffner et al.[36] reported risks for caesarean section by induction status, gestational age and maternal age stratified for parity in singleton pregnancies over 36 weeks of gestation. Maternal age 35 years or over was associated with an increased caesarean section rate among nulliparous women and maternal age 40 years or over was associated with an increased risk in multiparous women.[36] Similar increased caesarean section rates were reported by Gilbert et al.,[9] with a 47% caesarean section rate in nulliparous women aged 40 years or over compared with 22.5% in those aged 20–29 years. However, the authors acknowledged that a diagnosis of dystocia is physician derived and that they were unable to conclude what anxiety maternal age brought to clinical decision making on the part of the mother and the doctor.[9]

Extremes of maternal age

Few studies involve large numbers of the oldest mothers (aged 45 years or over). Simchen et al.[37] examined 123 mothers (55% of whom had received some form of

ART) aged 45 years or over, of whom 99 were aged 45–49 years and 24 were aged 50–64 years, and compared them with 5162 women within the general antenatal population giving birth at their centre. Ovum donation had been used in all pregnancies in women aged 50 years or over and in 13% of those aged 45 years or over. There were more multiple pregnancies in the women aged 45 years or over (23%) compared with the general population (3%). The finding of lower birth weights and earlier gestations at delivery in women aged 45 years or over compared with the rest of the antenatal population must be interpreted with this in mind. Sixty-three percent of those aged 50 years or over were hospitalised compared with 22% of those aged under 50 years ($P < 0.001$). Women aged 50 years or over gave birth at lower gestations to infants of lighter weight even after correction for plurality (but not gestation). The authors found no difference in hypertensive complications between those aged 50 years or over when compared with those aged 45 years or over, despite the higher proportion of women with ovum donation in the 50 years or over group. The numbers were small, however. The authors reported no stillbirths and that outcome was generally 'good'[37] but the small sample size may have influenced this.

Interventions for age as a risk factor

What seems clear is that older age strongly increases a woman's risk of stillbirth, miscarriage and ectopic pregnancy.[24] Higher pluralities are associated with the most complications and therefore represent the greatest risk.[26] Risks of other pregnancy complications depend on parity and on maternal coexisting morbidities. First-time mothers presenting before conception or in early pregnancy (following referral as a result of age being identified on risk factor screening) may wish to know the risk associated with their pregnancy[9] and, in the context of that increased risk, what interventions are available to improve outcome. Few studies have addressed interventions in older mothers where age is the only risk factor.

Unexplained stillbirths appear to increase with increasing gestation (Figure 13.7). In a UK population, the stillbirth rate has been reported as 0.86, 1.27, 1.55 and 2.12 per 1000 continuing pregnancies at 40, 41, 42 and 43 or more weeks of gestation, respectively, and the relative risk (with 95% CI) for stillbirth at 41, 42 and 43 or more weeks of gestation was 3.6 (2.5–5.2), 4.3 (2.5–7.6) and 6.0 (2.2–16.5), respectively, compared with the rate at 37 weeks.[38] The increase in stillbirths with rising gestation (see Figure 13.7), which is also seen in younger women, is magnified in older women (Figure 13.6).[10] In considering stillbirth, Hannah *et al.*[39] have shown that, in any pregnancy of 41 weeks or more of gestation, induction of labour resulted in lower rates of caesarean section than serial antenatal monitoring, with similar rates of perinatal morbidity and mortality. Given that women aged 40 years or over have a similar stillbirth risk at 39 weeks of gestation to that in women aged 25–29 years at 41 weeks,[26] perhaps interventions should be offered earlier.

Fretts *et al.*[40] reported that women aged 35 years or over would experience 5.2 unexplained fetal deaths per 1000 pregnancies between 37 and 42 weeks of gestation and discussed how best to intervene in women aged 35 years or over. They acknowledged that antepartum testing has a low sensitivity and estimated a value of 70% with a specificity of 90%; that is, 10% falsely positive and leading to unnecessary induction of labour, and 30% false negative and leading to fetal death in the interval before the next test. No specific test was assumed (that is, non-stress testing versus biophysical testing). The authors suggested that weekly antepartum testing (initiated during the 37th week), with delivery if abnormal or continuing pregnancy until 41 weeks if not, would avert

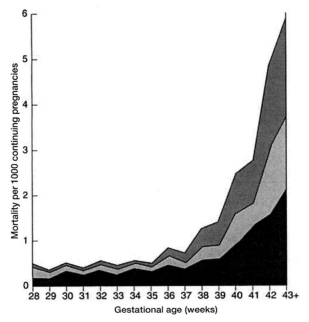

Figure 13.7 Summed mortality at each gestation per 1000 continuing pregnancies for the rate of stillbirth, neonatal death and post-neonatal death; reproduced with permission from Hilder et al.[38]

3.9 unexplained fetal deaths per 1000 pregnancies and would require 863 antepartum tests, 71 inductions and 14 additional caesarean sections to prevent one death.[40]

Hypertension and diabetes are two of the most common medical conditions to complicate pregnancy (7–10% and 3–5%, respectively). Historically, both of these conditions have been shown to be responsible for a significant proportion of fetal deaths. Policies of increased surveillance and intervention have been shown to reduce the risk of perinatal death in these conditions.[33,41]

The magnitude of the risk of stillbirth in older women is similar to that of women with hypertension and diabetes. Induction at 41 weeks of gestation in those aged 35 years or over requires 460–500 inductions to prevent one perinatal death.[40] No cost–benefit analysis has been performed. Neither the maternal age, for example 40 years or over, nor the gestation at which to intervene, for example more than 40 weeks, has been subjected to randomised controlled trials. Induction of labour in this age group may also have specific considerations compared with younger mothers. Heffner et al.[36] looked at the effect of maternal age on delivery after induction of labour and corrected for gestational age at delivery and coexisting medical disease. The authors reported that, compared with mothers aged under 35 years, mothers aged 40 years or over had an adjusted odds ratio for caesarean section after induction of labour of 1.98 (95% CI 1.49–2.63) in nulliparous women and 2.13 (95% CI 1.35–3.37) in multiparous women. For those aged 35–39 years, the figures were 1.97 (95% CI 1.69–2.30) in nulliparous and women 1.10 (95% CI 0.80–1.51) in multiparous women.[36] This suggests that intervention might reduce the risk of stillbirth but would inevitably increase caesarean section and maternal morbidity rates.

Policies of induction for the purpose of improving obstetric outcome (including late stillbirth) are employed in other conditions of pregnancy. In common with advanced maternal age, these risks may be small and the interventions not always robustly subjected to randomised controlled trials. Obstetricians must endeavour to remain consistent in the advice and interventions they offer to pregnant women. Until such time as a randomised controlled trial is available to guide practice, perhaps a pragmatic approach would be to be weigh an individual's composite risk based on other comorbidities or symptoms against the risks of induction.

The pregnant population is ageing, however (Figure 13.8). While the personal risk of adverse outcome with increased maternal age may be small for women with singleton pregnancies without comorbidities, the inevitable increasing burden of these problems to society and healthcare providers remains to be determined.

Conclusion

It is impossible (and wrong) for others to determine when it is the 'right' time for a woman, or couple, to have a baby. There may never be a perfect time. In an ideal world, one might expect that when the full complement of the right partner, finances and support are in place a woman may choose to have a baby. The definition of the right time may vary with personal, family, cultural and religious beliefs. Women who defer childbearing do so for many reasons, both within and outside their control.

Thanks to contraception and safe terminations of pregnancy, the timing of having a baby is more within an individual's choice than in the past, but female reproductive biology still determines outcome and should not be ignored.[14] Women need to be made aware of this. Once attending for antenatal care, expectations are high but older women face the unpleasant prospect of being advised of a poorer obstetric outcome

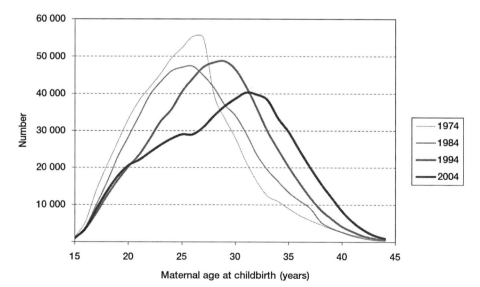

Figure 13.8 The age of mothers is increasing; source data: Office for National Statistics, 1974–2004; total number of births in 1974 = 639 885, 1984 = 636 818, 1994 = 664 726 and 2004 = 639 721; adapted with permission from Nwandison and Bewley[14]

than their younger counterparts, with no realistic strategies available to improve that outcome. This requires careful counselling, as anxiety itself is associated with worse pregnancy outcomes.[42–44] To consistently advise all women before pregnancy (that is, from school, through the media, in general practice and in family planning services) that the available data suggest that age 20–35 years remains the best age for childbearing, in terms of physiology and the most favourable maternal and fetal outcomes, would deliver the correct message and allow women to optimally plan their families in the light of their individual circumstances. Any societal pressures on women to defer childbearing beyond 35 years will come with a health consequence. Obstetricians and gynaecologists should advocate for policies that enable women to reproduce safely without personal cost to their education, careers, identity or their own or their offspring's health.

Acknowledgement

The authors would like to acknowledge the assistance of Dr M Nwandison in her contribution to this article.

References

1. Cleary-Goldman J, Malone FD, Vidaver J, Ball RH, Nyberg DA, Comstock CH, *et al.*; FASTER Consortium. Impact of maternal age on obstetric outcome. *Obstet Gynecol* 2005;105:983–90.
2. Ales KL, Druzin ML, Santini DL. Impact of advanced maternal age on the outcome of pregnancy. *Surg Gynecol Obstet* 1990;171:209–16.
3. Suzuki S. Obstetric outcomes in nulliparous women aged 35 and over with dichorionic twin pregnancy. *Arch Gynecol Obstet* 2007;276:573–5.
4. Young J, Trotman H, Thame M. The impact of antenatal care on pregnancy performance between adolescent girls and older women. *West Indian Med J* 2007;56:414–20.
5. Porreco RP, Harden L, Gambotto M, Shapiro H. Expectation of pregnancy outcome among mature women. *Am J Obstet Gynecol* 2005;192:38–41.
6. Sheiner E, Shoham-Vardi I, Hershkovitz R, Katz M, Mazor M. Infertility treatment is an independent risk factor for cesarean section among nulliparous women aged 40 and above. *Am J Obstet Gynecol* 2001;185:888–92.
7. Hoffman MC, Jeffers S, Carter J, Duthely L, Cotter A, González-Quintero VH. Pregnancy at or beyond age 40 years is associated with an increased risk of fetal death and other adverse outcomes. *Am J Obstet Gynecol* 2007;196;e11–13.
8. Jolly M, Sebire N, Harris J, Robinson S, Regan L. The risks associated with pregnancy in women aged 35 years or older. *Hum Reprod* 2000;15:2433–7.
9. Gilbert WM, Nesbitt TS, Danielsen B. Childbearing beyond age 40: pregnancy outcome in 24,032 cases. *Obstet Gynecol* 1999;93:9–14.
10. Reddy UM, Ko CW, Willinger M. Maternal age and the risk of stillbirth throughout pregnancy in the United States. *Am J Obstet Gynecol* 2006;195:764–70.
11. Donoso E, Carvajal JA. Maternal, perinatal and infant outcome of spontaneous pregnancy in the sixth decade of life. *Maturitas* 2008;59:381–6.
12. Salihu HM, Shumpert MN, Slay M, Kirby RS, Alexander GR. Childbearing beyond maternal age 50 and fetal outcomes in the United States. *Obstet Gynecol* 2003;102:1006–14.
13. Office for National Statistics. Maternities 1938–2004 [www.statistics.gov.uk/CCI/nscl.asp?ID=7542]; Births and fertility [www.statistics.gov.uk/CCI/nscl.asp?id=7434]; Birth statistics: Births and patterns of family building England and Wales (FM1) [www.statistics.gov.uk/statbase/Product.asp?vlnk=5768].
14. Nwandison M, Bewley S. What is the right age to reproduce. *Fetal Matern Med Rev* 2006;17:185–204.

15. Wang JX, Clark AM, Kirby CA, Philipson G, Petrucco O, Anderson G, *et al.* The obstetric outcome of singleton pregnancies following IVF/GIFT. *Hum Reprod* 1994;9:141–6.

16. Tan SL DP, Campbell S, Beral V, Risk B, Brinsden P, Mason B *et al.* Obstetric outcome of *in vitro* fertilization pregnancies compared with normally conceived pregnancie. *Am J Obstet Gynecol* 1992;167:778–84

17. Maman E LE, Levy A, Vardi H, Potashnik G. Obstetric outcome of singleton pregnancies conceived by *in vitro* fertilization and ovulation induction compared with those conceived spontaneously. *Fertil Steril* 1998;70:240–5.

18. Tallo CP, Vohr B, Oh W, Rubin LP, Seifer DB, Haning RV Jr. Maternal and neonatal morbidity associated with *in vitro* fertilization. *J Pediatr* 1995;127:794–800.

19. Bernasko J, Lynch L, Lapinski R, Berkowitz RL. Twin pregnancies conceived by assisted reproductive techniques: maternal and neonatal outcomes. *Obstet Gynecol* 1997;89:368–72.

20. Moise J LA, Armon Y, Gur I, Gale R. The outcome of twin pregnancies after IVF. *Hum Reprod* 1998;13:1702–5.

21. Bateman BT, Simpson LL. Higher rate of stillbirth at the extremes of reproductive age: a large nationwide sample of deliveries in the United States. *Am J Obstet Gynecol* 2006;194:840–5.

22. Luke B, Brown MB. Contemporary risks of maternal morbidity and adverse outcomes with increasing maternal age and plurality. *Fertil Steril* 2007;88:283–93.

23. Jacobsson B, Ladfors L, Milsom I. Advanced maternal age and adverse perinatal outcome. *Obstet Gynecol* 2004;104:727–33.

24. Stein Z, Susser M. The risks of having children in later life. *BMJ* 2000;320:1681–2.

25. Roberts CL, Tracy S, Peat B. Rates for obstetric intervention among private and public patients in Australia: population based descriptive study. *BMJ* 2000;321:137–41.

26. Nybo Andersen AM, Wohlfahrt J, Christens P, Olsen J, Melbye M. Maternal age and fetal loss: population-based register linkage study. *BMJ* 2000;320:1708–12.

27. Astolfi P, De Pasquale A, Zonta LA. Late paternity and stillbirth risk. *Hum Reprod* 2004;19:2497–501.

28. Henne MB, Zhang M, Paroski S, Kelshikar B, Westphal LM. Comparison of obstetric outcomes in recipients of donor oocytes vs. women of advanced maternal age with autologous oocytes. *J Reprod Med* 2007;52:585–90.

29. Smith GC, Fretts RC. Stillbirth. *Lancet* 2007;370:1715–25.

30. Wyatt PR, Owolabi T, Meier C, Huang T. Age-specific risk of fetal loss observed in a second trimester serum screening population. *Am J Obstet Gynecol* 2005;192:240–6.

31. Fretts RC, Duru UA. New indications for antepartum testing: making the case for antepartum surveillance or timed delivery for women of advanced maternal age. *Semin Perinatol* 2008;32:312–17.

32. Fretts RC, Schmittdiel J, McLean FH, Usher RH, Goldman MB. Increased maternal age and the risk of fetal death. *New Engl J Med* 1995;333:953–7.

33. Fretts RC. Etiology and prevention of stillbirth. *Am J Obstet Gynecol* 2005;193:1923–35.

34. Lewis G, editor. *Saving Mothers' Lives: Reviewing Maternal Deaths to Make Motherhood Safer 2003–2005. The Seventh Report on Confidential Enquiries into Maternal Deaths in the United Kingdom.* London: CEMACH; 2007.

35. Treacy A, Robson M, O'Herlihy C. Dystocia increases with advancing maternal age. *Am J Obstet Gynecol* 2006;195:760–3.

36. Heffner LJ, Elkin E, Fretts RC. Impact of labor induction, gestational age, and maternal age on cesarean delivery rates. *Obstet Gynecol* 2003;102:287–93.

37. Simchen MJ, Yinon Y, Moran O, Schiff E, Sivan E. Pregnancy outcome after age 50. *Obstet Gynecol* 2006;108:1084–8. Erratum in: *Obstet Gynecol* 2007;109:1002.

38. Hilder L, Costeloe K, Thilaganathan B. Prolonged pregnancy: evaluating gestation-specific risks of fetal and infant mortality. *Br J Obstet Gynaecol* 1998;105:169–73.

39. Hannah ME, Hannah WJ, Hellmann J, Hewson S, Milner R, Willan A. Induction of labor as compared with serial antenatal monitoring in postterm pregnancy – a randomized controlled trial. *New Engl J Med* 1992;326:1587–92.

40. Fretts RC, Elkin EB, Myers ER, Heffner LJ. Should older women have antepartum testing to prevent unexplained stillbirth? *Obstet Gynecol* 2004;104:56–64.

41. Crowther CA, Hiller JE, Moss JR, McPhee AJ, Jeffries WS, Robinson JS, *et al.* Effect of treatment of gestational diabetes mellitus on pregnancy outcomes. *New Engl J Med* 2005;352:2477–86.

42. Alder J, Fink N, Bitzer J, Hosli I, Holzgreve W. Depression and anxiety during pregnancy: a risk factor for obstetric, fetal and neonatal outcome? A critical review of the literature. *J Matern Fetal Neonat Med* 2007;20:189–209.

43. Wisborg K, Barklin A, Hedegaard M, Henriksen TB. Psychological stress during pregnancy and stillbirth: prospective study. *BJOG* 2008;115:882–5.

44. Glynn LM, Schetter CD, Hobel CJ, Sandman CA. Pattern of perceived stress and anxiety in pregnancy predicts preterm birth. *Health Psychol* 2008;27:43–51.

Chapter 14
The older mother and medical disorders of pregnancy

Mandish K Dhanjal

Introduction

Most medical diseases increase in prevalence with age. The average age of childbirth is rising in the UK, with the proportion of maternities in women aged 35 years or over increasing from 8% in 1985 to 19% in 2005, and continuing to rise.[1] Over the same period, the proportion of maternities in women aged 20–29 years fell from 64% to 44% (Figure 14.1). As women delay pregnancy until their 30s and 40s, more will embark on pregnancy with a pre-existing medical disorder. As the number of older pregnant women increases, more can also be expected to have a medical disorder diagnosed during pregnancy, increasing the requirement of specialist input and resources to care for them effectively.

Mortality statistics reveal that the main causes of death in women of childbearing age are cancer, circulatory diseases (mainly ischaemic heart disease and stroke), accidents and respiratory disease, with all except accidents increasing with age.[2] It can therefore be expected that these illnesses will become more prominent in maternal mortality statistics. Indeed, cardiac disease is now the most common cause of maternal death in the UK.[1]

The Confidential Enquiries into Maternal and Child Health (CEMACH) have been collecting data on maternal deaths in the UK since 1952. The trends show that maternal mortality has fallen dramatically since then.[1] However, since the 1991–93 period, the total maternal mortality has increased slightly and indirect deaths (which are mainly due to underlying medical or psychiatric causes) have become more frequent than direct deaths (which are related to pregnancy itself). An important factor behind this rise is advancing maternal age. Figures 14.2 and 14.3 show how the maternal death rate in women aged 40 years or over is three times higher than that in women aged under 25 years, and how deaths in pregnant women aged 40 years or over have increased by 50% since the 1991–93 period.

Other factors associated with the rise in maternal deaths include increasing numbers of women with obesity and medically complex pregnancies, both of which increase with age. Medical causes, including hypertension, heart disease and venous thromboembolism, now account for more than three-quarters of all maternal deaths.[1] Nearly one-quarter of pregnant women aged 45 years or over have a chronic medical

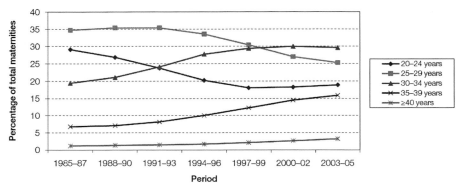

Figure 14.1 Percentage of total maternities by maternal age range in the UK, 1985–2005; data from Lewis[1]

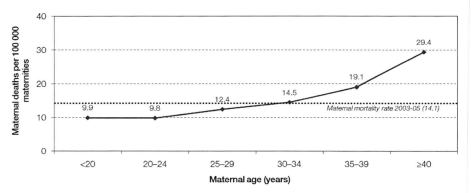

Figure 14.2 Maternal mortality rate by age in the UK, 2003–05; data from Lewis[1]

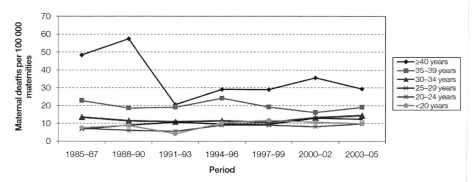

Figure 14.3 Maternal mortality rate by age in the UK, 1985–2005; data from Lewis[1]

disease.[3] The implications for ageing pregnant women are a greater likelihood of a high-risk pregnancy and, for local NHS providers, a need for increased resources with improved care pathways in primary and secondary care and more specialists who are trained to look after medical diseases in pregnancy.

This chapter covers the effect of age on the occurrence of systemic medical disorders that have an impact on pregnancy, such as hypertension, obesity, diabetes, ischaemic heart disease and cancer.

Hypertension

Hypertension is the most common medical complication in pregnancy, affecting 10–15% of maternities. Hypertensive complications of pregnancy are the second most common cause of maternal death in the UK, with 14% of direct deaths attributable to them.[1]

Hypertension in pregnancy is divided into three categories:

1. pre-existing hypertension (chronic hypertension) that predates pregnancy or occurs in the first 20 weeks of pregnancy and may be essential (that is, no identifiable cause) or secondary

2. pregnancy-induced hypertension – new-onset hypertension and proteinuria occurring after the 20th week of pregnancy

3. pre-eclampsia – new-onset hypertension and proteinuria (0.3 g/day or more) occurring after the 20th week of pregnancy; may be superimposed upon chronic hypertension.

Chronic hypertension

Blood pressure increases sharply with age (Figure 14.4).[4] Since 1993, there has been a general tendency for the mean systolic and diastolic blood pressure to fall in both sexes in England. Although the prevalence of hypertension continues to fall in women aged under 34 years, it has started to stabilise in women aged 35 years or over and even increase in women aged 45 years or over, which may reflect lifestyle changes (Figure 14.5).[5]

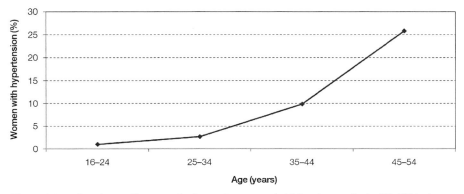

Figure 14.4 Prevalence of hypertension by age in women of childbearing age in the UK, 2006; data from the Joint Health Surveys Unit[4]

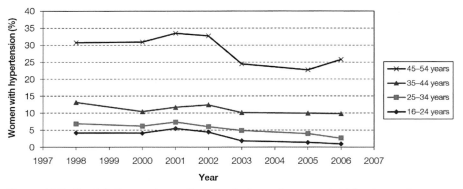

Figure 14.5 Trends in the prevalence of hypertension by age in women of childbearing age in England, 1998–2006; data from the National Centre for Social Research[5]

Risks associated with chronic hypertension include stroke, ischaemic heart disease and other vascular disease. A meta-analysis of prospective observational studies of blood pressure and mortality that included almost one million adults showed that, for adults aged 40–49 years, each 20 mmHg increase in the usual systolic blood pressure for that decade, or each 10 mmHg increase in the usual diastolic blood pressure for that decade, led to a greater than two-fold increase in the risk of death from stroke, ischaemic heart disease and other vascular causes.[6]

The risk of developing hypertension in pregnancy increases with advancing maternal age and it can result in severe fetal and maternal morbidity and mortality both in the pregnancy and in the future. The risk of developing chronic hypertension in women aged 40 years or over is up to five times higher in nulliparous women and up to nine times higher in multiparous women compared with those of similar parity aged 20–29 years.[7]

In the relatively short-term duration of a pregnancy, mild-to-moderate chronic hypertension will have a negligible impact on maternal wellbeing, although it does increase fetal morbidity and mortality. Chronic hypertension increases the risk of fetal growth restriction, doubles the risk of placental abruption and triples the risk of perinatal mortality.[8] Hypertension that is severe, associated with certain secondary causes such as phaeochromocytoma and aortic coarctation, or has already caused renal or significant vascular damage has a greater impact on maternal wellbeing than milder hypertension. Renal and vascular damage is more likely to have occurred in the older woman who may have had hypertension for a longer duration and who may also have developed other age-related risk factors such as diabetes and obesity. The maternal sequelae in these women are similar to those outside pregnancy and include ischaemic heart disease, haemorrhagic and ischaemic stroke, aortic dissection in those with a vulnerable vasculature and renal impairment that can be permanent and could result in end-stage renal failure.

Overall, the greatest risk of chronic hypertension in pregnancy is the development of superimposed pre-eclampsia, which occurs in 10% of those with mild chronic hypertension[9] at the beginning of pregnancy, in 52% of those with severe chronic hypertension at the beginning of pregnancy[10] and in 78% of those whose hypertension remains severe in the second half of pregnancy.[11]

Pregnancy-induced hypertension and pre-eclampsia

Numerous studies have shown that the risk of developing pre-eclampsia in those with a normal prepregnancy blood pressure increases with age.[11–16] A large population-based retrospective cohort study in California showed that the incidence of pre-eclampsia in women aged 40 years or over was approximately double that in women aged 20–29 years (Table 14.1).[11]

Data are now emerging on women in their late-40s and 50s who are healthy, with no pre-existing chronic medical conditions including hypertension or diabetes, and who conceive through *in vitro* fertilisation (IVF) and donor-egg programmes. They all show high rates of hypertension in pregnancy. One study found 9.1% of women aged 45–49 years developed hypertension in pregnancy, which doubled to 19% in those aged 50–60 years.[17] Another study of women aged 50–63 years gave an overall rate of 35% for the development of pre-eclampsia, but this reached 60% in the group of pregnant women aged 56 years or over. (Table 14.2).[18]

Age has a significant influence on the high rate of pre-eclampsia in these women but other factors include a large proportion of primigravidae (50%), and multiple pregnancies (25%), both of which are known to have an increased rate of pre-eclampsia compared with parous women and singleton pregnancies.[17–18] There is evidence to suggest that IVF itself in older women may contribute to the high pre-eclampsia rate. There is no difference in the rate of pre-eclampsia in women undergoing IVF with donor eggs compared with older women undergoing IVF with autologous eggs.[19] The rate of pre-eclampsia is higher in women undergoing IVF with donor eggs compared with older women conceiving spontaneously or age- and parity-matched women conceiving with in utero insemination of their partner's sperm.[20,21]

The number of women conceiving in their 50s may well increase in the future with the further development of assisted reproductive technologies (ART). Despite being

Table 14.1   Incidence of medical diseases with increased maternal age[11]

Disease	Incidence by maternal age			
	20–29 years ($n = 642\,525$)		≥40 years ($n = 24\,032$)	
	Primiparous	Multiparous	Primiparous	Multiparous
Chronic hypertension	0.3%	0.2%	1.6%	1.8%
Pre-eclampsia	3.4%	1.0%	5.4%	2.7%
Diabetes	0.5%	0.5%	1.4%	2.7%
Gestational diabetes	1.7%	1.6%	7.0%	7.8%

Table 14.2   Incidence of pre-eclampsia and gestational diabetes in women aged 50 years and older with donor oocytes; data from Paulson et al.[18]

Disease	Incidence by maternal age					
	50–55 years		56–63 years		All >50 years	
	n	%	n	%	n	%
Pre-eclampsia	8/30	26%	6/10	60%	14/40	35%
Gestational diabetes	4/30	13%	4/10	40%	8/40	20%

medically healthy at the onset of pregnancy, up to half of them will develop either pre-eclampsia or gestational diabetes (Table 14.2).

Pre-eclampsia, whether or not it is superimposed upon chronic hypertension, is associated with fetal risks of growth restriction, placental abruption and stillbirth[22] as well as maternal complications including HELLP syndrome (haemolytic anaemia, elevated liver enzymes and low platelet count), cerebrovascular accident, pulmonary oedema, renal failure, ischaemic heart disease and maternal death. In 2003–05 there were 18 deaths due to pre-eclampsia and eclampsia in the UK.[1] Ten of these deaths were due to intracranial haemorrhage that was a direct result of poor blood pressure control. It is important to tackle this, as intracranial haemorrhage now forms a large proportion of the deaths from hypertensive disease in pregnancy (Figure 14.6).[1,24–26] In the past, the emphasis has been on diastolic and mean arterial blood pressure control but maintaining a systolic blood pressure of less than 160 mmHg has been shown by a group in the USA to be very important in reducing morbidity and mortality from haemorrhagic stroke in pregnancy.[23] In their series, 23 of 24 pregnant women with pre-eclampsia had systolic blood pressures of 160 mmHg or above before their intracerebral bleed compared with only three of 24 women with pre-stroke diastolic blood pressures of 110 mmHg or above. Two-thirds of the women were aged 30 years or over and just over half of all the women with stroke died.

Future health consequences of hypertension in pregnancy

Older women are more likely to develop pre-eclampsia, which is not only an independent risk factor for developing ischaemic heart disease in pregnancy (see later) but also increases the risk of developing hypertension, ischaemic heart disease and stroke in the future.

In a prospective cohort study using data from the Royal College of General Practitioners (RCGP) oral contraceptive study, in the group of women who had never used oral contraceptives, the relative risk of future hypertension was 2.35 (95% CI 2.08–2.65) in parous women with previous pre-eclampsia compared with parous women without previous pre-eclampsia.[27] Interestingly, having an uncomplicated pregnancy at any age is protective against developing future hypertension, with such pregnancies having a lower incidence of subsequent hypertension than the general female population of similar age and race.

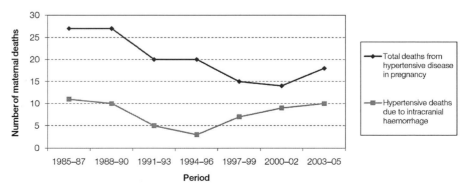

Figure 14.6 Hypertensive maternal deaths in the UK and the number due to intracranial haemorrhage, 1985–2005; data from Lewis[1,24–26]

In a study of 177 women with hypertensive disease in pregnancy who had subsequently died, death rates from ischaemic heart disease were increased (RR of dying 1.47; 95% CI 1.05–2.02) compared with that expected from analysis of population data from public health and census reports during the corresponding periods of time. The risk of dying from ischaemic heart disease was greatest in those with eclampsia (RR 2.61; 95% CI 1.11–6.12), followed by those with pre-eclampsia (RR 1.90; 95% CI 1.02–3.52), compared with those with hypertension alone.[28] The RCGP oral contraceptive study showed that in parous women with pre-eclampsia, the overall risk of ischaemic heart disease was 1.65 compared with parous women without pre-eclampsia, and the RR of acute myocardial infarction was 2.24.[27]

A retrospective cohort study from Scotland using hospital discharge data showed an adjusted hazard ratio of 2.0 (95% CI 1.5–2.5) for the association between pre-eclampsia and later ischaemic heart disease in the mother, which increased to 4.5 (95% CI 2.7–7.4) if the pre-eclampsia was associated with preterm birth, and further increased to 7.0 (95% CI 3.3–14.5) if the pre-eclampsia was associated with preterm birth and fetal growth restriction.[29]

Another retrospective cohort study in Aberdeen that was not based on patient recall confirmed that women with hypertension in pregnancy were at increased risk of hypertension but did not find such a strong association with ischaemic heart disease as was the case with stroke. The study found that long-term cardiovascular risks were greater for women with pre-eclampsia than for those with pregnancy-induced hypertension.[30]

Obesity

Obesity and its complications are an emerging serious public health concern across the developed world. The classification of obesity is shown in Table 14.3.[31,32]

The rates of overweight (body mass index [BMI] 25–29.9 kg/m^2) and obesity (BMI 30 kg/m^2 or more) have dramatically increased in the UK general population since the mid-1980s. The incidence of obesity increases significantly with age, particularly after the menopause in women. Among women of childbearing age, there was an approximately 50% increase in obesity from 1993 to 2003 (Figure 14.7).[1,4,26,34] One-third of women aged 35–54 years were overweight and one-quarter were obese in 2003. Forecasters have predicted a further 20% rise in the number of women who are obese in this age group by 2010 based on projections of a continued rise.[33]

The Health Survey for England has released figures from 2006 that show a slowdown in the rising rates of obesity in women, with prevalence rates actually

Table 14.3 Classification of obesity

BMI (kg/m²)	NICE classification (2006)[31]	Health Survey for England definition (2006)[32]
<18.5		Underweight
18.5–24.9	Healthy weight	Normal
25–29.9	Overweight	Overweight
30–34.9	Obesity I	Obese
35–39.9	Obesity II	
≥40	Obesity III	Morbidly obese

BMI = body mass index; NICE = National Institute for Health and Clinical Excellence

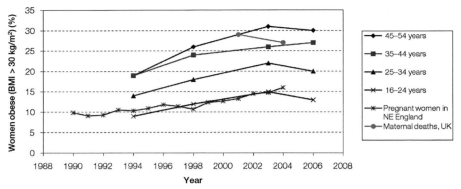

Figure 14.7 Prevalence of obesity in women of childbearing age in England, in pregnant women in north-east England and in women who had a maternal death in the UK; data from Lewis,[1,26] Joint Health Surveys Unit[4] and Heslehurst *et al.*[34]

having fallen in women aged 16–34 years and 45–54 years.[4] They have continued to rise at a steady rate in women aged 35–44 years and, if this continues, the expected prevalence of obesity in this age group by 2010 will be 28.5%.[33]

Maternal weight at the start of pregnancy is following the same rising trends of overweight and obesity as seen in the general population. This was first evidenced by a study in the USA that showed an increase in maternal booking weight of 20% over a period of 20 years, and specifically a doubling in the proportion of obese women with a BMI over 29 kg/m^2 from 16.3% in 1980 to 36.4% in 1999.[35] They also showed a concomitant increase in maternal and perinatal morbidity attributable to obesity. There is no formal system of national data collection for BMI status at booking in pregnant women in the UK, although the UK Obstetric Surveillance System (UKOSS) has started collecting data on women with a BMI of 50 kg/m^2 or more or maternal weight of 140 kg or more at any stage in pregnancy.[36] Several retrospective studies have been published showing similar increasing trends of obesity in pregnant women in the UK, albeit less than seen in the USA.[37–39] They show that the rise in maternal obesity is at a greater rate than can be explained by age alone.

A study from Cardiff showed that between 1990 and 1999 the incidence of obesity at booking increased from 3.2% to 8.9%.[37] Anecdotally, it was reported that by 2004 one-third of their pregnant population was obese. A smaller study in Glasgow found that 9.4% of pregnant women in 1990 were obese at booking (less than 15 weeks of gestation) and that this had doubled to 18.9% in 2002–04.[38]

A study in north-east England showed that obesity at booking (less than 16 weeks of gestation) rose from 9.9% to 16.0% between 1990 and 2004.[34] The rate of rise of maternal obesity was similar to that seen in all women of childbearing age in the general population of England, although the incidence of maternal obesity was lower than that of the general population (Figure 14.7). This lower incidence is reflected in other studies too and is probably due to the reduced fertility and increased risk of miscarriage in women who are obese.[39] The women who were obese were older, more parous and lived in more socially deprived areas. Assuming that the trend of maternal obesity is to increase at the same rate, the authors predicted that 22% of pregnant women will be obese by the end of 2010 and that the proportion of mothers with an ideal BMI (18.5–24.9 kg/m^2) will fall from 65% in 1990 to 47% by 2010.

Maternal obesity is associated with increased maternal and fetal morbidity and mortality due to increased pregnancy loss and medical and intrapartum complications. The increased maternal risks include hypertensive disease, gestational diabetes, thromboembolism, infection, cardiac disease and postpartum haemorrhage. Older mothers are more obese than younger mothers and are more likely to have these complications

Obese women are more likely to have chronic hypertension[40] and pregnant women who are obese are twice as likely as those of normal weight to develop pregnancy-induced hypertension,[41,42] with women who are morbidly obese having a three-fold increased risk (12.3%).[42] A systemic review of the association between maternal BMI and pre-eclampsia has shown that risk of pre-eclampsia typically doubled with each 5–7 kg/m² increase in prepregnancy BMI.[43] This relation persisted in studies that excluded women with chronic hypertension, diabetes or multiple gestations, or after adjustment for other confounders. This suggests that a 1 unit increase in BMI would result in an approximately 0.6% increase in the incidence of pre-eclampsia.[38] The risks of venous thromboembolism are doubled in pregnant women who are obese compared with those of normal weight.[44] Gestational diabetes is increased two- to three-fold in women who are obese.[42,44]

Obesity has been reported as becoming an important factor in maternal death. Figure 14.7 shows how a greater percentage of women whose death is related to pregnancy are obese compared with the general population.[1] Figure 14.8 shows that women who are overweight or obese have a greater risk of maternal death than women who are of normal weight. Over half the maternal deaths in 2003–05 were in obese women.[1] In the three most common medical causes of maternal death (thromboembolism, hypertensive disease and cardiac disease), one-half to two-thirds of the women who died were overweight or obese and 10–20% were classified as morbidly obese with a BMI of 40 kg/m² or more (Table 14.4).[1]

Offspring of mothers who are overweight or obese are at increased risk of themselves becoming overweight or obese as children or adults.[45] A retrospective cohort study in the USA of over 8400 children showed that maternal obesity in the first trimester resulted in a 2.4- to 2.7-fold increase in prevalence of obesity in the offspring at age 2, 3 and 4 years compared with the children of mothers with a normal BMI.[46]

The cost of obesity to the NHS was approximately £1 billion in 2003 and it is predicted that the annual cost to the economy would be £3.6 billion if the present

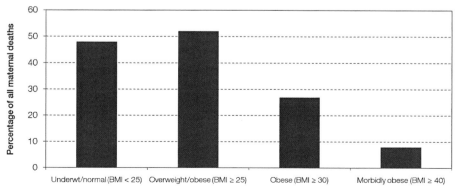

Figure 14.8 Body mass index (BMI) of maternal deaths in the UK, 2003–05, UK; data from Lewis[1]

Table 14.4   BMI of women who died of the most common medical causes in pregnancy in the UK, 2003–05; data from Lewis[1]

Medical cause of maternal death	Underweight/normal, BMI < 25 kg/m² n (%)	Overweight/obese, BMI ≥ 25 kg/m² n (%)	Obese, BMI ≥ 30 kg/m² n (%)	Morbidly obese, BMI ≥ 40 kg/m² n (%)
Thromboembolism (n = 31)[a]	11 (35)	20 (65)	14 (45)	6 (19)
Pre-eclampsia/eclampsia (*n* = 18)[a]	9 (50)	9 (50)	3 (17)	2 (11)
Cardiac disease (n = 42)[a]	13 (31)	29 (69)	15 (36)	5 (12)

[a] number of women in whom BMI was known

trend continues.[47] The trend of rising obesity in older pregnant women is continuing. As the proportion of older pregnant women increases, a greater degree of obesity will be seen as more of them are obese than younger women. This will lead to a further increase in maternity costs of care.

Diabetes

The prevalence of diabetes increases substantially with age. It has also been increasing dramatically over the past 15 years due to changing lifestyles, with increasing obesity as well as an increasing contribution from particular minority ethnic groups.[3] Figure 14.9 shows a doubling in the prevalence of diabetes in perimenopausal women and younger women. These changes are yet to be seen in women of older childbearing age, but a similar increase is anticipated in this group as the younger cohort ages and due to the effect of obesity, which is still increasing in women aged 35–44 years.[3,4] The prevalence of diabetes in women aged 15–44 years was estimated at 1% (0.68% type 1, 0.36% type 2) in the UK in 2004.[48] Type 2 diabetes was previously considered a disease of middle age but, with the obesity epidemic, children and adolescents are increasingly being diagnosed.[49]

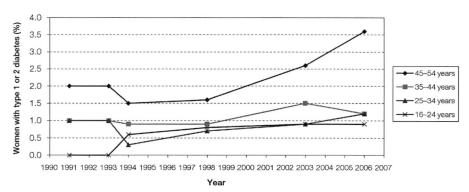

Figure 14.9   Prevalence of self-reported diabetes by age in women in England, 1991–2006; data from Dildy *et al*.[3]

Pre-existing diabetes (type 1 and 2 diabetes)

Diabetes affects 2–5% of pregnant women in the UK. Approximately 87.5% of these are estimated to be due to gestational diabetes, 7.5% due to type 1 diabetes and 5% due to type 2 diabetes.[50] In 2002–03, 0.38% of pregnant women had pre-existing diabetes in the UK (0.27% type 1, 0.11% type 2).[51] This is lower than in the general population, which may reflect the reduced fertility and increased miscarriage rates in women with diabetes.[50] The proportion of pregnant women with type 2 diabetes varies widely across the regions, accounting for between 13.3% and 44.5% of the total births to women with pre-existing diabetes (Figure 14.10). These differences are largely accounted for by the higher ethnic diversity and/or social deprivation in those areas with higher rates of type 2 diabetes. Women with type 2 diabetes are older and more likely to have had previous children. These data help inform us of the regions where diabetes, particularly type 2 diabetes, is likely to increase as the population in these areas delays childbirth.

There is a lack of data on trends in pre-existing diabetes in pregnancy in the UK. A retrospective analysis of clinical databases and birth certificates in Southern California found 2784 pregnant women with pre-existing diabetes. The authors showed that the prevalence of pre-existing diabetes had increased across all reproductive age groups since 1999 (Figure 14.11).[52] Unfortunately, data on BMI were not available.

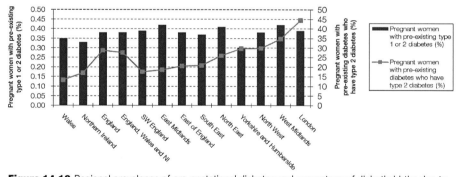

Figure 14.10 Regional prevalence of pre-gestational diabetes and percentage of diabetic births due to type 2 diabetes in England, Wales and Northern Ireland, 2002–03; data from CEMACH[51]

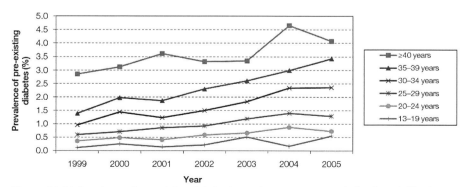

Figure 14.11 Prevalence of pre-existing diabetes by age in pregnant women in Southern California, 1999–2005; data from Lawrence et al.[52]

Diabetes is a significant risk factor for pregnancy, with maternal risks including worsening diabetic control, an acceleration in microvascular disease (specifically diabetic retinopathy and diabetic nephropathy) and a higher chance of operative delivery. The 2002–03 CEMACH report found that only 18% of women with pre-gestational diabetes had a spontaneous labour compared with 69% in the general population in England and Wales.[1] Thirty-nine percent were induced, mainly routinely because of maternal diabetes, and usually before 39 weeks of gestation. There was a high caesarean section rate of 67.4% in women with diabetes compared with 22% in the general population.[51] Fetal risks include miscarriage, congenital malformations, macrosomia, shoulder dystocia, neonatal hypoglycaemia and perinatal death.[50]

Gestational diabetes

The incidence of gestational diabetes also increases with age. There is a lack of data as to the prevalence of gestational diabetes in the UK but the average prevalence across England and Wales has been estimated as 3.5%.[50] There is a two- to five-fold increase in the prevalence of gestational diabetes in women aged 40 years or over compared with women in their 20s (Table 14.1).[11,12,15,16,53,54] Parity does not increase the risk of gestational diabetes in older women.[11,12]

Like type 1 and type 2 diabetes, the incidence of gestational diabetes has been increasing over the past 15 years, again due to rising obesity rates and an increasing contribution from certain minority ethnic groups. A retrospective cohort study examining certain hospital databases and a diabetes registry in Northern California found over 14 000 pregnant women diagnosed with gestational diabetes. They showed that, for all age groups, there had been an increase in the incidence of gestational diabetes over 10 years.[54] The rate increased by 30% for women aged 35–49 years between 1991 and 2000 (Figure 14.12). The Southern California group had performed a similar retrospective study between 1999 and 2005 and found that the incidence of gestational diabetes in their population had stabilised although the incidence of pre-existing diabetes in that cohort continued to increase.[52] Neither of these two studies provided data on BMI. Across the USA, the incidence of gestational diabetes continued to increase in all reproductive age groups between 1989 and 2004, with an increase from 1.9% in 1989 to 4.2% in 2004. In women aged 35 years or over, the rate had doubled to reach approximately 8% in 2004.[55]

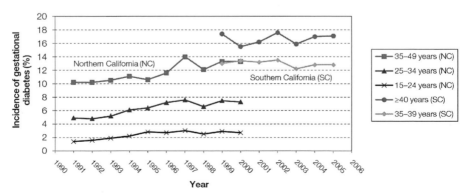

Figure 14.12 Incidence of gestational diabetes by age in California, USA, 1991–2005; data from Lawrence *et al.*[52] and Ferrara *et al.*[54]

Healthy women aged 50 years or over who have been rigorously screened to exclude medical diseases to undergo donor egg programmes have a 20% chance of developing gestational diabetes (Table 14.2).[18] This rate doubles in women aged 55 years or over. Few data exist on the incidence of medical disease in women who have spontaneous pregnancies over the age of 50 years. In a very small study of seven pregnant women over the age of 50 years, one women developed gestational diabetes.[56]

Gestational diabetes has been shown to have important consequences for the fetus and neonate, with increased levels of morbidity compared with women without diabetes and compared with women with gestational diabetes who have been intensively treated.[50,57]

It is recommended that all women with diabetes be seen regularly for antenatal care in a joint obstetric/diabetic clinic.[51] An anticipated rise in gestational and type 2 diabetes would result not only in an increased need for more capacity within current joint obstetric/diabetic clinics, but also in more interventional deliveries.

Future consequences of maternal diabetes include an increased incidence of obesity and diabetes in their offspring.[58] Additionally, gestational diabetes is associated with an up to 70% chance of the mother developing type 2 diabetes within 10 years.[59] A systematic review has shown that the incidence of developing type 2 diabetes increased most rapidly in the first 5 years after pregnancy.[59] This has implications for surveillance for type 2 diabetes in these women and their children by their primary care physicians.

Coronary heart disease

The incidence of acquired heart disease increases with age, reflecting the increasing acquisition of risk factors with time. These include avoidable or remediable risk factors, such as smoking, obesity, type 2 diabetes and hypercholesterolaemia, and largely unavoidable risk factors, such as development of hypertension, non-obesity-linked diabetes and a family history of heart disease.

Coronary heart disease is the main cause of death in the UK. One in six women die from coronary heart disease but the death rate has fallen by more than 50% in the UK since the late 1970s (Figure 14.13).[60,61] Approximately 40% of this decrease has been due to the combined effects of modern cardiological treatments, including thrombolysis, aspirin, angiotensin-converting enzyme (ACE) inhibitors, statins and

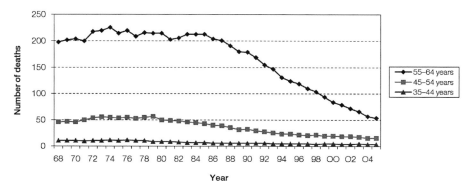

Figure 14.13 Deaths in women from coronary heart disease by age in the UK, 1968–2005; data from Allender *et al.*[60] and Office for National Statistics[61]

coronary artery bypass surgery, and almost 60% due to a reduction in major risk factors, particularly smoking.[62]

Between 1995 and 2005 there was a slowing of the reduction in mortality from coronary heart disease in women of childbearing age compared with the falls seen in older women. The death rate in women aged 35–44 years fell by 20% compared with a 56% fall in deaths in women aged 55–64 years. Indeed, the death rate in women aged 35–44 years remained static between 2001 and 2005.[60,61] This may reflect a stabilisation of risk factors in this age group. For example, there was only a 7% fall in smoking in women aged 35–49 years compared with an 18% fall in women aged 50–59 years between 2000 and 2005.[60]

This broader picture of improvement is not reflected in the available maternity statistics. The incidence of cardiac disease has been increasing in pregnant women and it is now also the most common cause of maternal death overall in the UK. Myocardial infarction, mostly due to ischaemic heart disease, and dissection of the thoracic aorta are the leading causes of maternal cardiac death.[1] In comparison with all women of childbearing age, where the death rates from coronary heart disease are now stabilising, the incidence of maternal deaths from ischaemic causes of coronary heart disease has increased since 1997–99 (Figure 14.14), with maternal deaths from myocardial infarction increasing markedly with age (Figure 14.15).

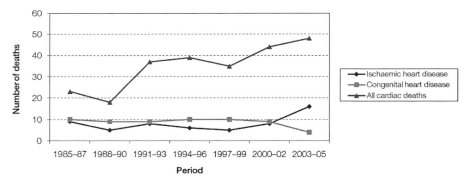

Figure 14.14 Maternal deaths from ischaemic and congenital heart disease in the UK, 1985–2005; data from Lewis[1,24–26]

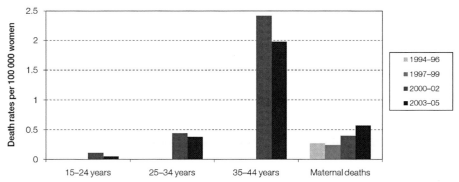

Figure 14.15 Maternal deaths and deaths in women of childbearing age from myocardial infarction in the UK, 2000–2005, UK; data from Lewis[1,24–26]

Few data exist as to the prevalence of myocardical infarction in pregnancy in the UK. The UKOSS is currently collecting data across all maternity units in the UK on antenatal myocardial infarction.[36] There are two population-based retrospective studies from the USA that show that the incidence of myocardial infarction in pregnant women is on an increasing trend.[63,64] A Californian study performed over 10 years showed that the incidence of myocardial infarction had increased from 1.4 per 100 000 maternities in 1991 to 4.1 per 100 000 maternities by 2001 (average 2.8 per 100000).[63] A USA-wide study between 2000 and 2002 showed a further increase to 6.2 per 100 000 maternities, which was 3–4 times higher than that the general population.[64,65] The authors suggested that the increased incidence of myocardial infarction with time was due to an increased detection of previously undetected small events through the use of troponin testing, and an increase in maternal age of pregnant women who have more cardiovascular risk factors. Both studies found age to be an independent risk factor for myocardial infarction, with an odds ratio of 4.5 for a woman aged 40 years or over compared with age 21–25 years. Other independent variables were the presence of chronic hypertension, diabetes, thrombophilia, severe pre-eclampsia or eclampsia. There was an increased propensity for myocardial infarctions to occur in the antenatal or intrapartum period. These women had poorer outcomes than those diagnosed postnatally.

Reported myocardial infarction case fatality rates in the USA fell from rates as high as 37% in older studies[66] to 7.3% in a 1991–2001 study,[63] with a further decline to 5.1% in a 2000–2002 study.[64] This improvement was because of developments in diagnosis and treatment, including newer treatments such as angioplasty and insertion of stents. Almost 50% of the women in the 2000–2002 study had cardiac catheterisation performed.

As women delay pregnancy until their 40s they are more likely to accrue risk factors such as hypertension, obesity, diabetes and pre-eclampsia that will put them at risk of having a myocardial infarction in pregnancy. Even without these risk factors, they are at an increased risk of coronary heart disease, which should be borne in mind when women in their 50s and 60s undergo ART with donor eggs. It is anticipated that the number of women suffering myocardial infarction in pregnancy will continue to rise and thus it is imperative that diagnosis in pregnancy is further improved. Obstetricians and cardiologists should be made aware that urgent coronary angiography should not be withheld in pregnant women. Percutaneous coronary intervention should be made available to all pregnant women with acute myocardial infarction, which may well lead to further improvements in case fatality rates.

Cancer

There was a 32% increase in the incidence of cancer in women in the UK over the 30 years between 1975 and 2004.[67–69] This was double the increase seen in men over the same period (Figure 14.16).

The rates have stabilised over the past decade and have remained constant in women of reproductive age (Figure 14.17).[70] Figures 14.17 and 14.18 show the effect of age on cancer diagnosis.

Few data exist on the occurrence of cancer in pregnancy in the UK. A population-based retrospective analysis of data from the California Cancer Registry from 1991 to 1999 gives an incidence of approximately 1 in 1000 of cancer in pregnancy and within 12 months of delivery.[71] In a previous analysis of their data from 1992 to 1997, this group showed that maternal age was the most significant risk factor for development

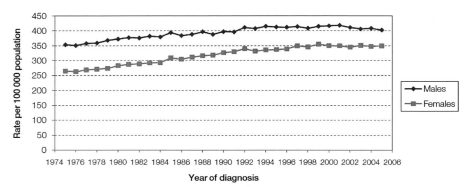

Figure 14.16 Age-standardised incidence rates of all cancers excluding non-melanoma skin cancer in the UK, 1975–2004; data from Office for National Statistics,[67] GRO for Scotland[68] and Northern Ireland Cancer Registry[69]

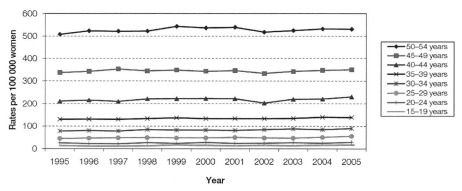

Figure 14.17 Incidence of all cancers by age in women excluding non-melanoma skin cancer in England, 1995–2005; data from Office for National Statistics[70]

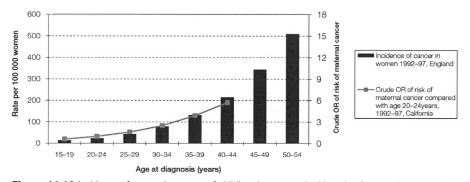

Figure 14.18 Incidence of cancer in women of childbearing age and odds ratio of cancer in pregnant women, 1992–1997; data from Office for National Statistics[70] and Smith *et al*.[72]

of cancer in pregnancy, with an almost six-fold increase in cancer in the women aged 40 years or over compared with those aged 20–24 years.[72] (Figure 14.18). The group did not compare their data with that of the general population, but other authors have estimated that the incidence of cancer in pregnancy is half that for nonpregnant women of a similar age.[73] Suggested explanations for this reduced incidence in pregnancy include women with a cancer diagnosis deliberately avoiding pregnancy, women in early pregnancy with an aggressive cancer opting for a termination of pregnancy, delays in diagnosis either due to screening (for example, cervical smears, colposcopy, radiological investigations or invasive procedures such as gastroscopy) being postponed until after pregnancy or suggestive symptoms being inappropriately attributed to pregnancy rather than malignancy. The last two explanations are supported by the fact that two-thirds of the diagnoses of maternal malignancy in the Californian data set were made postpartum.

The most common cancers, which accounted for 64% of the total, were cancer of the breast (0.193/1000), thyroid (0.144/1000) and cervix (0.12/1000), melanoma (0.087/1000) and Hodgkin's disease (0.054/1000). In the 2003–05 CEMACH report in the UK, there were 82 maternal deaths due to malignancy, which was much higher than in previous years because of improved ascertainment through the Office for National Statistics linkage system.[1] The Enquiry showed that, despite breast cancer being more common, there were more deaths from gastrointestinal malignancy and lung cancer, with similar numbers of deaths from cancer of the breast, brain, blood and melanoma. It was of note that perinatal and clinical outcomes were worse when a diagnosis of cancer was made within 3 months of delivery. Iatrogenic preterm delivery to allow earlier maternal treatment may have accounted for some of this adverse perinatal outcome.

As women delay pregnancy, an increase in cancer diagnoses in pregnancy and postpartum can be expected.

Conclusion

Maternal age is rising in the UK and women are accordingly at increasing risk of developing a medical illness either before they conceive, during pregnancy itself or postpartum. The incidence of hypertension, obesity, diabetes, ischaemic heart disease and cancer increases with age and is generally two- to five-fold greater in women over the age of 40 years compared with women in their 20s, both in the general population and in pregnancy. The overall increase in maternal and fetal morbidity and mortality from advancing maternal age has a significant impact on maternity services. The UK government has recently focused on bringing maternity care into the community but with the older pregnant woman we must recognise that there is a greater likelihood of her having a high-risk pregnancy and at least part of her care should be undertaken in a hospital setting.

We must be vigilant for diseases that were previously very uncommon in pregnancy, such as myocardial infarction, as their occurrence is set to increase.

Women contemplating delaying pregnancy should be informed of the health consequences of this and advised that completion of childbearing in their 20s will greatly reduce their obstetric and medical risks. A growing number of women are requesting ART to conceive in their 40s and 50s. They should also be informed of the greatly increased risks of developing pre-eclampsia and gestational diabetes and how these diseases can have an impact on their pregnancy and that they increase the chances that they and their children will develop cardiovascular morbidity, obesity and diabetes in the future.

References

1. Lewis G, editor. *Saving Mothers' Lives: Reviewing Maternal Deaths to Make Motherhood Safer 2003–2005. The Seventh Report on Confidential Enquiries into Maternal Deaths in the United Kingdom.* London: CEMACH; 2007.

2. Office for National Statistics. *Mortality Statistics, Deaths Registered in 2006. Review of the Registrar General on deaths in England and Wales 2006.* London: HMSO; 2008 [www.statistics.gov.uk/downloads/theme_health/DR-2006/DR_06Mort_Stats.pdf].

3. Dildy GA, Jackson GM, Fowers GK, Oshiro BT, Varner MW, Clark SL. Very advanced maternal age: pregnancy after age 45. *Am J Obstet Gynecol* 1996;175:668–74.

4. Joint Health Surveys Unit. *Health Survey for England 2006. Cardiovascular Disease and Risk Factors.* Leeds: The Information Centre; 2008.

5. National Centre for Social Research. *Health Survey for England 2006. Latest Trends.* Leeds: The Information Centre; 2008 [www.ic.nhs.uk/statistics-and-data-collections/health-and-lifestyles-related-surveys/health-survey-for-england/health-survey-for-england-2006-latest-trends].

6. Prospective Studies Collaboration. Age-specific relevance of usual blood pressure to vascular mortality: a meta-analysis of individual data for one million adults in 61 prospective studies. *Lancet* 2002;360:1903–13.

7. Gilbert WM, Nesbitt TS, Danielsen B. Childbearing beyond age 40: pregnancy outcome in 24,032 cases. *Obstet Gynecol* 1999;93:9–14.

8. Ferrer RL, Sibai BM, Mulrow CD, Chiquette E, Stevens KR, Cornell J. Management of mild chronic hypertension during pregnancy: a review. *Obstet Gynecol* 2000;96:849–60.

9. Sibai BM, Abdella TN, Anderson GD. Pregnancy outcome in 211 patients with mild chronic hypertension. *Obstet Gynecol* 1983;61:571–6.

10. Sibai BM, Anderson GD. Pregnancy outcome of intensive therapy in severe hypertension in first trimester. *Obstet Gynecol* 1986;67:517–22.

11. Vigil-De Gracia P, Montufar-Rueda C, Smith A. Pregnancy and severe chronic hypertension: maternal outcome. *Hypertens Pregnancy* 2004;23:285–93.

12. Bianco A, Stone J, Lynch L, Lapinski R, Berkowitz G, Berkowitz RL. Pregnancy outcome at age 40 and older. *Obstet Gynecol* 1996;87:917–22.

13. Weerasekera DS, Udugama SG. Pregnancy at 40 and over: a case–control study in a developing country. *J Obstet Gynaecol* 2003;23:625–7.

14. Callaway LK, Lust K, McIntyre HD. Pregnancy outcomes in women of very advanced maternal age. *Aust N Z J Obstet Gynaecol* 2005;45:12–16.

15. Diejomaoh MF, Al-Shamali IA, Al-Kandari F, Al-Qenae M, Mohd AT. The reproductive performance of women at 40 years and over. *Eur J Obstet Gynecol Reprod Biol* 2006;126:33–8.

16. Delbaere I, Verstraelen H, Goetgeluk S, Martens G, De Backer G, Temmerman M. Pregnancy outcome in primiparae of advanced maternal age. *Eur J Obstet Gynecol Reprod Biol* 2007;135:41–6.

17. Antinori S, Versaci C, Panci C, Caffa B, Gholami GH. Fetal and maternal morbidity and mortality in menopausal women aged 45–63 years. *Hum Reprod* 1995;10:464–9.

18. Paulson RJ, Boostanfar R, Saadat P, Mor E, Tourgeman DE, Slater CC, *et al.* Pregnancy in the sixth decade of life: obstetric outcomes in women of advanced reproductive age. *JAMA* 2002;288:2320–3.

19. Krieg SA, Henne MB, Westphal LM. Obstetric outcomes in donor oocyte pregnancies compared with advanced maternal age in *in vitro* fertilization pregnancies. *Fertil Steril* 2008;90:65–70.

20. Henne MB, Zhang M, Paroski S, Kelshikar B, Westphal LM. Comparison of obstetric outcomes in recipients of donor oocytes vs. women of advanced maternal age with autologous oocytes. *J Reprod Med* 2007;52:585–90.

21. Salha O, Sharma V, Dada T, Nugent D, Rutherford AJ, Tomlinson AJ, *et al.* The influence of donated gametes on the incidence of hypertensive disorders of pregnancy. Hum Reprod 1999;14:2268–73.

22. Ray JG, Burrows RF, Burrows EA, Vermeulen MJ. MOS HIP: McMaster outcome study of hypertension in pregnancy. Early Hum Dev 2001;64:129–43.

23. Martin JN Jr, Thigpen BD, Moore RC, Rose CH, Cushman J, May W. Stroke and severe pre-eclampsia and eclampsia: a paradigm shift focusing on systolic blood pressure. *Obstet Gynecol* 2005;105:246–54.

24. Drife J, Lewis G, editors. *Why Mothers Die. Report on Confidential Enquiries into Maternal Deaths in the United Kingdom 1994–96.* London: The Stationery Office; 1998.

25. Lewis G, editor. *Why Mothers Die 1997–1999. The Fifth Report of the Confidential Enquiries into Maternal Deaths in the United Kingdom.* London: RCOG Press; 2001.

26. Lewis G, CEMACH. *Why Mothers Die 2000–2002 – The Sixth Report of Confidential Enquiries into Maternal Deaths in the United Kingdom.* London: RCOG Press; 2004.

27. Hannaford P, Ferry S, Hirsch S. Cardiovascular sequelae of toxaemia of pregnancy. Heart 1997;77:154–8.

28. Jónsdóttir LS, Arngrímsson R, Geirsson RT, Sigvaldason H, Sigfússon N. Death rates from ischemic heart disease in women with a history of hypertension in pregnancy. *Acta Obstet Gynecol Scand* 1995;74:772–6.

29. Smith GC, Pell JP, Walsh D. Pregnancy complications and maternal risk of ischaemic heart disease: a retrospective cohort study of 129,290 births. Lancet 2001;357:2002–6.

30. Wilson BJ, Watson MS, Prescott GJ, Sunderland S, Campbell DM, Hannaford P, *et al.* Hypertensive diseases of pregnancy and risk of hypertension and stroke in later life: results from a cohort study. BMJ 2003;326:845.

31. National Institute for Health and Clinical Excellence. *Obesity: the Prevention, Identification, Assessment and Management of Overweight and Obesity in Adults and Children.* London: NICE; 2006 [www.nice.org.uk/guidance/CG43].

32. Information Centre for Health and Social Care. *Statistics on Obesity, Physical Activity and Diet: England, 2006.* Leeds: Information Centre; 2006.

33. Zaninotto P, Wardle H, Stamatakis E, Mindell J, Head J. *Forecasting Obesity to 2010.* London: Department of Health and Joint Health Surveys Unit, National Centre for Social Research; 2006 [www.dh.gov.uk/en/Publicationsandstatistics/Publications/PublicationsStatistics/DH_4138630].

34. Heslehurst N, Ells LJ, Simpson H, Batterham A, Wilkinson J, Summerbell CD. Trends in maternal obesity incidence rates, demographic predictors, and health inequalities in 36,821 women over a 15-year period. BJOG 2007;114:187–94.

35. Lu GC, Rouse DJ, DuBard M, Cliver S, Kimberlin D, Hauth JC. The effect of the increasing prevalence of maternal obesity on perinatal morbidity. *Am J Obstet Gynecol* 2001;185:845–9.

36. Knight M, Kurinczuk JJ, Spark P, Brocklehurst P. *UKOSS Annual Report 2007.* Oxford: National Perinatal Epidemiology Unit; 2007.

37. Usha Kiran TS, Hemmadi S, Bethel J, Evans J. Outcome of pregnancy in a woman with an increased body mass index. BJOG 2005;112:768–72.

38. Kanagalingam MG, Forouhi NG, Greer IA, Sattar N. Changes in booking body mass index over a decade: retrospective analysis from a Glasgow Maternity Hospital. BJOG 2005;112:1431–3.

39. Balen AH, Anderson RA; Policy & Practice Committee of the BFS. Impact of obesity on female reproductive health: British Fertility Society, Policy and Practice Guidelines. *Hum Fertil (Camb)* 2007;10:195–206.

40. Kannel WB, Brand N, Skinner JJ Jr, Dawber TR, McNamara PM. The relation of adiposity to blood pressure and development of hypertension. The Framingham study. Ann Intern Med 1967;67:48–59.

41. Abrams B, Parker J. Overweight and pregnancy complications. *Int J Obes* 1988;12:293–303.

42. Weiss JL, Malone FD, Emig D, Ball RH, Nyberg DA, Comstock CH, *et al.*; FASTER Research Consortium. Obesity, obstetric complications and cesarean delivery rate – a population-based screening study. *Am J Obstet Gynecol* 2004;190:1091–7.

43. O'Brien TE, Ray JG, Chan WS. Maternal body mass index and the risk of pre-eclampsia: a systematic overview. Epidemiology 2003;14:368–74.

44. Sebire NJ, Jolly M, Harris JP, Wadsworth J, Joffe M, Beard RW, *et al.* Maternal obesity and pregnancy outcome: a study of 287,213 pregnancies in London. *Int J Obes Relat Metab Disord* 2001;25:1175–82.

45. Parsons TJ, Power C, Logan S, Summerbell CD. Childhood predictors of adult obesity: a systematic review. *Int J Obes Relat Metab Disord* 1999;23 Suppl 8:S1–107.

46. Whitaker RC. Predicting preschooler obesity at birth: the role of maternal obesity in early pregnancy. Pediatrics 2004;114:e29–36.

47. Comptroller and Auditor General. *Tackling Childhood Obesity – The First Steps.* London: The Stationery Office; 2006.

48. Diabetes UK. *Diabetes in the UK 2004.* London: Diabetes UK; 2004.

49. Rosenbloom AL, Silverstein JH, Amemiya S, Zeitler P, Klingensmith GJ. Type 2 diabetes mellitus in the child and adolescent. ISPAD clinical practice consensus guidelines 2006–2007. *Pediatr Diabetes* 2008;9:512–26.

50. National Collaborating Centre for Women's and Children's Health. *Diabetes in Pregnancy: Management of Diabetes and Its Complications from Preconception to the Postnatal Period.* London: RCOG Press; 2008.

51. Confidential Enquiry into Maternal and Child Health: *Pregnancy in Women with Type 1 and Type 2 Diabetes in 2002–03, England, Wales and Northern Ireland.* London: CEMACH; 2005.

52. Lawrence JM, Contreras R, Chen W, Sacks DA. Trends in the prevalence of preexisting diabetes and gestational diabetes mellitus among a racially/ethnically diverse population of pregnant women, 1999–2005. *Diabetes Care* 2008;31:899–904.

53. Solomon CG, Willett WC, Carey VJ, Rich-Edwards J, Hunter DJ, Colditz GA, *et al.* A prospective study of pregravid determinants of gestational diabetes mellitus. *JAMA* 1997;278:1078–83.

54. Ferrara A, Kahn HS, Quesenberry CP, Riley C, Hedderson MM. An increase in the incidence of gestational diabetes mellitus: Northern California, 1991–2000. *Obstet Gynecol* 2004;103:526–33.

55. Getahun D, Nath C, Ananth CV, Chavez MR, Smulian JC. Gestational diabetes in the United States: temporal trends 1989 through 2004. *Am J Obstet Gynecol* 2008;198:525.e1–5.

56. Narayan H, Buckett W, McDougall W, Cullimore J. Pregnancy after fifty: profile and pregnancy outcome in a series of elderly multigravidae. *Eur J Obstet Gynecol Reprod Biol* 1992;47:47–51.

57. Crowther CA. Hiller JE. Moss JR, McPhee AJ, Jeffries WS, Robinson JS. Effect of treatment of gestational diabetes mellitus on pregnancy outcomes. N Engl J Med 2005;352:2477–2486.

58. Metzger BE. Long-term outcomes in mothers diagnosed with gestational diabetes mellitus and their offspring. *Clin Obstet Gynecol* 2007;50:972–9.

59. Kim C, Newton KM, Knopp RH. Gestational diabetes and the incidence of type 2 diabetes: a systematic review. *Diabetes Care* 2002;25:1862–8.

60. Allender S, Peto V, Scarborough P, Boxer A, Rayner M. *Coronary Heart Disease Statistics.* London: BHF; 2007 [www.heartstats.org/datapage.asp?id=6799].

61. Office for National Statistics. *Mortality Statistics, Deaths Registered in 2002–2005. Review of the Registrar General on Deaths in England and Wales by Cause Sex and Age 2002–2005.* Series DH2 Nos.29–32 [www.statistics.gov.uk/statbase/Product.asp?vlnk=618].

62. Unal B, Critchley JA, Capewell S. Explaining the decline in coronary heart disease mortality in England and Wales between 1981 and 2000. *Circulation* 2004;109:1101–17.

63. Ladner HE, Danielsen B, Gilbert WM. Acute myocardial infarction in pregnancy and the puerperium: a population-based study. *Obstet Gynecol* 2005;105:480–4.

64. James AH, Jamison MG, Biswas MS, Brancazio LR, Swamy GK, Myers ER. Acute myocardial infarction in pregnancy: a United States population-based study. Circulation 2006;113:1564–71.

65. Petitti DB, Sidney S, Quesenberry CP Jr, Bernstein A. Incidence of stroke and myocardial infarction in women of reproductive age. Stroke 1997;28:280–3.

66. Hankins GD, Wendel GD Jr, Leveno KJ, Stoneham J. Myocardial infarction during pregnancy: a review. *Obstet Gynecol* 1985;65:139–46.

67. Office for National Statistics. *Mortality Statistics: Cause. England & Wales, 2006.* Vol. DH2 No.32. London: TSO; 2006.

68. General Register Office for Scotland. *Scotland's Population 2006 – The Registrar General's Annual Review of Demographic Trends.* Edinburgh: GRO for Scotland; 2007.

69. Northern Ireland Cancer Registry. Cancer Mortality in Northern Ireland, 2006 [http://www.qub.ac.uk/research-centres/nicr/Data/OnlineStatistics/].

70. Office for National Statistics. *Cancer Statistics Registrations: Registrations of Cancer Diagnosed in 1992–2005, England.* Series MB1 no.25–36, 1998–2008. [www.statistics.gov.uk/statbase/Product.asp?vlnk=8843].

71.   Smith LH, Danielsen B, Allen ME, Cress R. Cancer associated with obstetric delivery: results of linkage with the California cancer registry. *Am J Obstet Gynecol* 2003;189:1128–35.
72.   Smith LH, Dalrymple JL, Leiserowitz GS, Danielsen B, Gilbert WM. Obstetrical deliveries associated with maternal malignancy in California, 1992 through 1997. *Am J Obstet Gynecol* 2001;184:1504–12.
73.   Drife JO. The contribution of cancer to maternal mortality. In: O'Brien PM, McLean AB, editors. *Hormones and Cancer: Proceedings of an RCOG Study Group.* London: RCOG; 2000.

Chapter 15

The ageing mother and medical needs

Discussion

Dimitrios Nikolaou: Two excellent presentations. Many women think that if they optimise their health, somehow they just will 'get away with it' – do you agree?

Mandish Dhanjal: It is difficult to tease out the data. Maybe if you look at the egg donation pregnancies because they are obviously a healthy group of women. Hypertension and diabetes, etc., have all been excluded. Yet they have much greater risk.

Susan Bewley: Thank you very much for two excellent talks. I took away two points. One is around framing age as an individual's problem – because when we reach 30 we cannot go back to be being 20 – as opposed to a public health problem. With those very dramatic shifts in women rightwards (see Figure 13.8, page 137), if 600 000–700 000 women giving birth annually are on average 3 years older than their counterparts were 20–30 years ago, the whole UK childbearing population is almost 2 million reproductive years older! There is a tension between the individual woman, and not making her anxious, and the public health problem – which needs naming. I would like your comments. The second point is directed to the fertility experts here. Do you think there is an age, even with a healthy, marathon-running, vitamin-taking woman that we should say 'Actually, it is unethical to get you pregnant because of the maternal risks'? Albeit the risk of death is small, you are making women pregnant and they might die.

Mandish Dhanjal: With regard to the public health, yes, it is a very important message. I think it has started to get out. Certainly with the last Confidential Enquiry into Maternal Deaths,[1] there was a lot of interest in maternal age and obesity. I had not realised that the maternal mortality rate had slowed down and that is very interesting. With regard to high age, the data clearly show that there are vastly increased risks. We are talking about a small group of women and the data are muddied by multiple pregnancy – 25% of the [ovum recipient] women have multiple pregnancy. Fifty percent were in their first pregnancy. We know that first pregnancy increases the risks of pre-eclampsia. But women giving birth over the age of 50 is something we need to think of in a social context as well. I do not know whether there are comments from the reproductive endocrinologists …

Stephen Hillier: I was intrigued by your recommendation that you should positively counsel that it is better to have children in your 20s. I am speaking as a non-clinical reproductive endocrinologist who is the father of two daughters, one of whom is a medic in her early 30s who still has not had a delivery and the other is busy in the City. I would offer them as case studies of the reality of what middle-class young women are doing with their lives now. I do not think you can really offer that as a practical recommendation

Anna Kenyon: But are women aware? If I were 20 and I wanted to plan my life in the way that I plan my career (and maybe your daughters are planning their careers), where would we find that information easily? The messages out there seem to be 'Don't worry about this. You will get pregnant when you're 35, when you're 40. The technology is there. We can help you'. I wonder whether we could infuse the information that people have access to with this little bit of information. I accept that I am just like your daughter in terms of delay. We should not stigmatise women by saying 'You have to have children now'. It would just be nice to feel that there is that information and so women can't get to 35 and say 'I didn't know, and maybe if I had known I would have done things differently.'

Stephen Hillier: I absolutely agree with that. I was also intrigued by the point you made about the ethics of making women pregnant at high age. Both the point that you just made about recommending the 20s and the point made ethically are redolent of the HFEA [Human Fertilisation and Embryology Authority] and the advice that you give mothers when you're doing assisted conception procedures. The risks that you are knowingly making someone pregnant at a certain age, as a fertility specialist, have to be matched against the fact that women do get pregnant at that age. That is a normal human right. Women do get pregnant in their 50s and then ethically how can you say 'No, we will not treat you because of a high risk of death'?

Susan Bewley: It is very tough and no one is discounting the pain of childlessness. There are some issues for doctors, the general public and policy makers, though, which are about making it easier both to be a parent and to be successful in the City or in medicine, or whatever. Many things have nothing to do doctoring at all. They are to do with the way society works. However, if a GP hands out the pill for 20 years, contracepting a woman through her fertile years, and then she turns up age 45 or so, there must be a question about the appropriate use of medical resources and the appropriate advice from obstetricians and gynaecologists. We see the results on our labour wards. We see those near-misses with maternal death. I had a labour ward day at St Thomas' not so long ago, when four babies were lost on the same day from two IVF twin pregnancies miscarrying at 23 and 24 weeks. You see in your clinics the terrible pain of repeated miscarriage and infertility. The treatments that you have do not work most of the time. I just think obstetricians and gynaecologists can't be indifferent to the social trend. I am not saying we should go and 'nanny' women about it but, these two talks have just demonstrated that there is a clash. As the age of the pregnant population moves upwards they will bump into middle-age disease. Sadly, I do not think the advice is controversial.

David Barlow: The speakers understandably referred to the risks of pre-eclampsia increasing – a figure of 60% was quoted for the over-50s. Pre-eclampsia is a very broad church. What sort of pre-eclampsia are you referring to? You get the pre-eclampsia defined in hospital by the fact that blood pressure went over the threshold and not much else happened. I am very conscious of the pre-eclampsia issue. Since you are reminiscing, I will reminisce. My late-20s daughter-in-law had fulminating pre-eclampsia at 26 weeks and delivered our first grandchild last November. At 900 g he spent 3 months in the intensive care, and happily is fine as far as we can judge at 10 months of age. That's the extreme end that really matters an awful lot, as does

HELLP syndrome [haemolysis, elevated liver enzymes, low platelets]. Are a lot of these 60% simply because of blood pressure threshold? Do you have the information?

Mandish Dhanjal: Yes. About two-thirds have mild to moderate pre-eclampsia and one-third have severe pre-eclampsia.

David Barlow: OK. The figure jumped out, but in an awful lot that doesn't seem to matter.

Mandish Dhanjal: But do not forget that pre-eclampsia is not just hypertension. It is also proteinuria and usually requires admission of the woman to hospital for the rest of the duration of her pregnancy. I am not talking about pregnancy-induced hypertension, which is different.

David Barlow: That's what I was trying to clarify.

Peter Braude: Susan, Melanie and I got into trouble the first time we went down this line of telling people what to do with their lives.[2] I think it is very important that you can't take that view … and there is an issue to do with autonomy.

Susan Bewley: We did not tell people what to do! We just said that this is the secure, healthy age range.

Peter Braude: There are two important messages that confuse the issue. One is that we give all the figures in the number of women and the percentage change. We are not actually talking about the real numbers, which are small. That is why reproductive medicine specialists say 'Well, it is a good idea to put two embryos, and get one family from twins to start with'. Because the real risk in terms of numbers is timing and there is a lot of time and that is not how you should always think of it. But for the person who has a choice, will we say 'Have no kids because you are too old' or 'Have some kids but take the risks'? I do not think there is any doubt what they will do. The second point that Steve Hillier brought out beautifully is that women over 50 do not get babies on their own. There is a misconception in the press. You read it all the time – and I collect the HELLO! and OK! magazine articles which show these wonderful women at 47, 'we've had twins' – and not a sausage mentioned that they must have had egg donation. So there is this misconception that women can wait forever because, look, they're 50 and having babies! That is the message we have to give out: that says you can't do it forever and when you come to 35, 36, 37+ you are going to struggle. The women that you read about in the glam mags are doing it by egg donation. That is not easy and it is expensive.

Anna Kenyon: That's true. I was doing a patient-style literature research, put 'advanced maternal age' in Google and found a website for older mothers extolling the virtues of reproducing at an older age. Their headline is a picture of seven celebrities, all in very glamorous poses, aged 46, or with twins, and there is no mention of ART [assisted reproductive technology].

Mandish Dhanjal: The only thing that we know for certain is that many pregnancies in older women are unplanned.

Siladitya Bhattacharya: Two slightly unconnected things. Whenever data are presented on increased maternal risks, infertility and the treatment thereof are always separated. It makes excellent epidemiological and statistical sense to adjust for that. But in reality, these women are going to be older. Therefore their risks remain their risks. So the clinical interpretation should take that into account and not try to separate out age and the effect of infertility treatment. The second is to join in on the comment about the ideal age for reproduction and how that message gets across. There needs to be a lot of more work on understanding the barriers as to why women don't have children between the ages of 20 and 35. Career and so on has been mentioned but there are other things. One is obviously this unrealistic faith in the joys of assisted reproduction and what it can deliver, and you have alluded to that. And the second one is very simple: women do not find a partner they could have babies with. I think that needs to be taken into account because, in the somewhat sparse literature on the subject, this is something that jumps out.[3] The other problem is trying to get this knowledge across to a population of teenagers essentially, in a climate where teenage pregnancy is still seen as a huge problem.

Kate Brian: Did you say that you thought the multiple rate was possibly muddying the figures? Given what we saw yesterday about the really quite alarming multiple rates, particularly in women in their mid- to late 40s, how significant do you think that is? If we really cut that multiple rate do you think it might make a significant difference to your outcome?

Anna Kenyon: I am sure it would, definitely. Obviously, the rate of twinning goes up with age even without ART. Those ones we are unlikely to control, but certainly among the ART group. In the graphs that I showed you (Figures 13.3 and 13.4, page 129), plurality has a worse effect on outcome than age. This is what is in the HFEA document[4] and what Professor Braude said yesterday about 'One at a time'.[5]

Mandish Dhanjal: And it would certainly have an impact on hypertension and gestational diabetes, which are both known to be increased in twins.

Anna Kenyon: Maybe prepregnancy counselling in the IVF units will come into it very strongly. When people have struggled long and hard to get pregnant, the thought of having two at once would be incredibly attractive. I can see that. But if women knew the actual costs of that, plus their individual comorbidities … Perhaps we could come up with an individualised risk for that woman. She may say 'Yes, I know, thank you very much. I still want my family.' Well that's her choice. Probably they do want that pregnancy at any cost, but they need to know.

Peter Braude: The information is actually available because there was a document on the risks of assisted reproduction.[6] When you produce something like that, there is a patient information document that goes with it so that should have been available.

Dimitrios Nikolau: Actually, this may be a recommendation, just as we have for women considering hysterectomy or whatever, for older women who go to fertility clinics to seek formal preconception counselling

Roger Gosden: We do that.

William Ledger: A couple of comments. The first is that we are we are in the middle of an HFEA initiative supported by the British Fertility Society to replace one embryo in younger women who are having IVF or ART.[5] I think we have may have missed a trick. In my view, the group who should be targeted quite strongly with this initiative are the older women who are having donor oocytes. We have not extended, or proposed, the policy to that group, but some of the morbidity would be reduced if the older group were having one baby at a time instead of two. That's something maybe to take away, or a very solid recommendation to make: that all donor oocytes should be single embryo transfer. We have seen the data and their pregnancy success rates are the same as for a 25-year-old even if the recipient happens to be 45 because it is the quality of the egg, rather than the uterus, as we heard very eloquently yesterday. [See Section 2 on the basic science of reproductive ageing.] The second thing was the sadness I felt yesterday when Dr Botting was presenting because miscarriage is not included in national statistics. What we've heard from Anna is that 50% of pregnancies in the over-40-year-olds are lost. Therefore all the slides we see with the increasing number of live births in the over 40s are actually only a fraction of the number of wanted pregnancies. The demographic trend is actually greater than we think – because the number of pregnancies does not match the number of live births. That is something else to come out in the recommendations.

Melanie Davies: The clinical data as presented are a real challenge for the maternity services. I think we could usefully spend some time thinking about the implications for the government, hospital trusts and ourselves in the way that we organise services to accommodate this increased demand from older women, which is predicted to increase in the next decade.

Mandish Dhanjal: I agree. The importance, of course, is that with more diseases developing, more women are going to require care in the hospital, whereas the government's ambition is to move deliveries into the community and it does not sit nicely with their policies.

Gordon Smith: Yes. In terms of the consequences, we tend to talk about the mothers whom David alluded to in his personal story. But if you look at the public health significance, the number of women dying each year from pre-eclampsia is actually the same as the number of women in the UK dying from malaria! The major public health impact is the generation of extreme preterm deliveries of babies who then have lifelong problems with their health and education, etc., and also the morbidity and mortality associated with that. I think it is particularly important to look at the preterm babies in the context of age. Anna, you mentioned the effect of age on prematurity but there are two major generators of prematurity: spontaneous preterm birth rate and elective preterm deliveries as a consequence of complications such as pre-eclampsia. Could you find from the literature whether this association with advanced age tended to be a combination of those two, or whether it was more elective deliveries for pre-eclampsia?

Anna Kenyon: Some studies have separated out spontaneous versus iatrogenic prematurity. Because the most statistically robust studies are large retrospective ones from national data registries, they often cannot tease it out. It is very difficult to determine the effect of age. It comes back to what Mandish said about how you have to make assumptions about pre-eclampsia. What we would say is that a third of pre-eclampsia is severe and those preterm deliveries are iatrogenic. I do not think one study teased that out. It is a mixture of two. Of course multiple pregnancies deliver preterm. Then there's also obstetrician and patient anxiety about delivering children at high age. In running the recurrent prematurity clinic that we have at St Thomas', for example, I do not get the impression that age alone prompts those risk factors. But then, of course, in terms of coming into pregnancy, women accumulate comorbidities which of themselves may lead them to deliver earlier. I am not sure I have a concise answer to the question but it is an important point.

Diana Mansour: I see lots of women who delay having their first child and use contraception for many years and I think they are aware of what risks they are putting themselves at and they feel constant pressure on them. I think you've got to be very aware how we put messages across because often women think it's actually worse than what we are stating: infertility as well as the obstetric issues. The other comment I had was around your diabetes data. I was fascinated that Scotland was missed off but also London has quite a high prevalence for diabetes or gestational diabetes. Is that purely due to age or are there other factors?

Mandish Dhanjal: It is age, ethnicity and social deprivation. Scotland was not missed off.... I thought it was on the end of the slide but maybe I missed it off inadvertently. It was split into England, Wales and Scotland.

Anna Kenyon: I accept that women perhaps know about the reduction in their fertility with age but I wonder whether they know about the obstetric risks?

Diana Mansour: And they do not know them in absolute terms. I think it gives us pause for thought and it is worthwhile that it is publicised. Then it's a matter of how you put it across. We had a formal complaint when a doctor had wanted to bring this up and the woman found it insulting.

Anna Kenyon: Age is a very difficult thing to discuss sensitively in antenatal clinics also. Women might get referred for obstetric opinion and input with 'age over 35' as a risk factor. But actually, once you meet someone who is pregnant she has already done better than the nonpregnant 35-year-old. She may have been through a number of miscarriages and struggled to get where she is. To then sit with her in the clinic and say 'Dread it, because here you go, you've got this and that risk' without offering realistic solutions in terms of how to reduce it….. You know this is the time she wants to go to the clinic and say 'Fantastic, haven't I done well? I'm pregnant!'

Maya Unnithan: Apart from targeting women, is there any responsibility that you can share more widely? Perhaps another issue that needs to be considered is the way in which the women sought medical intervention. There is advertising shown. And clearly you can't have a celebration about successsful medical achievements on the one hand, where some women are being treated, and then many people can't get access.

Susan Bewley: Two comments and a question. No woman should be bullied into a pregnancy when, or if, she does not want to – we should support that very strongly. However, we should not be indifferent to the effect of age and making this general public knowledge. It seems to me OK to have those graphs showing falling fertility with age and increasing miscarriages and complications on the J-shaped curves (see Figure 21.1, page 228) available in family planning clinics. There are the facts in front of you. Family planning used to be about planning families – now it's merely about contraception – that's a nice old-fashioned virtue to go back to. Secondly, Gordon points out that the real numbers of maternal mortality are very small. That is only because obstetricians work fantastically hard to keep them low! For every woman who dies, at least a hundred others go to intensive care,[7] and several thousands will have a severe morbidity of childbirth such as a hospital admission, complication, induction or caesarean section – which vary with age in the same J-shaped graph way. So there is a huge burden of morbidity. Pregnancy is not merely about the baby – of course, the aim is having a baby – but every time a baby is born a new mother is created and she has to be in good mental and physical health, supported by the people around her. It is that social support which brings me to the question which I'll leave in the air. This comes from the surveys about what it is that makes women delay.[8,9] What women say is that they have not met the right person and so forth. This begs a question that

I would like the older men here who want to become grandfathers to think about: were men more suitable in the past? Or are women demanding something different of them nowadays? [laughter]

References

1. Lewis G, editor. *Saving Mothers' Lives: Reviewing Maternal Deaths to Make Motherhood Safer 2003–2005. The Seventh Report on Confidential Enquiries into Maternal Deaths in the United Kingdom.* London: CEMACH; 2007.
2. Bewley S, Davies M, Braude P. Which career first? *BMJ* 2005;331:588–9.
3. Maheshwari A, Porter M, Shetty A, Bhattacharya S. Women's awareness and perceptions of delay in childbearing. *Fertil Steril* 2008;90:1036–42.
4. Human Fertilisation and Embryology Authority. *One Child at a Time: Reducing Multiple Births after IVF.* Report of the Expert Group on Multiple Births after IVF. London: HFEA; 2006.
5. Oneatatime website [www.oneatatime.org.uk].
6. Royal College of Obstetricians and Gynaecologists. *Perinatal Risks Associated with IVF.* Scientific Advisory Committee Opinion Paper 8. London: RCOG Press; 2007.
7. Bewley S, Wolfe C, Waterstone M. Severe maternal morbidity in the UK. In: MacLean AB, Neilson J, editors. *Maternal Morbidity and Mortality.* London: RCOG Press; 2002. p. 132–46.
8. Robinson GE, Garner DM, Gare DJ, Crawford B. Psychological adaptation to pregnancy in childless women more than 35 years of age. *Am J Obstet Gynecol* 1987;156:328–33.
9. Mothers 35 Plus website. Older mothers – facts and figures [www.mothers35plus.co.uk/intro. htm].

Section 4

The outcomes:
children and mothers

Chapter 16
What is known about children born to older parents?

Alastair Sutcliffe and Yasmin Baki

Introduction

In developed countries, there has been an undeniable trend towards later childbearing. In 1968, the average maternal age at first birth in the UK was 23 years. In 2007, data from the Office for National Statistics[1] revealed that the average age was between 30 and 31 years. In 1985, 7.9% of births in England and Wales were in women aged 35 years or over but by 1995 this statistic had increased to 11.8%.[2] This dramatic shift towards voluntary postponement of motherhood beyond the age of 30 years reflects the changing role of women in society. Historical changes such as the introduction of the contraceptive pill in the early 1960s, subsequent abortion legislation and the advent of amniocentesis and improved antenatal and obstetric care have allowed this societal move to occur. Increasing economic opportunities for women and rising divorce rates have led to the concept of the 'working mother' becoming increasingly the norm. The development of assisted reproductive technologies (ART) has resulted in the traditional perceptions of childbearing capability being changed, with, for example, a woman in Romania giving birth at the age of 66 years.

In contrast with this, studies show that the biomarker age of fertility is 38 years, with a 2–3 times increased risk of permanent childlessness in women aged 38 years or over compared with those under 30 years. Defining 'the older mother' is problematic as studies use varying cut-off points. More recent studies use 38 years as the biomarker age.[3] There is a paucity of literature in this area regarding outcomes for children of older mothers. Most studies focus on a restricted time period during infancy and a narrow range of parent and child outcomes, and do not account for the confounding effects of fertility problems and marital/partnership issues.

What factors distinguish older mothers' personal attributes?

Older first-time mothers are not a random population.[4] There are specific associations within this group that need to be addressed to understand the trend towards delayed motherhood. They are a more autonomous group and less orientated towards parenthood than younger mothers who have more traditional views. They tend to be university graduates and have high-status employment and therefore have higher socio-economic status than average. They are also likely to be more geographically mobile than younger women, living further away from their extended families and relying more on friends for support. Personality traits identified in older mothers include resilience, hardiness and less dependence on others. So, in general, older mothers exhibit maturity, well-developed problem-solving skills, have a stable committed relationship with a partner and are financially secure.[2]

The complexity of multiple factors influencing women's decisions regarding the timing of motherhood operate at individual, family and societal levels and also interact across levels. Benzies et al.[5] questioned a range of women and identified the common issues listed below.

Individual factors:

- Independence. The importance of establishing independence through education, secure employment and financial stability was evident in women aged 35 years or over.
- Family motivation.
- Readiness. Women who had delayed childbirth felt ready as they did not feel they were 'missing anything' and felt they had satisfied their personal goals.
- Projecting the life plan. A mental plan for their life, integrating their intended age at childbearing with their child's life transitions, was another common theme.
- The biological clock. Women aged 30 years or over were aware of the risks of declining fertility with increasing age but were confident that ART was available to assist them. The risks of ART, such as multiple births and preterm labour, and of childlessness were largely not considered and older women still favoured education, career and other personal goals before starting a family.
- Chronic health problems were linked to infertility across the age groups.
- Stable relationship. Security in partnership was critical to women because they wanted support in childrearing but with increasing age the urgency to have a child could override the need to have a stable relationship. Some women had previous failed relationships or marriages before they found a suitable partnership for having a child; others were aware of the risk of 'missing the boat'.

Familial factors:

- Partner readiness.
- Financial stability. This influenced the older age group more strongly than younger mothers.
- Family of origin. Families are now more geographically distant. Women were influenced by their family's expectations for grandchildren that were both implicit and explicit and they were also influenced by the timing of their own mother's childbearing. There was a positive association between mother's and daughter's parity and the desirability of pregnancy, suggesting an attitudinal role in the previous generation.

Societal factors:

- Social acceptability of delayed childbearing. Societal expectations for personal independence before motherhood was perceived by women to allow older motherhood to become more normative and not feel 'out of sync' with on-time mothers. In fact, younger mothers felt prejudiced against and that society viewed them as 'bad mothers' who had been robbed of opportunities for education and the acquisition of material things.

- Divorce rates. An awareness of the high rates of divorce among women further supported the view that women should be self-sufficient.
- Social policy. Parental benefits such as maternity benefits were not found to be influential but more flexible employment patterns and social changes relating to male participation in childrearing were more relevant.

The risks

Conception, pregnancy and childbirth in older mothers involve increased physical risks to both the mother and the offspring (Box 16.1). After the age of 31 years, the probability of conception falls rapidly and older women take longer to conceive and are more likely to require reproductive assistance. Age-related decline in the quality of oocytes results in increased egg donation in ART in older women. Couples who have ART are on average 5 years older than those who conceive spontaneously. Advanced maternal age, particularly in the late 30s and beyond, is associated with an increased risk of miscarriage. Advanced paternal age is also associated with a deteriorating sperm count and therefore difficulties in conceiving. ART itself can be unsuccessful, particularly in older women, or, at the other extreme, can result in multiple pregnancy. ART is also associated with a 30% greater risk of birth defects, particularly imprinting disorders such as Beckwith–Wiedemann syndrome, compared with the baseline population.[6,7] Even after the hurdles of conception and pregnancy are overcome, fetal and neonatal risks remain, as listed in Box 16.1.

Although pregnancies in women aged 35 years or over are often labelled 'high risk', they generally have good pregnancy outcomes with few maternal age effects related to obstetric outcome. Older mothers are physically healthier than in the past and chronic health problems in this group are better managed. They are also likely to have fewer children than midlife gravidas of the past, thus avoiding the complications

---

Box 16.1   The risks of conception, pregnancy and birth in older parents[6–11]

Conception:
- Reproductive difficulties. Greater egg donation in ART in older women
- Longer time to conceive
- Increased risk of miscarriage
- *In vitro* fertilisation (IVF) failure or multiple pregnancy
- Older fathers – poor sperm count

Gestation and labour:
- More complications – bleeds in pregnancy, pre-eclampsia
- Increased risk of caesarean section
- Greater concomitant pre-existing medical problems such as hypertension and diabetes.

Fetal and neonatal:
- Increased morbidity and mortality
- Higher odds of trisomy, mitochondrial DNA disorders
- Higher risks of new inheritable mutation disorders in older men as spermatozoa are more vulnerable to mutational changes
- Older fathers – association with autism and schizophrenia

of increased parity. There are increased rates of caesarean section in women aged 35 years or over. It is not clear whether this is due to maternal choice or concern on the part of professionals exceeding actual medical indications. Data from the Leicester Motherhood Project[12] illustrated that older women were aware of the increased risk associated with pregnancy and were more likely to opt for serum screening for Down syndrome. Older mothers received more assessments in pregnancy than younger women – for example, they were more likely to have more than one ultrasound during pregnancy – but infant outcomes did not differ. In addition, they were more aware that their baby's life was at risk during labour and delivery than were younger women.

Older mothers show less attachment to the fetus in mid-pregnancy but in late pregnancy attachment is comparable with that of on-time mothers. This is possibly explained by greater anxiety in pregnancy in older women related to increased risk, and which may also be linked to healthcare professionals' influence or their own maturity in realising that childbirth involves risk. Lower expectations and increased appreciation of and satisfaction with staff care may reflect this anxiety. Less optimal maternal–fetal attachment secondary to anxiety may result in delayed psychological preparation for the baby. The study by Windridge and Berryman,[12] although limited by a small sample size, showed the impact of the expectation of a 'high-risk' pregnancy on older mothers.

The study by McMahon et al.[13] that looked at age effects in psychosocial wellbeing in pregnancy in couples who had undergone ART, showed higher scores for hardiness in older mothers that may be protective in managing stresses related to obstetric risk. Hardiness was inversely related to anxiety and depression throughout pregnancy. Ego resilience and behaviour-related measures of self-efficacy reflecting psychological maturity in older mothers can be protective but it is not known whether this effect remains beyond childbirth. Older mothers felt a lack of preparation for the material needs of the baby and a tendency to put aside thoughts of being a mother but younger infertile women were more likely to have irrational idealistic cognitions about pregnancy and parenthood. Thus, older mothers' 'lower identification with motherhood' may in fact be more realistic and adaptive of the challenges of parenthood.[14] Conversely, this could be interpreted as a reluctance to engage with enormous life change, as illustrated by many older mothers' approach to motherhood as a project to be managed with a determination that the baby would fit into and not disrupt their established lifestyle.

Older mothers have a breadth of life experience and wisdom not available to younger mothers. They are also likely to have better financial and social resources. Hofferth's maternal maturity hypothesis[15] reflects that experience allows older mothers to have already developed coping strategies to deal with obstacles faced and they are able to draw on this in the context of motherhood. Older mothers' self-awareness is also demonstrated by the fact that compared with younger women they take fewer risks in the perinatal period. For example, they are less likely to smoke or take illicit substances and more likely to plan their pregnancy, have a good diet, gain weight appropriately, begin prenatal care earlier in pregnancy and breastfeed than younger women. Generally, they take a more cautious approach to pregnancy and early infancy, balancing against the risks previously referred to.

Parenting

Very little research exists that specifically focuses on parenting and child outcomes in older parent families. Most research in this area is in the context of ART. The 1995 paper by Colpin *et al.*[16] controversially postulated that the child may act as a constant reminder of previous infertility, possibly acting as a 'narcissistic injury' or creating asymmetry in the marital relationship. This view contrasts with the more conventional perspective that the child is seen as very 'precious'.[17] Thus, after a long period of infertility, parents are overprotective, with exaggerated expectations of the child and difficulty in adapting to childrearing. It has also been reported that a child conceived by ART may be perceived as different by the family's social network. Despite this, Van Balen's review[17] of the existing small-size studies of the development of children conceived by ART showed no negative difference in parent–child relationships or in children's psychological development. In fact, mothers who became pregnant with ART reported more pleasure in their children, more warmth towards them and more parental competence than naturally fertile mothers.[18] Mothers in the ART group also reported less stress and fathers were more involved in this group compared with naturally conceiving controls but this may reflect a tendency for the ART group to report socially desirable responses. Colpin's small study[16] based in Belgium showed that, at age 2–3 years, *in vitro* fertilisation (IVF) mothers in employment were less able to allow their children autonomy in problem-solving tasks than naturally conceiving mothers. In contrast, Gibson's Australian study[19] did not corroborate these findings and showed no differences in parent–child attachment or maternal sensitivity, structuring or hostility during free play. Fathers in the IVF group in Gibson's study expressed lower self-esteem and less marital satisfaction than fathers in the natural conception group but adjustment and parenting were not different.

A large multi-site European study[20] compared children conceived by ART (IVF or intracytoplasmic sperm injection, ICSI) with naturally conceived controls, focusing on family functioning and the children's socio-emotional development. Assessments included the Bene–Anthony family relations test,[21] which allows the child to attribute 16 positive and 16 negative feelings to their mother, father, sibling or nobody, represented by cardboard shapes attached to a posting box base. An additional eight items reflected dependence (for example, who helps you get dressed?). As expected, maternal and paternal age were significantly older in the ART group, allowing some comparison of older and younger parents. Mothers, but not fathers, with children conceived through ICSI were less committed to their work role and more to their parenting role, seeing themselves primarily as a mother. Negating their role in the outside world in order to commit to parenting may lead to regret as chances of career development recede but as yet there is no evidence of resentment in this context. ICSI mothers were less hostile and aggressive about their child than naturally conceiving mothers, possibly reflecting overprotective tendencies by suppressing negative feelings about their child. In adolescence, when independence is being established and teenagers have different emotional and behavioural issues compared with younger children, this may have challenging implications. No difference was found in marital difficulties, mental health problems or marital stress between the two groups. No strains were identified in marital or parent–child relationships and no increased risk of negative socio-emotional impact for parents or children.

Maternal age is likely to be associated with different domains of parenting and parenting outcomes. Three distinct parenting theories exist:

1. The 'intuitive parenting' theory[22] suggests that age bears no fixed relation to parenting. It predicts that some parenting cognitions and practices proceed automatically as unconscious and habitual features of parenting (trait conceptualisation of parenting). First-time mothers of all ages engage in a repertoire of parenting practices, including nurturing, physical and social

practices, to meet the fundamental needs of the newborn, that are not linked to maternal age.

2. The second model suggests that age has a linear relationship to parenting. In one respect, there is increased risk in pregnancy and prenatal and perinatal outcomes in ageing mothers but, conversely, increased maturity, experience, understanding and financial capital are positive associations with age. Increasing maternal age is linearly related to greater satisfaction with parenting, greater time commitment to parenting and more optimal observed parenting, controlling for confounding demographic and psychosocial factors.[23] Maternal age is consistently positively associated with richer, more responsive and more abundant talk to infants and toddlers. Rowe *et al.*[24] hypothesised that older mothers may hold different beliefs about child development than younger women and have more experience in communicating in general and thus speak more frequently and with a more diverse vocabulary with their children.

3. Thirdly, Rossi's 'timing of events' model of parenting[25] suggests a curvilinear relationship between age and parenting, such that having a child early or very late was age-inappropriate and off-time compared with age-appropriate on-time births. For example, a U-shaped relationship between maternal age and maternal provision of the material environment was shown in the study by Bornstein *et al.*[26] Both younger and older mothers allowed less exploratory opportunities than the mothers in the middle of the distribution.

In reality, mothers are heterogeneous where age effects are concerned. In their early 20s, adults begin to shift their 'centre of gravity' from their family of origin to their own home base and in their 30s typically develop roots and settle down.[27] Women who time their first birth in their 20s take on the role of parent well before resolution of their own separation and establishment of individuality from their family of origin occurs.[28] Ego strength and maturity are also both associated with responsivity and reciprocity towards infants.[29] Bornstein's data[26] indicate that, for some parenting outcomes, the benefits of maternal maturity reach a plateau at around the age of 30 years, possibly because personality traits tend to stabilise around then. Neugarten[30] stated that in middle age an executive facet to personality develops that is characterised by an increase in an individual's capacity to navigate complex environments and multiple pressures in both personal and interpersonal experiences. Thus the features of parenting may stabilise once certain personality and cognitive functions mature.

Childbearing and rearing

The first months of a newborn's life represent a period of critical adjustment in multiple aspects of parenting. There is a heightened awareness of biological and medical perinatal concerns and parents need support systems to offer help and information and also to aid individual self-definition in the new role. Primiparous women confront the necessity and responsibility of caring for the infant themselves.[31] Social support refers to emotional, instrumental and informational resources available to individuals through relationships with family, friends and others. Support positively influences maternal parenting adjustment, especially in the first few months of the baby's life. Socially supported mothers are less harried, feel less overwhelmed, have fewer competing demands on their time and are therefore more available to their babies.[32] Support from extended families decreases with increasing maternal age, as they are more likely to be involved and supportive of younger mothers with little or no spousal support. Mothers who perceive the father as providing social support have better mental and physical health than those with less support, and their infants also fare better.[33]

Older women possess more life experience and information and therefore may feel more psychologically ready to assume the responsibilities of childrearing. More parenting knowledge is seen in older mothers who reportedly interact with their children in more positive, affectionate, stimulating, sensitive and verbal ways.[23] Despite this, parents who delay first births may lack the capacity and stamina to meet the demands of caregiving, given the decline in physical fitness and health with age. Mothers' perception of their baby's maladjustment in the first month were also linearly correlated with maternal age.[34] Despite the fact that all babies were born at term and healthy, Bornstein's data[26] showed that, with increasing age, mothers perceived infants as more difficult or possibly had more difficulty in coping with the challenges associated with newborn adjustment compared with younger mothers.

The relationship

Older couples are likely to have been in a longer term partnership, on average 3–5 years longer, than younger couples, creating an altered parenting context. Again, there is little research in this area but recent studies have shown that older mothers expressed less warmth towards their partner and perceived less warmth from their partner than younger women. Similarly, older fathers also expressed less warmth to their partner and perceived less warmth from them. This may be due to a continued decline in expressed warmth, love and affection over the course of a relationship.[20] This is a time-related change in the couple relationship rather than one due to parenting at older age.[35] In addition, older mothers and fathers demonstrate more depressive symptoms. In older mothers, depressive symptoms may be menopause related, with greater vasomotor symptoms, sleep disturbance and sexual dysfunction.[20]

Older mothers are likely to be in partnership with older fathers. There is inadequate research on men's experience in this context. It is known that older fathers are more highly involved in parenting and that older mothers share more parenting tasks and rely more significantly on their partner in early infancy. In the study by McMahon et al.[13] in families using ART, male partners in ART families reported lower marital satisfaction, and lower levels of self-esteem were recorded in infertile men than women. Partners of older women also had a more negative social orientation in pregnancy relating to the quality of the relationship, interest in sex and social boredom. In contrast to previous research regarding longer partnership in older couples, in this ART-based study older couples had been in their relationship for less time than younger couples before trying to get pregnant. Potentially, pregnancy early in the relationship compromised marital quality for older men.

The child

Few data on child outcomes in families with older mothers exist beyond infancy. Fergusson and Woodward[36] showed that maternal chronological age at birth uniquely predicts positive educational and psychosocial outcomes in children at 18 years of age, even when controlling for childrearing and home environment. In general, increasing maternal age tended to be associated with more nurturant, supportive and stable home environments. There is no evidence that increasing maternal age is associated with poorer child outcomes or wellbeing in early/middle childhood or psychosocial advantage or disadvantage for children.[13,20] In fact, older mothers provide more sensitivity and richer cognitive experiences in infants than younger mothers. The interaction between maternal age and parenting is not merely related to the timing of events but is highly complex and nuanced.

The long-term considerations in older mothers conceiving by egg donation are issues regarding disclosure to the child and the desire for and capacity to achieve further children, and health-related issues may also emerge as parents move into the fifth decade of life. More research is required, particularly in middle childhood and adolescence, to determine the long-term impact of older parenting and to address the issues raised by young adults caring for their older parents or dealing with early bereavement.

References

1. Office of National Statistics. *Birth Statistics.* Series FM1 no. 35. London: ONS; 2007.
2. Berryman J, Thorpe K , Windridge K. *Older Mothers: Conception, Pregnancy and Birth After 35.* London: Pandora; 1995.
3. Collins J, Croignani PG. Fertility and ageing. *Hum Reprod Update* 2005;11:261–76.
4. Bewley S, Davies M, Braude P. Which career first? *BMJ* 2005;331:588–9.
5. Benzies K, Tough S, Tofflemire K, Frick C, Faber A, Newburn-Cook C. Factors influencing women's decisions about timing of motherhood. *J Obstet Gynecol Neonatal Nurs* 2006;35:625–33.
6. Sutcliffe AG, Ludwig M. Outcomes of assisted reproduction. *Lancet* 2007;370:351–9.
7. Anpananthar A, Sutcliffe AG. Congenital anomalies and assisted reproductive technology. In: Rizk BRMB, Garcia-Velasco JA, Sallam HN, Makrigiannakis A, editors. *Infertility and Assisted Reproduction.* Cambridge: Cambridge University Press; 2008. p. 684–94.
8. Tarin JJ, Brines J, Cano A. Long term effects of delayed parenthood. *Hum Reprod* 1998;13:2371–6.
9. Weiser M, Reichenberg A, Werbeloff N, Kleinhaus K, Lubin G, Shmushkevitch M, *et al.* Advanced parental age at birth is associated with poorer social functioning in adolescent males: shedding light on a core symptom of schizophrenia and autism. *Schizophr Bull* 2008;34:1042–6.
10. Zammit S, Allebeck P, Dalman C, Lundberg I, Hemmingson T, Owen MJ. Paternal age and risk for schizophrenia. *Br J Psychiatry* 2003;183:405–8.
11. Bray I , Gunnell D, Davey Smith G. Advanced paternal age: how old is too old? *J Epidemiol Community Health* 2006;60:851–3.
12. Windridge KC, Berryman JC. Women's experiences of giving birth after 35. *Birth* 1995;26:16–23.
13. McMahon C, Gibson FL, Allen JL, Saunders D. Psycholosocial adjustment during pregnancy for older couples conceiving through assisted reproductive technology. *Hum Reprod* 2007;22:1168–74.
14. Carolan M. 'Doing it properly': The experience of first time mothering over 35 years. *Health Care Women Int* 2005;26:764–87.
15. Hofferth SL. The children of teen childbearers. In: Hofferth SL, Hayes CD, editors. *Risking the Future: Adolescent Sexuality, Pregnancy and Childbearing.* Washington, DC: National Academy Press; 1987. p. 174–206.
16. Colpin H, Demyttenaere K, Vandemeulebroeke L. New reproductive technology and the family: the parent–child relation following *in vitro* fertilisation. *J Child Psychol Psychiatry* 1995;36:1429–41.
17. Van Balen F. Development of IVF children. *Dev Rev* 1998;18:30–46.
18. Golombok S, Brewaeys A, Cook R, Giavazzi MT, Guerra D, Manovani A, *et al.* The European study of assisted reproductive families: family functioning and child development. *Hum Reprod* 1996;11:2324–31.
19. Gibson FL, Ungerer JA, McMahon CA, Leslie GI, Saunders DM. The mother–child relationship following *in vitro* fertilisation (IVF): infant attachment, responsivity and maternal sensitivity. *J Child Psychol Psychiatry* 2000;41:1015–23.
20. Barnes J, Sutcliffe AG, Kristoffersen I, Loft A, Wennerholm U, Tarlatzis BC. The influence of assisted reproduction on family functioning and children's socio-economic development: results from a European study. *Hum Reprod* 2004;19:1480–7.
21. Bene E. *Manual for the Family Relations Test.* 2nd ed. Slough: NFER; 1985.
22. Papousek H, Papousek M. Intuitive parenting. In: Bornstein MH, editors. *Handbook of Parenting: Vol. 2. Biology and Ecology of Parenting.* 2nd ed. Mahwah: Erlbaum; 2002. p. 183–203.

23. Ragozin A, Basham R, Crnic K, Greenberg M, Robinson N. Effects of maternal age on parenting role. *Dev Psychol* 1982;18:627–34.
24. Rowe ML, Pan BA, Ayoub C. Predictors of variation in maternal talk to children: a longitudinal study of low income families. *Parenting: Science and Practice* 2005;5:285–310.
25. Rossi MW. Life-span theories and women's lives. *Signs: J Women Culture Soc* 1980;6:4–32.
26. Bornstein MH, Putnick DL, Suwalsky JTD, Gini M. Maternal chronological age, prenatal and perinatal history, social support, and parenting of infants. *Child Dev* 2006;77:875–92.
27. Smith J, Baltes PB. Life-span perspectives on development. In: Bornstein MH, Lamb ME, editors. *Developmental Psychology: an Advanced Textbook*. 4th ed. Mahwah: Erlbaum; 1999. p. 47–72.
28. Walter CA. The timing of motherhood: The challenge to social workers. *Child Adolesc Social Work* 1989;6:231–44.
29. Cowan CP, Cowan PA. *When Partners Become Parents: the Big Life Change for Couples*. New York: Basic Books; 1992.
30. Neugarten BL. The awareness of middle age. In: Neugarten BL, editor. *Middle Age and Aging*. Chicago: University of Chicago Press; 1968. p. 93–8.
31. Bornstein MH. Parenting infants. In: Bornstein MH, editor. *Handbook of Parenting: Vol.1. Children and Parenting*. 2nd ed. Mahwah: Erlbaum; 2002. p. 3–43.
32. Crnic KA, Greenberg MT. Minor parenting stresses with young children. *Child Dev* 1990;61:1628–37.
33. Levitt MJ, Weber RA, Clark MC. Social network relationships as sources of maternal support and well-being. *Dev Psychol* 1986;22:310–16.
34. Mirowsky J. Parenthood and health: The pivotal and optimal age at first birth. *Social Forces* 2002;81:315–49.
35. Van Laningham J, Johnson DR, Amato P. Marital happiness, marital duration and the U-shaped curve: evidence from a five-wave panel study. *Social Forces* 2001;79:1313–41.
36. Fergusson DM, Woodward LJ. Maternal age and educational and psychosocial outcomes in early adulthood. *J Child Psychol Psychiatry* 1999;40:479–89.

Chapter 17
Consequences of changes in reproductive patterns on later health in women: a life course approach

Gita Mishra and Rachel Cooper

Introduction

This chapter presents a life course approach to the study of how changes in the reproductive patterns of women may affect their future health. A life course approach examines how biological, behavioural and social factors throughout life (and across generations) act independently, cumulatively and interactively to influence reproductive function.[1] Reproductive health throughout a woman's life is influenced by factors *in utero*, in childhood and in the adult environment as well as by intergenerational factors. Reproductive health also acts as a marker for her underlying health and her propensity to suffer from chronic diseases in later life.[1]

Considerable changes in reproductive patterns have occurred over the past few decades, with women having children at later ages and achieving smaller family sizes.[2] However, there have also been secular changes in other factors that influence health in later life. For example, many countries, including the UK, the USA and Australia, have experienced a rise in the prevalence of obesity[3] and a decline in rates of hormone replacement therapy (HRT) use.[4–6] This chapter concludes with a discussion of the implications for research aimed at predicting health in later life and with some recommendations for how future studies should be conducted.

Reproductive function

A woman's reproductive function cannot be directly measured but is instead indicated by a range of reproductive events and characteristics that occur across her reproductive life. Menarche heralds the beginning of a female's reproductive life and menopause signals its end, as defined by the initiation and termination of menses.

Three major themes have emerged from a recent review of the literature on the early life predictors of age at menarche, namely the effects of body size, social circumstances and exposure to unfavourable psychological circumstances.[7] Specifically, the main early life factors associated with early menarche have been established as:

- higher growth rate during childhood[8,9]
- higher childhood socio-economic position[10–14]

■ family conflict and parental divorce[15–17]

■ presence of a stepfather[18]

■ exposure to stressors during or shortly before menarcheal age.[19,20]

In addition, there is evidence for a positive correlation between mother's and daughter's age at menarche.[21]

While the relationships between many adult environmental factors and timing of menopause have been investigated, only cigarette smoking and nulliparity have consistently been related to an earlier menopause.[22–27] Some studies have also found a relationship between adult socio-economic position and the timing of menopause, with those women of lower position experiencing earlier menopause than women of higher position.[28–31] In contrast, and highlighting the importance of a life course perspective on reproductive function, a number of studies have established the link between early life factors and early menopause; these include not having been breastfed, poor early growth, poor socio-economic conditions in childhood, poor cognitive abilities and parental divorce in childhood.[32,33] Family and twin studies have also indicated that the genetic effect on timing of menopause is considerable, with estimates of heritability ranging from 30% to 85%.[34,35] This is supported by evidence from cross-sectional and cohort studies that a woman's age at menopause is strongly associated with her mother's reported age at menopause.[24,25,33,34,36–38]

As the timing of menarche and menopause determines the duration of a woman's reproductive life, they are important markers of reproductive function. Between these two events, however, her reproductive capacity or fecundity is not constant. This is because, as women age, their reproductive systems also age and the quantity and quality of oocytes are constantly declining. Furthermore, exposures to endogenous hormones that influence fertility are constantly changing. While there is variation in the age at which women reach each stage of reproductive life, it is estimated that women are subfertile (that is, they fail to achieve conception within 12 months of attempting) by an average age of 31 years and are sterile by an average age of 41 years.[39] On average, at the age of 46 years women begin to experience menstrual cycle irregularity, which directly precedes menopause, when ovulation and hence menstruation cease entirely.

Identifying the various stages of reproductive life

It is less easy to recognise when women have reached the intermediate stages of their reproductive life, since these are not associated with events that are as clearly defined as menarche and menopause. There are, however, a range of other reproductive events, such as childbirth, and reproductive characteristics, including menstrual regularity and complications during pregnancy, that act as markers of reproductive function and help define what stage in her reproductive life a woman has reached. The various components of a woman's reproductive function are associated with each other and with other factors across life, and even with the reproductive characteristics of previous generations.[21]

Studies have also found positive correlations across generations for age at first parenthood and family size.[21]

Reproductive health as sentinel of chronic disease

Reproductive health, from menarche to menopause, is not only understood as integral to women's overall health and wellbeing but is increasingly recognised as a sentinel of chronic disease in later life.[1,32,40] For example, earlier menarche and later menopause are associated with higher risk of breast cancer[41,42] and may also be associated with an increased risk of endometrial cancer.[43–45] Earlier menarcheal age may also be a risk factor for adult obesity but has minimal impact on cardiovascular risk.[1,46,47]

Until recently, the increased cardiovascular risk in women that is associated with early menopause has been proposed as a consequence of the deprivation of endogenous estrogen.[48] However, the lack of positive benefit of HRT on cardiovascular events in two large-scale clinical trials (Women's Health Initiative, and Heart and Estrogen/progestin Replacement Study, HERS)[49,50] has raised doubts on both the benefit of HRT to prevent cardiovascular events in postmenopausal women and the direction of causality between menopause and cardiovascular risk.[51] In a recent study using data from the Framingham Heart Study, Kok and colleagues found that, for premenopausal women, a higher level of total serum cholesterol, higher blood pressure and higher body weight were associated with an earlier age at menopause. Their study thus supports the view that, since the ovaries are highly vascularised organs, ischaemic damage to the ovaries during reproductive life may induce early menopause.[51]

Osteoporosis and associated fractures are characterised by low bone mineral density and are a major cause of mortality and morbidity. Studies have shown that earlier menarche,[52,53] later menopause and a long reproductive life (the time period between these two events) are all associated with higher bone mineral density.[53,54] It is therefore worth noting that, while longer duration of exposure to reproductive hormones may increase the risk of some cancers such as breast cancers, they are protective against other conditions such as osteoporosis.

In addition to age at menarche and at menopause, other reproductive characteristics such as the health of the mother during pregnancy may also act as a marker of her health in later life. Women with a history of adverse pregnancy outcomes, including pre-eclampsia, pregnancy-induced hypertension, gestational diabetes, preterm delivery and having had low-birthweight babies, appear to be at increased risk of coronary heart disease in later life.[55]

The reproductive characteristics discussed above serve as an illustrative rather than an exhaustive list of the more established relationships, as there are many other health outcomes that are in some way related to reproductive function.

Common risk factors and mechanism

The relationships between reproductive characteristics and chronic diseases in later life observed in the examples above could also be the result of common risk factors that have a direct influence on both reproductive characteristics and chronic diseases.[56] For instance, poor early growth, having a low socio-economic background in childhood and smoking are established risk factors for early menopause and also for coronary heart disease. Therefore, the relationships between age of menopause and coronary heart disease may merely reflect earlier exposures in childhood and adolescence that are the direct determinants of chronic disease, rather than age of menopause being a direct risk factor in its own right. Similarly, fetal programming may be associated with preterm birth, low birth weight and an increased risk of coronary heart disease.[55]

Changing patterns of reproductive function

Menarche

The average age at menarche in Western European countries is currently estimated as being in the range 12.0–13.5 years.[57] Records suggest that there has been a secular decline in age at menarche in industrialised countries since the mid-19th century, when average age at menarche was 15–17 years.[58,59] This decline has been attributed to improvements in the nutritional status, socio-economic conditions and general health of populations. Analyses of data from the second half of the 20th century indicate that in many countries, including the USA, China, Brazil and Mexico, the average age at menarche has continued to decrease, although possibly at slower rates than previously.[57,59,60] However, there is wide variation between countries in the rates of decline and evidence suggests that average age at menarche may have reached a plateau in some countries, including Denmark, the Netherlands, Norway, Belgium and Italy.[57,58] In spite of the link between body size and age at reaching puberty, a study published in 2004 found no evidence for an association between the secular rise in the prevalence of obesity and the decline in average age at menarche.[60]

Menopause

Menopause usually occurs between ages 40 and 60 years,[22,34,61] with the most reliable estimates indicating that the median age at menopause in current populations in western industrialised countries is between 48 and 52 years.[23] While secular changes in age at menopause are less well documented than those for age at menarche, there is some evidence to suggest that over the course of the 20th century there have been modest increases in average age at menopause.[62–64]

Trends in childbearing

The decrease in age at menarche and increase in age at menopause over the last century have resulted in women from more recent generations having, on average, slightly longer reproductive lives than earlier generations. However, changes in patterns of childbearing in the second half of the 20th century have been more dramatic and potentially more important when considering later life health outcomes. When examining demographic trends over the course of the 20th century, it can be seen that the average age of women at childbearing and the fertility rate fluctuate from year to year and trends have not always continued in the same direction. For example, early in the 20th century there was a general decline in the average age at childbearing, from approximately 29.5 years in 1900 to 26.5 years in 1977 in France.[65]

More recently, in countries across the developed world, an important and consistent trend has been the increase in average age of women at childbearing.[65,66] Data from England and Wales analysed by the Office for National Statistics[66] show that the average age of women at childbearing increased from 26.4 years in 1976 to 28.9 years in 1998, with increasing proportions of births occurring to mothers in their 30s and 40s. This pattern is also found in other industrialised countries.[65] The general trend has continued over the past decade in England and Wales, such that in 2004 the fertility rate of women aged 30–34 years overtook that of women aged 25–29 years who have traditionally had higher fertility rates.[2] These increases in the average age at childbearing are not the result of women having more children and thus extending the period of time during which they are having children, but rather they result from women delaying the start of childbearing to later ages. As a consequence, women are having fewer children over the reproductive lifespan. Data from England and Wales show that women born in 1931 had an average of 2.34 liveborn children whereas those women born in 1961 had only 1.96 children.[2]

This shift in the patterns of childbearing are related to a range of cultural and social changes that have occurred in the last few decades of the 20th century. These include improvements in the educational opportunities available to women, their increased participation in the labour force, changing patterns of marriage and cohabitation, and the reduced link between marriage and childbearing (44% of births in England and Wales in 2006 were outside marriage).[2] They are also strongly related to the increased availability and acceptability of effective methods of contraception, which have given women far more control over their own fertility.

By delaying childbearing until their 30s when their fecundity has begun to decline, women are more likely to be subfertile.[39,65] Thus, the reductions seen in total achieved family size may not only be the result of couples choosing to have fewer children but may also be a consequence of the increased likelihood for women who postpone childbearing until their 30s to experience delays in conception. Furthermore, the prevalence of pregnancy-induced complications is much greater in women aged 40 years or over.[67]

Use of assisted reproductive technologies

The difficulty in conceiving naturally for those women who delay childbearing may have also contributed to the increased use of assisted reproductive technologies (ART), such as *in vitro* fertilisation. The rise in popularity of these treatments over the past two decades reflects both the increasing demand for fertility treatments but also their wider acceptability and availability. The number of multiple births reported has increased in recent years, with 15.3 maternities with multiple births per 1000 women giving birth reported in England and Wales in 2006 compared with 13.8 in 1996.[2] This has been attributed by some to the greater use of ART,[68] and is supported by evidence that multiple births are increasing at higher rates among older women.[2]

Can we predict future trends in chronic disease?

To predict future trends in chronic disease for women based on their changing patterns of reproductive characteristics, we need to consider the trends of other risk factors linked to reproductive health and health in later life (Figure 17.1).

Obesity

Over recent decades an increasing proportion of the global population has become overweight or obese.[3] Not only is obesity linked to an array of chronic diseases in later

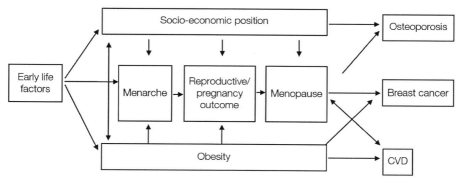

Figure 17.1   The causes and consequences of reproductive ageing: life course approach; CVD = cardiovascular disease

life but it is also associated with early puberty, aberrant menstrual patterns, decreased contraceptive efficacy, ovulatory disorders, an increased miscarriage rate and worse outcomes from ART.[69]

Hormone therapy use

Another potentially important trend has been the change in the use of exogenous hormones. HRT was widely used by women until around 2002 when a number of trials, including the Women's Health Initiative,[50] showed that the harmful effects of HRT use outweighed the benefits that had previously been found in observational studies. After the publication of these results, the use of HRT declined rapidly[4–6] and changes in the practice of prescribing HRT have been implemented whereby fewer women now receive this treatment for preventive health.

Other risk factors

Apart from impacting on health, social inequalities are also linked to differences in reproductive characteristics, such as earlier first births for women from low socio-economic classes.[70] Risks associated with smoking are well understood but the recent legislation across the European Union[71] to ban smoking in public places and work environments may impact on baseline exposure levels to tobacco smoke not seen in recent generations of women. Similarly, other environmental factors may also have a role not previously identified, for instance changes in exposure to both the level and type of pollutants. Many social trends have also emerged relatively recently, such as increasing levels of binge drinking in women, with their effects yet to be fully revealed over the lifespan.[72]

When predicting the likely impact of these trends on health in later life, we need to consider how their effects may act independently, cumulatively or interactively. For instance, reproductive factors detrimental for one chronic disease may be beneficial or protective to another.[1] Moreover, life course research is often based on cohort studies that may have followed a generation of women from birth through to the postmenopausal years (or obtained similar data from recall), so the relevant trends may have occurred when the cohort of women being studied were past their childbearing years. We thus face a complex challenge in predicting the long-term health of women, based on the finding of research on the reproductive health of previous generations, when the factors affecting current women are so different and changing rapidly.

Future research

A life course perspective is essential when characterising the factors affecting reproductive health, especially as they act from early life and previous generations through to environmental and behavioural factors in adulthood. Such a perspective is also important for understanding the impact of reproductive function on health in later life. Three major secular trends have occurred in recent decades: changing reproductive behaviour and technology, rising levels of obesity, and a decline in HRT use. Other trends are manifesting in the lives of younger women, for which it is difficult to apply the findings of previous studies.

In attempting to address these issues, the future study of reproductive health would benefit from a more integrated approach incorporating information from across the life course and intergenerational and family data. Family-based studies (intergenerational, sibling and twin studies) across the life course can be used to test specific causal mechanisms and life course models, as they can help us to understand whether the timing of risk factors (critical and sensitive periods) are important and the role of heritability.[73] By moving beyond associations to understanding the underlying mechanisms that determine reproductive health and the relationships with chronic disease, we will strengthen our ability to predict outcomes and make timely interventions that can benefit current and future generations of young women.

References

1. Rich-Edwards J. A life course approach to women's reproductive health. In: Kuh D, Hardy R, editors. *A Life Course Approach to Women's Health*. Oxford: Oxford University Press, 2002: p. 23–43.
2. Office for National Statistics. Annual update: Births in England and Wales, 2006. *Popul Trends* 2007;130(Web supplement):1–5.
3. Government Office for Science. *Tackling Obesities: Future Choices – Project Report*. Foresight Programme. Runcorn: Department for Innovation, Universities & Skills; 2007.
4. Mishra G, Kok H, Ecob R, Cooper R, Hardy R, Kuh D. Cessation of hormone replacement therapy after reports of adverse findings from randomized controlled trials: evidence from a British birth cohort. *Am J Public Health* 2006;96:1219–25.
5. Usher C, Teeling M, Bennett K, Feely J. Effect of clinical trial publicity on HRT prescribing in Ireland. *Eur J Clin Pharmacol* 2006;62:307–10.
6. de Jong-van den Berg, Faber A, van den Berg PB. HRT use in 2001 and 2004 in the Netherlands – a world of difference. *Maturitas* 2006;54:193–7.
7. Mishra GD, Tom SE, Cooper R, Kuh D. Early life circumstances and their impact on subsequent reproductive health: a review. *Womens Health* 2009;5:175–90.
8. dos Santos Silva I, De Stavola BL, Mann V, Kuh D, Hardy R, Wadsworth ME. Prenatal factors, childhood growth trajectories and age at menarche. *Int J Epidemiol* 2002;31:405–12.
9. Blell M, Pollard TM, Pearce MS. Predictors of age at menarche in the Newcastle Thousand Families Study. *J Biosoc Sci* 2008;40:563–75.
10. Attallah NL, Matta WM, El Mankoushi M. Age at menarche of schoolgirls in Khartoum. *Ann Hum Biol* 1983;10:185–8.
11. Billewicz WZ, Fellowes HM, Thomson AM. Menarche in Newcastle upon Tyne girls. *Ann Hum Biol* 1981;8:313–20.
12. Ulijaszek SJ, Evans E, Miller DS. Age at menarche of European, Afro-Caribbean and Indo-Pakistani schoolgirls living in London. *Ann Hum Biol* 1991;18:167–75.
13. Rao S, Joshi S, Kanade A. Height velocity, body fat and menarcheal age of Indian girls. *Indian Pediatr* 1998;35:619–28.
14. Oduntan SO, Ayeni O, Kale OO. The age of menarche in Nigerian girls. *Ann Hum Biol* 1976;3:269–74.
15. Bogaert AF. Age at puberty and father absence in a national probability sample. *J Adolesc* 2005;28:541–6.
16. Bogaert AF. Menarche and father absence in a national probability sample. *J Biosoc Sci* 2008;40:623–36.
17. Romans SE, Martin JM, Gendall K, Herbison GP. Age of menarche: the role of some psychosocial factors. *Psychol Med* 2003;33:933–9.
18. Mendle J, Turkheimer E, D'Onofrio BM, Lynch SK, Emery RE, Slutske WS, *et al*. Family structure and age at menarche: a children-of-twins approach. *Dev Psychol* 2006;42:533–42.
19. Pesonen AK, Raikkonen K, Heinonen K, Kajantie E, Forsen T, Eriksson JG. Reproductive traits following a parent–child separation trauma during childhood: a natural experiment during World War II. *Am J Hum Biol* 2008;20:345–51.
20. Mul D, Oostdijk W, Drop SL. Early puberty in adopted children. *Horm Res* 2002;57:1–9.
21. Morton SM, Rich-Edwards J. How family based studies have added to understanding the life course epidemiology of reproductive health. In: Lawlor D, Mishra G, editors. *Family Matters:*

Designing, Analysing and Understanding Family Based Studies in Life Course Epidemiology. Oxford: Oxford University Press; 2009. p. 295–315.

22. Bromberger JT, Matthews KA, Kuller LH, Wing RR, Meilahn EN, Plantinga P. Prospective study of the determinants of age at menopause. *Am J Epidemiol* 1997;145:124–33.

23. Hardy R, Kuh D, Wadsworth M. Smoking, body mass index, socioeconomic status and the menopausal transition in a British national cohort. *Int J Epidemiol* 2000;29:845–51.

24. van Asselt KM, Kok HS, Der Schouw YT, Grobbee DE, te Velde ER, Pearson PL, *et al.* Current smoking at menopause rather than duration determines the onset of natural menopause. *Epidemiology* 2004;15:634–9.

25. Cramer DW, Xu H, Harlow BL. Does 'incessant' ovulation increase risk for early menopause? *Am J Obstet Gynecol* 1995;172:568–73.

26. Discigil G, Gemalmaz A, Tekin N, Basak O. Profile of menopausal women in west Anatolian rural region sample. *Maturitas* 2006;55:247–54.

27. Hardy R, Kuh D. Reproductive characteristics and the age at inception of the perimenopause in a British National Cohort. *Am J Epidemiol* 1999;149:612–20.

28. Do KA, Treloar SA, Pandeya N, Purdie D, Green AC, Heath AC, *et al.* Predictive factors of age at menopause in a large Australian twin study. *Hum Biol* 1998;70:1073–91.

29. Shinberg DS. An event history analysis of age at last menstrual period: correlates of natural and surgical menopause among midlife Wisconsin women. *Soc Sci Med* 1998;46:1381–96.

30. Torgerson DJ, Avenell A, Russell IT, Reid DM. Factors associated with onset of menopause in women aged 45–49. *Maturitas* 1994;19:83–92.

31. Wise LA, Krieger N, Zierler S, Harlow BL. Lifetime socioeconomic position in relation to onset of perimenopause. *J Epidemiol Community Health* 2002;56:851–60.

32. Hardy R, Mishra G, Kuh D. Life course risk factors for menopause and diseases in later life. In: Keith L, editor. *Menopause, Postmenopause and Ageing*. London: Royal Society of Medicine Press; 2005. p. 11–19.

33. Mishra G, Hardy R, Kuh D. Are the effects of risk factors for timing of menopause modified by age? Results from a British birth cohort study. *Menopause* 2007;14:717–24.

34. Kok HS, van Asselt KM, van der Schouw YT, Peeters PH, Wijmenga C. Genetic studies to identify genes underlying menopausal age. *Hum Reprod Update* 2005;11:483–93.

35. van Asselt KM, Kok HS, Pearson PL, Dubas JS, Peeters PH, te Velde ER, *et al.* Heritability of menopausal age in mothers and daughters. *Fertil Steril* 2004;82:1348–51.

36. de Bruin JP, Bovenhuis H, van Noord PA, Pearson PL, van Arendonk JA, te Velde ER, *et al.* The role of genetic factors in age at natural menopause. *Hum Reprod* 2001;16:2014–18.

37. Murabito JM, Yang Q, Fox C, Wilson PW, Cupples LA. Heritability of age at natural menopause in the Framingham Heart Study. *J Clin Endocrinol Metab* 2005;90:3427–30.

38. Torgerson DJ, Thomas RE, Reid DM. Mothers and daughters menopausal ages: is there a link? *Eur J Obstet Gynecol Reprod Biol* 1997;74:63–6.

39. Broekmans FJ, Knauff EA, te Velde ER, Macklon NS, Fauser BC. Female reproductive ageing: current knowledge and future trends. *Trends Endocrinol Metab* 2007;18:58–65.

40. Barsom SH, Dillaway HE, Koch PB, Ostrowski ML, Mansfield PK. The menstrual cycle and adolescent health. *Ann N Y Acad Sci* 2008;1135:52–7.

41. Kelsey JL, Gammon MD, John EM. Reproductive factors and breast cancer. *Epidemiol Rev* 1993;15:36–47.

42. Hsieh CC, Trichopoulos D, Katsouyanni K, Yuasa S. Age at menarche, age at menopause, height and obesity as risk factors for breast cancer: associations and interactions in an international case–control study. *Int J Cancer* 1990;46:796–800.

43. Wernli KJ, Ray RM, Gao DL, De Roos AJ, Checkoway H, Thomas DB. Menstrual and reproductive factors in relation to risk of endometrial cancer in Chinese women. *Cancer Causes Control* 2006;17:949–55.

44. Xu WH, Xiang YB, Ruan ZX, Zheng W, Cheng JR, Dai Q, *et al.* Menstrual and reproductive factors and endometrial cancer risk: Results from a population-based case–control study in urban Shanghai. *Int J Cancer* 2004;108:613–19.

45. Pettersson B, Adami HO, Bergstrom R, Johansson ED. Menstruation span – a time-limited risk factor for endometrial carcinoma. *Acta Obstet Gynecol Scand* 1986;65:247–55.

46. Harris MA, Prior JC, Koehoorn M. Age at menarche in the Canadian population: secular trends and relationship to adulthood BMI. *J Adolesc Health* 2008;43:548–54.

47. Kivimaki M, Lawlor DA, Smith GD, Elovainio M, Jokela M, Keltikangas-Jarvinen L, et al. Association of age at menarche with cardiovascular risk factors, vascular structure, and function in adulthood: the Cardiovascular Risk in Young Finns study. *Am J Clin Nutr* 2008;87:1876–82.

48. Matthews KA, Meilahn E, Kuller LH, Kelsey SF, Caggiula AW, Wing RR. Menopause and risk factors for coronary heart disease. *N Engl J Med* 1989;321:641–6.

49. Hulley S, Grady D, Bush T, Furberg C, Herrington D, Riggs B, et al. Randomized trial of estrogen plus progestin for secondary prevention of coronary heart disease in postmenopausal women. Heart and Estrogen/progestin Replacement Study (HERS) Research Group. *JAMA* 1998;280:605–13.

50. Rossouw JE, Anderson GL, Prentice RL, LaCroix AZ, Kooperberg C, Stefanick ML, et al. Risks and benefits of estrogen plus progestin in healthy postmenopausal women: principal results from the Women's Health Initiative randomized controlled trial. *JAMA* 2002;288:321–33.

51. Kok HS, van Asselt KM, van der Schouw YT, van der Tweel I, Peeters PH, Wilson PW, et al. Heart disease risk determines menopausal age rather than the reverse. *J Am Coll Cardiol* 2006;47:1976–83.

52. Ito M, Yamada M, Hayashi K, Ohki M, Uetani M, Nakamura T. Relation of early menarche to high bone mineral density. *Calcif Tissue Int* 1995;57:11–14.

53. Li HL, Zhu HM. [Relationship between the age of menarche, menopause and other factors and postmenopause osteoporosis]. *Zhonghua Fu Chan Ke Za Zhi* 2005;40:796–8.

54. Osei-Hyiaman D, Satoshi T, Ueji M, Hideto T, Kano K. Timing of menopause, reproductive years, and bone mineral density: a cross-sectional study of postmenopausal Japanese women. *Am J Epidemiol* 1998;148:1055–61.

55. Sattar N, Greer IA. Pregnancy complications and maternal cardiovascular risk: opportunities for intervention and screening? *BMJ* 2002;325:157–60.

56. Kuh D, Hardy R. A life course approach to women's health: linking the past, present, and future. In: Kuh D, Hardy R, editors. *A Life Course Approach to Women's Health.* Oxford: Oxford University Press; 2002. p. 397–412.

57. Parent AS, Teilmann G, Juul A, Skakkebaek NE, Toppari J, Bourguignon JP. The timing of normal puberty and the age limits of sexual precocity: Variations around the world, secular trends, and changes after migration. *Endocr Rev* 2003;24:668–93.

58. Ong KK, Ahmed ML, Dunger DB. Lessons from large population studies on timing and tempo of puberty (secular trends and relation to body size): The European trend. *Mol Cell Endocrinol* 2006;254:8–12.

59. Kaplowitz P. Pubertal development in girls: secular trends. *Curr Opin Obstet Gynecol* 2006;18:487–91.

60. Demerath EW, Towne B, Chumlea WC, Sun SS, Czerwinski SA, Remsberg KE, et al. Recent decline in age at menarche: The fels longitudinal study. *Am J Hum Biol* 2004;16:453–7.

61. van Noord PA, Dubas JS, Dorland M, Boersma H, te VE. Age at natural menopause in a population-based screening cohort: the role of menarche, fecundity, and lifestyle factors. *Fertil Steril* 1997;68:95–102.

62. Flint M. Is there a secular trend in age of menopause? *Maturitas* 1978;1:133–9.

63. Flint MP. Secular trends in menopause age. *J Psychosom Obstet Gynaecol* 1997;18:65–72.

64. Rodstrom K, Bengtsson C, Milsom I, Lissner L, Sundh V, Bjourkelund C. Evidence for a secular trend in menopausal age: a population study of women in Gothenburg. *Menopause* 2003;10:538–43.

65. Baird DT, Collins J, Egozcue J, Evers LH, Gianaroli L, Leridon H, et al. Fertility and ageing. *Hum Reprod Update* 2005;11:261–76.

66. Botting B, Dunnell K. Trends in fertility and contraception in the last quarter of the 20th century. *Popul Trends* 2000;100:32–9.

67. Seoud MA, Nassar AH, Usta IM, Melhem Z, Kazma A, Khalil AM. Impact of advanced maternal age on pregnancy outcome. *Am J Perinatol* 2002;19:1–8.

68. Collins J. Global epidemiology of multiple birth. *Reprod Biomed Online* 2007;15:45–52.

69.   Lash MM, Armstrong A. Impact of obesity on women's health. *Fertil Steril* 2008 Apr 12 [Epub ahead of print].

70.   Imamura M, Tucker J, Hannaford P, da Silva MO, Astin M, Wyness L, *et al.* Factors associated with teenage pregnancy in the European Union countries: a systematic review. *Eur J Public Health* 2007;17:630–6.

71.   Boessen S, Maarse H. The impact of the treaty basis on health policy legislation in the European Union: a case study on the tobacco advertising directive. *BMC Health Serv Res* 2008;8:77.

72.   Jefferis BJ, Manor O, Power C. Social gradients in binge drinking and abstaining: trends in a cohort of British adults. *J Epidemiol Community Health* 2007;61:150–3.

73.   Lawlor DA, Mishra GD. *Family Matters: Designing, Analysing and Understanding Family Based Studies in Life Course Epidemiology*. Oxford: Oxford University Press; 2009.

Chapter 18
The outcomes: children and mothers

Discussion

Stephen Hillier: This distribution of age of onset of menopause – you gave a median but there were two populations. Is that statistically significant?

Gita Mishra: Yes. The actual distribution you saw is skewed. That's the observed distribution and it is definitely not a normal distribution. So, we think that distribution fits these data well. It turns out that this skewed distribution is a mixture of two distributions; one distribution is normal with an early age of menopause around 40, and the other one is normal with a mean age around 50. If you simulate these data with normal distribution with these two and you mix it, a third and two-thirds, you get a distribution that fits the observed distribution perfectly.

Stephen Hillier: Perhaps this is a naïve question, but have you tried to relate any of the other factors independently to the two groups to see whether there is any difference?

Gita Mishra: Yes. We found a lot of early factors determine you to be in this [earlier] distribution and there was an interaction. For instance, the mother's age of menopause: if the mother had a very early age menopause the person was more likely to be in the earlier distribution. Weight at 2 years: if a child was lighter at 2 years old then she is more likely to be in the first distribution. And the other thing that was quite surprising was the effect of parental divorce.

Stephen Hillier: That is interesting. You showed another graph showing that in this lifelong study sterility and fertility kicked in before the menopause. You implied that there was a causative effect of divorce on menopause. But isn't it more likely that people get divorced because they are having reproductive problems that portend the menopause?

Gita Mishra: You are absolutely right to question it. This study was done in 1946. Remember the women are already born; it's in the 1950s that their parents are having a divorce. The way we see this is that the children are being put into a stressful situation at earlier in life. Similarly, if they came from a parental manual background they had earlier menopause. What we think is that something early in their life, the stressful environment, must have triggered something in the rate of decline of all oocytes. We don't know but these are all very early developmental factors that tend to affect later life.

Donna Dickerson: Wonderful insight. I have a question for each of you please. Does the effect for divorce also hold for death of a parent? And do you think that the reasons are the same?

Gita Mishra: Yes it does. You are absolutely right because one of our hypotheses is putting them under early stress. And so we did look at both factors: the death of their parents when they were a child, or the divorce, or both. The numbers were not that great so we put them together. We looked at both separately and then combined. Exactly the same effect. So, stress does play a part.

Donna Dickerson: And for Alastair, let us go to the lesser degree of warmth that partners share with each other compared with the considerable degree of warmth they share with the child. Can I cynically suggest that's because they are married longer? [laughter]

Alastair Sutcliffe: That is one suspicion.

Donna Dickerson: Or is it possibly also that because they have become more used to an autonomous lifestyle or more independent? Do you have any other ideas or hypotheses why this is?

Alastair Sutcliffe: Married longer was the thing I thought of, but it's speculation.

David Barlow: A question to each speaker about the very same issue about the older couples and the analyses you are reporting. Fertility services are working a lot with these older couples who are looking for a pregnancy because they're reformulated relationships and so if you get success you will be able to have kids, but they often have baggage and a background of other families and other offspring. Can your research disentangle those two situations? I wonder whether you can disentangle offspring.

Alastair Sutcliffe: I will go back to the literature and look at the important point about confounders. They might be on the second relationship.

David Barlow: Gita, the issue of menopause we heard in your analysis – if women have hysterectomies, how did you handle that?

Gita Mishra: In my chapter, I looked at the age of natural menopause. We have done a lot of analyses, competitive risks analyses, where we looked at those who went through natural menopause and compared them with others; that is, those on HRT [hormone replacement therapy] (because you can't actually tell what their age of menopause is). There is a third group of women that had hysterectomy. So, we have done series of competitive risks analyses and work on hysterectomy because these women already have high risk of cardiovascular disease. We have written them up[1] – this was really about natural menopause.

Roger Gosden: This is an observation addressed to the convenors more than the speakers. I had some concern that the final report would be totally pessimistic and also I was worried about the perceptions of professional and business women. They might feel that this report did not reflect all of their experiences as older mothers, where they are, of course, an over-represented group. I thought Alastair's presentation was the first time we actually addressed this question and try to find something positive to say. One of the ways we could perhaps deal with this in a recommendation draws on this point. I also found in my trawl of the literature that there is very little good research on parenting, the experiences of parenting and outcomes of parenting for older parents. I think a call for more research in this area would be very desirable.

William Ledger: Is there a relationship between the age of menarche and the age of menopause? I didn't quite catch that in your presentation.

Gita Mishra: There isn't.

William Ledger: This lack of a relationship fits with what others have shown, but it is not what most women think. They think if they started their periods early, they will finish early. My other question is about the data linking HRT discontinuation with breast cancer. It seems to me, knowing a little bit about the biology of cancer, that there is usually a long latent phase before cancer becomes detectable clinically. Doesn't it surprise you that there is such a sudden decrease in the number of cancers so soon after the decline in HRT use? One would assume there would be a longer lag phase.

Gita Mishra: There isn't any work that's been done linking the two. The only study that's come up is the Australian one.[2] They say that if they adjust for everything they do find a decrease in the rate of cancer. It takes a while for the effect to kick in. But that's what they've shown and it would be interesting to see what's the aetiology

William Ledger: We have to wait a few more years to see the trend.

David Barlow: There are insufficient data around the world to know, but if it is showing anything it's probably an accelerated effect on estrogen receptor-positive cancer rather than HRT having a role in initiation. Many who argue one way or the other about initiation would accept acceleration. If you're pulling out something that causes acceleration then you might well find the rate falling quite quickly, as opposed to when the cancer has started.

Diana Mansour: Depending on the state, the USA and Australia don't have a call–recall breast screening programme. I think we will see some better data from Scandinavia and ourselves.

Maya Unnithan: Did you find stigma for older mothers? And how does that affect their relationships with their children?

Alastair Sutcliffe: I think the stigma is with the child rather than on the parents themselves. When they go to school and they report things like 'my parents were older than other people', 'being mistaken for grandparents' – that kind of thing. These were just quotes from children.

Peter Braude: Talking about the question about breast cancer and older age, what you proposed is not new. I am reminded about talking to Roger Gosden and Roger Short at the Royal Society in 1974.[3] With the evolution of reproduction, women may go to menopause. The natural state for women is lactation. Menstruation all the time is completely unphysiological. That breasts are exposed to cyclical estrogen and progesterone for so many years is a completely artificial phenomenon, not natural. This may be one of the factors that influence or increase the risk of breast cancer. You can have the pill, maybe change your lifestyle, or use different kinds of contraception which totally change the lifelong exposure to estrogen or progesterone.

Susan Bewley: Alastair, you talked about adverse childhood events and I've been impressed by the excellent American ACE study [Adverse Childhood Experiences] which shows the long-term devastating effects of the loss of a parent, whether by death, divorce or prison.[4] Is there a way to understand whether children themselves are binding or stressing to a relationship? Parenting must be different in an unwanted, unsupported pregnancy as opposed to a wanted and planned pregnancy, and different again in those pregnancies that are neither – the happy accidents. Is there any evidence about whether a child would bind parents more warmly or drive them apart even in a relationship with a wanted child?

Alastair Sutcliffe: They are ways of looking at child stress – in total we used about eight like these and you can see how the child made the checklist. We can also measure child stress in relation to the stresses within a relationship in the family. I am not sure that such issues have been specifically studied to date.

Susan Bewley: Sometimes we go to weddings and say 'Oh, it will never last!' [laughter] Is there any work on the prediction of relationships that will stick or not? I ask because of that devastating effect on the children, accepting that there's probably nothing you could do about it. You've seen wiser, older people being cooler together but sticking to the child. And this is very reassuring, as Roger said. Now that we lead controlled, autonomous lives when we can choose children, are there predictive factors for the stable setting, years down the line, for the benefit of those children?

Alastair Sutcliffe: There is a lot of evidence about what makes a relationship successful or not – socio-economic status and a whole variety of things. I am not sure there is any relation to how many children you have and at what age you have them. There's certainly a need for research.

Melanie Davies: There's a lot of good news, also, is there not, around parenting and family stability for assisted conception children as well? Susan Golombok's work on egg donation,[5] and also single women,[6] although not specifically about older women, did have very good short-term data about outcome. Gita, is this is the only cohort study or are there other comparable data? There was another cohort who are now in their 70s.[7] They went through school exams and the best predictor of menopause was cognitive function in childhood.

Gita Mishra: Yes, there are other cohorts with comparable data, such as the British birth cohorts: the 1958 birth cohort, the 1970 birth cohort and the millennium birth cohort. There are also other cohorts based on participants from a particular area, such as ALSPAC [Avon Longitudinal Study of Parents and their Children] and the Aberdeen children of the 1950s study. However, the 1946 cohort is one of the oldest-running studies with detailed data on women's health.

Finbarr Martin: I'm a geriatrician. You made a wonderful observation and I'd also like to ask a question about your relationship between the early menopause group and degenerative diseases in old age. As you'll know, you chose to record parental divorce, but the association with the time of death from many degenerative diseases, when talking about cardiovascular-respiratory, is very closely associated with parental divorce for certain cohorts, particularly where that is associated with social status and socio-economic level. It seems likely to me that that will be another example of that same specific phenomenon. Although you might call it stress, it may actually perhaps be something slightly different from stress and not fully explained by socio-economics but partly by that – and that is the observation. The other question is that you mentioned early menopause being the earliest sign of ageing, but it is complicated by the fact that many things, such as sarcopenia and osteoporosis, a lot of processes are associated potentially with estrogens but there are maybe some things that are not. I wonder whether there are any early observations of instances of other age-related phenomena (for example, cataracts) occurring earlier in old age in women who experienced an early menopause. This would seem to me to be a necessary condition to suggest that early menopause is indicative of general ageing rather than specifically ovarian ageing.

Gita Mishra: One of the drawbacks is that we do not have clinical/biological data during the menopause. We have anthropometric data such as blood pressure. In the ideal world we would have obtained data before they hit menopause. Then we could see what happens, whether they were really showing signs of degenerative diseases. Results from our study[8] have shown that women with higher cognitive ability have later menopause.

References

1. Kuh D, Langenberg C, Hardy R, Kok H, Cooper R, Butterworth S, Wadsworth ME. Cardiovascular risk at age 53 years in relation to the menopause transition and use of hormone replacement therapy: a prospective British birth cohort study. *BJOG* 2005;112:476–85.

2. Canfell K, Banks E, Moa AM, Beral V. Decrease in breast cancer incidence following a rapid fall in use of hormone replacement therapy in Australia. *Med J Aust* 2008;188:641–4.

3. Short RV. The evolution of human reproduction. *Proc R Soc Lond B Biol Sci* 1976;195:3–24.

4. Centers for Disease Control and Prevention. *Adverse Childhood Experiences Study* [www.cdc.gov/ nccdphp/ace/index.htm].

5. Golombok S, Murray C, Brinsden P, Abdalla H. Social versus biological parenting: family functioning and the socioemotional development of children conceived by egg or sperm donation. *J Child Psychol Psychiatry* 1999;40:519–27.

6. Golombok S, Tasker F, Murray C. Children raised in fatherless families from infancy: family relationships and the socioemotional development of children of lesbian and single heterosexual mothers. *J Child Psychol Psychiatry* 1997;38:783–91.

7. Kuh D, Butterworth S, Kok H, Richards M, Hardy R, Wadsworth ME, Leon DA. Childhood cognitive ability and age at menopause: evidence from two cohort studies. *Menopause* 2005;12:475–82.

8. Kok HS, Kuh D, Cooper R, van der Schouw YT, Grobbee DE, Wadsworth ME, *et al*. Cognitive function across the life course and the menopausal transition in a British birth cohort. *Menopause* 2006;13:19–27.

Section 5

Future fertility insurance: screening, cryopreservation or egg donors?

Chapter 19
Screening for early ovarian ageing

Abha Maheshwari, Ahmed Gibreel and Siladitya Bhattacharya

Introduction

Ovarian ageing is thought to be caused by a decrease in the number of primordial follicles and/or a decline in the quality of the oocytes within them. Oocyte numbers within the fetal ovary peak at 20 weeks of gestation, subsequently falling to 1–2 million at birth. Thereafter, the rate of atresia within the oocyte pool remains relatively constant until the age of 37.5 years, when there is an accelerated diminution in oocyte numbers, which fall to around 1000 at menopause (51 years).[1] However, incipient ovarian senescence may start many years earlier, and one in 100 women can expect to experience premature menopause before the age of 40 years.[2] It has been suggested that there is a 13-year window between the beginning of an accelerated phase of follicular atresia (age 38 years) and menopause itself (age 51 years), during which menstrual cyclicity is maintained but fecundity is significantly reduced.[3] Thus, a woman who enters natural menopause at the age of 45 years could have begun the process of accelerated atresia (early ovarian ageing) at the age of 32 years. It is this period of silent ovarian ageing that offers a window for appropriate screening. In this chapter, we consider the rationale for ovarian reserve testing, examine the attributes of an ideal test and review the predictive value of a number of common tests. We conclude by discussing the suitability of these tests for inclusion in a screening strategy for early ovarian ageing.

Rationale for tests of ovarian ageing

Age is acknowledged to be the single most important determinant of fertility in women. However, the presence of significant variability in reproductive performance among women of the same age underlines the need for accurate tests for biological ovarian age. This is particularly relevant at the present time, when increasing numbers of women choosing to defer childbirth face a potential future risk of subfertility due to early ovarian ageing. The term 'ovarian ageing' is used interchangeably with 'compromised ovarian reserve', where ovarian reserve relates to the functional potential of the ovary and reflects the number and quality of oocytes within it. A number of tests of ovarian reserve have been developed to meet the following clinical needs:

■ **Prediction of early ovarian ageing**. Tests that predict the risk of early ovarian ageing in a general population are particularly relevant for women choosing to delay their first pregnancy. Ideally, the tests should indicate whether a woman is at a higher risk of decline in fertility than could be predicted from age alone. These tests may be particularly useful in assessing women at risk of early ovarian failure following ovarian surgery, chemotherapy or radiotherapy.

■ **Management of women attending subfertility clinics**. Tests that predict the chances of pregnancy and live birth (with or without treatment) are helpful in deciding whether to proceed with assisted reproductive technologies (ART). These tests can also help in the selection of the most appropriate treatment and the optimal dose of gonadotrophins for ovarian stimulation.

Assessing the quality of a test of ovarian reserve

The key features of a diagnostic test for ovarian reserve are described in Table 19.1.[4] A positive likelihood ratio (LR+) above 10 represents a highly accurate test and an LR+ of 5–10 a moderately accurate test. LR+ values of 2–5 suggest a test with poor accuracy, 1–2 very poor accuracy and 1 indicates a worthless test. A receiver operating characteristic (ROC) curve depicts the continuing relationship between sensitivity and specificity with shifting threshold values for a given test. The area under an ROC curve (AUC) provides information on the discriminatory capacity of the test. Values of 1.0 imply a perfect test while a value of 0.5 indicates complete lack of discrimination. From a clinical perspective, the most relevant outcome that a test must predict should be live birth or, at the very least, pregnancy. However, most available tests have tended to focus on surrogate outcomes such as ovarian response, as defined by the number of oocytes retrieved in an *in vitro* fertilisation (IVF) cycle.

What are the available tests of ovarian reserve?

A number of tests have been used to predict ovarian ageing/poor ovarian reserve (Box 19.1). Despite the large number of tests in current use, an ideal test has yet to be developed. The most comprehensive systematic review for tests of ovarian reserve concluded that an IVF cycle itself may be a more reliable predictor of ovarian response to stimulation than any of the existing tests.[5] For the purpose of this chapter, we have concentrated on the predictive value of four of the most commonly used tests.

Table 19.1   Important features of a diagnostic test for ovarian reserve; reproduced with permission from Jain *et al.*[4]

Feature	Question addressed
Sensitivity	How good is this test at picking up women who cannot conceive?
Specificity	How good is this test at correctly excluding women who can conceive?
Positive predictive value	If a woman has an abnormal test, what is the probability that she cannot conceive?
Negative predictive value	If a woman has a normal test, what is the probability that she can conceive?
Likelihood ratio of a positive test	How much more likely is an abnormal test to be found in a woman who cannot conceive than in a woman who can?
Likelihood ratio of a negative test	How much more likely is a normal test to be found in a woman who can conceive than in a woman who cannot?

Box 19.1	Tests of ovarian reserve

1. Basal serum follicle-stimulating hormone (FSH)
2. Basal serum estradiol
3. Basal luteinising hormone (LH)/FSH ratio
4. Basal serum inhibin B level
5. Serum anti-müllerian hormone level
6. Basal ovarian volume
7. Antral follicle count
8. Ovarian stromal blood flow
9. Ovarian biopsy
10. Clomifene citrate challenge test (CCCT)
11. Gonadotrophin-releasing hormone (GnRH) agonist stimulation test (GAST)
12. Exogenous FSH ovarian reserve test (EFORT)

Basal serum follicle–stimulating hormone

Early follicular phase fluctuations in follicle-stimulating hormone (FSH) reflect the balance between ovarian steroid production, peptide inhibition and hypothalamic–pituitary drive. Basal serum FSH is an indirect measure of the size of the follicle cohort and is regulated by a variety of factors, including inhibins, activins, estradiol and follistatins.[6] Appropriate timing of FSH measurement is important but this is difficult for women with irregular periods, such as those with polycystic ovary syndrome (PCOS). In addition, intercycle and intersample variations (within assay and between assays) can confound test results.[7] Most IVF units tend to use basal serum FSH levels (measured on day 3 of the menstrual cycle) as an indicator of ovarian responsiveness but the available evidence does not suggest that it has high predictive value.[8] Defining an abnormal test result is problematic, as a wide range (4–25 iu/ml) in cut-off values are in use.[9] The limitations of serum FSH in this context are now recognised[10] and its use as a routine test in the prediction of IVF outcome has been questioned.[9]

Away from assisted reproduction, the role of day 3 FSH in the evaluation of ovarian reserve in young healthy women is even more limited.[8] Elevated FSH levels in younger women may be related to receptor polymorphisms rather than reduced ovarian reserve.[11] Although relatively simple to perform, basal serum FSH does not accurately diagnose poor ovarian reserve until high cut-off values are used and the test has very limited capacity in terms of predicting pregnancy.[5]

Antral follicle count

The antral follicle count (AFC) is the number of small ovarian follicles measuring 2–10 mm in diameter visualised by transvaginal ultrasound scan. An age-related decline in the AFC has been observed[12] and AFC has attracted considerable interest in recent years as a test of ovarian reserve. A systematic review has demonstrated the superiority of AFC over basal FSH in the prediction of poor ovarian response[13] but interpreting AFC results can be challenging. Definitions of what constitutes an antral follicle have tended to vary, with cited diameters ranging from 2–10 and 2–5 mm. Moreover, there is considerable variation in terms of what is considered to be a normal count.[13] There can also be a degree of intercycle variability in AFC,[14–16] especially in young women and in women with large numbers of antral follicles. A low AFC in young, infertile but ovulatory women should be interpreted with caution as this may not necessarily indicate poor ovarian reserve.

It has been suggested that AFC is better than either age or FSH in predicting pregnancy in older women aged between 38 and 44 years,[17] but not in a general population of women undergoing IVF.[5] In a systematic review by Gibreel et al. in 2008,[18] the likelihood ratio of a positive test to predict nonpregnancy at a cut-off value of fewer than four antral follicles (AFC < 4) was 7.77 (95% CI 2.20–27.45). However, it is very rare to find values as low as this in young, regularly cycling women.

Serum inhibin B

Inhibin is a heterodimeric glycoprotein consisting of α and β subunits. There are two distinct molecular forms of the β subunit, βA and βB, and, when combined with an α subunit, these form inhibin A and inhibin B, respectively. Inhibin B is mainly produced by the granulosa cells in growing follicles and offers a more immediate assessment of ovarian activity than other serum tests. A fall in day 3 inhibin B levels may predict poor ovarian reserve before the expected rise in day 3 FSH.[19–21] The highest sensitivity (81%) and specificity (81%) for prediction of oocyte yield in IVF was obtained at a cut-off value of 56 pg/ml.[25] The odds ratio for clinical pregnancy was 6.8 (95% CI 1.8–25.6) in women with basal serum inhibin B levels of more than 45 pg/ml compared with women with lower levels.[26]

However, not all studies support the use of inhibin B as a predictive marker in IVF.[22,23] Serum levels are influenced by total body fat content and follicles of women who are obese produce less inhibin B those those in their lean counterparts.[24] In addition, there is a lack of universal agreement regarding appropriate cut-off values for predicting poor response; these have been reported to vary from 45 to 105.3 pg/ml.

Serum antimüllerian hormone

Antimüllerian hormone (AMH), also known as müllerian inhibiting substance, belongs to a superfamily of dimeric glycoproteins that are structurally related to transforming growth factor-beta (TGFβ). It is produced by granulosa cells of recruited ovarian follicles before they become sensitive to FSH.[6] AMH regulates follicle recruitment, thus preventing depletion of the entire primordial follicle pool at once.[27] As serum AMH levels decline with advancing female age, it has therefore been identified as a predictor of ovarian response and ovarian reserve.[28–31] AMH is the only marker of ovarian reserve that can be tested for in both follicular and luteal phases of the cycle, although cut-off levels in both phases need to be standardised. AMH levels have been found to be two to three times higher in women with PCOS, making it difficult to find a cut-off value for poor ovarian reserve without a significant overlap with normal values.[32–34]

A number of studies have commented on the fact that AMH appears to be a good test for ovarian response but less successful in predicting pregnancy.[35–38] Interpretation of test results is confounded by the fact that the definition of poor ovarian response varies[39] and there is no consensus on appropriate cut-off values for an abnormal test. The summary ROC curve (Figure 19.1a) for prediction of nonpregnancy runs close to the line of equality, indicating that the test has little predictive value for pregnancy. Comparison with AFC indicates that AMH behaves in a very similar manner in terms of prediction of poor response as well as nonpregnancy (Figure 19.1b). Overall, AMH has a number of advantages as a screening test. Its level corresponds well with AFC, it remains constant throughout the menstrual cycle and it has superior intercycle reproducibility compared with FSH and AFC.[40–43]

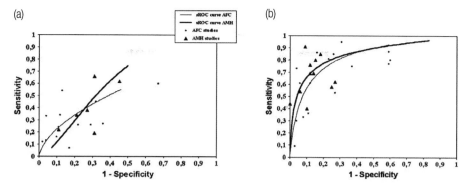

Figure 19.1 Summary receiver operating characteristic curves: (a) accuracy of predictions of nonpregnancy; (b) accuracy of prediction of poor response; reproduced with permission from Broer *et al.*[40]

Other tests

The clomifene citrate challenge test (CCCT), gonadotrophin-releasing hormone (GnRH) agonist stimulation test (GAST) and exogenous FSH ovarian reserve test (EFORT) have not been found to be useful, even in women undergoing ART.[44] Ovarian biopsy is too invasive to be part of routine screening. Early follicular ovarian volume can be a good screening test for prediction of poor response, but only at extreme values of less than 3 cm^3.[45] The ovarian stromal blood flow test is far from standardised, in terms of technique, reference standard and cut-off values.[17] The serum estradiol and luteinising hormone (LH)/FSH ratio tests are hardly ever used in routine clinical practice, either singly or together.

Combinations of tests and multivariate models

Combinations of various tests have not been shown to be more effective in predicting reproductive outcomes in ART, early ovarian ageing or its rate than individual tests.[46,47] Multivariate models (Figure 19.2) for the prediction of ovarian response in women undergoing IVF display no advantage over AFC alone.[48] No data are available regarding the capacity of these models to predict robust outcomes such as pregnancy and live birth. Moreover, it is recommended that age should be considered as a variable in all the tests that are used.[49]

Table 19.2 summarises data from a systematic review[5] published in 2006. Although results of more recent studies are not included, this summary table demonstrates the range of (cut-off) values used in the literature to define abnormality for a number of common tests of ovarian reserve. It also underlines the wide variation in likelihood ratios of a positive test both for prediction of poor response and pregnancy in an IVF cycle. This reflects the uncertainty within the current literature regarding interpretation of test results.

Most primary studies of tests of ovarian reserve are based on women undergoing ART. It has been argued that these tests provide an individualised prognosis to these women. Given the relatively low livebirth rate of 20–30%[50] per IVF treatment, most women with 'normal' test results are unlikely to have a successful treatment outcome. As a consequence, most of the evaluative work on these tests has relied on surrogate reference standards such as the number of eggs retrieved. The number

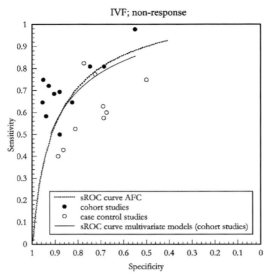

Figure 19.2 Receiver operating characteristic space with reported sensitivities and specificities of the multivariate models; reproduced with permission from Verhagen et al.[48]

of antral follicles is related to the size of the primordial follicle pool, and ovarian response to stimulation should reflect ovarian reserve. However, oocyte quantity does not necessarily represent quality – a critical parameter that none of the available tests is able to address.

Commercially available tests of ovarian reserve

Internationally, a number of 'fertility prediction tests' have been marketed which arebased on a combination of some of the above tests. These have been mainly developed within an IVF setting, using data on outcomes of ovarian stimulation. In terms of assessing the likelihood of IVF success, their accuracy in terms of predicting clinically relevant outcomes (pregnancy and live birth) is either poor or unknown. Used outside their original context, these tests are not particularly effective in predicting current or future levels of ovarian ageing in a general population of women concerned about their reproductive potential.

Table 19.2 Summary of predictive value (that is, likelihood ratio [LR] of a positive test) for prediction of poor response and nonpregnancy; data from Broekmans et al.[5]

Test	Range of cut-off values	Range of LR of a positive test for prediction of poor response	Range of LR of a positive test for prediction of nonpregnancy
Basal FSH (iu/ml)	4–25	0–21.4	0.4–13.6
Basal AFC	<4 to <10	1.3–19.7	0.8–3.6
Basal inhibin B (pg/ml)	<45 to <105.3	1.3–6.9	0.9–5.2
Serum AMH (micrograms/l)	<0.1 to <0.3	5.6–8.2	1.7–2.2

AFC = antral follicle count; AMH = antimüllerian hormone; FSH = follicle-stimulating hormone

Can we develop a screening strategy for early ovarian ageing?

Criteria for an effective screening strategy are shown in Box 19.2. It is clear from our analysis that poor ovarian reserve does not fulfil the criteria of a condition for which a screening programme can be developed. We are uncertain about the population to be screened (whether this should include all women, women attending general infertility clinics or those undergoing ART, or a high-risk population, including those with a history of ovarian surgery, radiation, chemotherapy or early menopause in close family members). Other uncertainties include lack of agreement on:

■ when screening should start
■ which tests should be used (bearing in mind that the best available tests can only successfully predict ovarian response in women undergoing IVF)
■ frequency of testing
■ appropriate cut-off values for test results
■ clinical response to an abnormal test result in the absence of an effective intervention.

Conclusion

As a clinical condition, early ovarian ageing does not, as yet, satisfy accepted criteria for screening. There is little evidence to support the use of currently available ovarian reserve tests for screening for early ovarian ageing. As the results of most published studies are based on a population of women undergoing ART, they cannot be extrapolated to a general population. The more successful tests are able to predict ovarian response to a gonadotrophin stimulation regimen in an IVF cycle (that is, the number of eggs retrieved). None of the available tests or combinations of tests has been shown to predict pregnancy or live birth with sufficient accuracy.

Serum AMH concentration and AFC are two increasingly popular tests of ovarian reserve in the context of IVF treatment. These tests can predict oocyte yield but not oocyte quality or pregnancy.[45,52–54] It is possible that an IVF cycle itself may be a more accurate, albeit invasive, test of a woman's current reproductive potential, as it permits direct information on oocytes, embryos, implantation and livebirth rates.

Box 19.2   Criteria for a successful screening strategy; reproduced with permission from Beaglehole[51]

Diagnostic test:
• sensitive and specific
• safe and acceptable
• simple and cheap
• reliable

Disease:
• serious
• high prevalence of preclinical stage
• natural history understood
• long period between first signs and overt disease

Diagnosis and treatment:
• facilities are adequate
• effective, acceptable and safe treatment is available

References

1. Faddy M, Gosden R, Gougeon A, Richardson S, Nelson J. Accelerated disappearance of ovarian follicles in mid-life: implications for forecasting menopause. *Hum Reprod* 1992;7:1342–6.
2. van Noord P, Dubas J, Dorland M, Boersma H, te Velde E. Age at natural menopause in a population based screening cohort: the role of menarche. *Fertil Steril* 1997;68:95–102.
3. Nikolaou D, Templeton A. Early ovarian ageing: a hypothesis. Detection and clinical relevance. *Hum Reprod* 2003;18:1137–9.
4. Jain T, Soules MR, Collins JA. Comparison of basal follicle-stimulating hormone versus the clomiphene citrate challenge test for ovarian reserve screening. *Fertil Steril* 2004;82:180–5.
5. Broekmans F, Kwee J, Hendriks D, Mol B, Lambalk C. A systematic review of tests predicting ovarian reserve and IVF outcome. *Hum Reprod Update* 2006;12:685–718.
6. te Velde E, Pearson P. The variability of female reproductive ageing. *Hum Reprod Update* 2002;8:141–54.
7. Lambalk C, de Koning C. Interpretation of elevated FSH in the regular menstrual cycle. *Maturitas* 1998;30:215–20.
8. Wolff EF, Taylor HS. Value of the day 3 follicle-stimulating hormone measurement. *Fertil Steril* 2004;81:1486–8.
9. Bancsi L, Broekmans F, Mol B, Habbema J, te Velde E. Performance of basal follicle-stimulating hormone in the prediction of poor ovarian response and failure to become pregnant after *in vitro* fertilization: a meta-analysis. *Fertil Steril* 2003;79:1091–100.
10. Sharara FI, Scott RT, Seifer DB. The detection of diminished ovarian reserve in infertile women. *Am J Obstet Gynecol* 1998;179:804–12.
11. Schipper I, de Jong FH, Fauser BC. Lack of correlation between maximum early follicular phase serum follicle stimulating hormone concentrations and menstrual cycle characteristics in women under the age of 35 years. *HumReprod* 1998;6:1442–8.
12. van Rooij IA, Broekmans FJ, Scheffer GJ, Looman CW, Habbema JD, de Jong FH, *et al*. Serum antimullerian hormone levels best reflect the reproductive decline with age in normal women with proven fertility: a longitudinal study. *Fertil Steril* 2005;83:979–87.
13. Hendriks DJ, Mol BW, Bancsi LF, Te Velde ER, Broekmans FJ. Antral follicle count in the prediction of poor ovarian response and pregnancy after *in vitro* fertilization: a meta-analysis and comparison with basal follicle-stimulating hormone level. *Fertil Steril* 2005;83:291–301.
14. Scheffer GJ, Broekmans FJ, Dorland M, Habbema JD, Looman CW, te Velde ER. Antral follicle counts by transvaginal ultrasonography are related to age in women with proven natural fertility. *Fertil Steril* 1999;72:845–51.
15. Bancsi LF, Broekmans FJ, Looman CW, Habbema JD, te Velde ER. Impact of repeated antral follicle counts on the prediction of poor ovarian response in women undergoing *in vitro* fertilization. *Fertil Steril* 2004;8:35–41.
16. Elter K, Sismanoglu A, Durmusoglu F. Intercycle variabilities of basal antral follicle count and ovarian volume in subfertile women and their relationship to reproductive ageing: a prospective study. *Gynecol Endocrinol* 2005;20:137–43.
17. Klinkert ER, Broekmans FJ, Looman CW, Habbema JD, te Velde ER. The antral follicle count is a better marker than basal follicle-stimulating hormone for the selection of older patients with acceptable pregnancy prospects after *in vitro* fertilization. *Fertil Steril* 2005;83:811–14.
18. Gibreel A, Maheshwari A, Bhattacharya S, Johnson N. Ultrasound ovarian reserve tests, a systematic review of diagnostic accuracy. *Hum Fertil (Camb)* 2009 (in press).
19. Danforth DR, Arbogast LK, Mroueh J, Kim MH, Kennard EA, Seifer DB, *et al*. Dimeric inhibin: a direct marker of ovarian ageing. *Fertil Steril* 1998;70:119–23.
20. Seifer DB, Scott RT, Bergh PA, Arbogast LK, Friedman CI, Mack CK, *et al*. Women with declining ovarian reserve may demonstrate a decrease in day 3 serum inhibin B before a rise in day 3 follicle stimulating hormone. *Fertil Steril* 1999;72:63–5
21. Fried G, Remaeus K, Harlin J, Krog E, Csemiczky G, Aanesen A, *et al*. Inhibin B predicts oocyte number and the ratio IGF-I/IGFBP-1 may indicate oocyte quality during ovarian hyperstimulation for *in vitro* fertilization. *J Assist Reprod Genet* 2003;20:167–76.

22. Hall JE, Welt CK, Cramer DW. Inhibin A and inhibin B reflect ovarian function in assisted reproduction but are less useful at predicting outcome. *Hum Reprod* 1999;14:409–15.

23. Creus M, Penarrubia J, Fabregues F, Vidal E, Carmona F, Casamitjana R, *et al*. Day 3 serum inhibin B and FSH and age as predictors of assisted reproduction treatment outcome. *Hum Reprod* 2000;15:2341–6.

24. Tinkanen H, Blauer M, Laippala P, Tuohimaa P, Kujansuu E. Correlation between serum inhibin B and other indicators of the ovarian function. *Eur J Obstet Gynecol Reprod Biol* 2001;94:109–13.

25. Ficicioglu C, Kutlu T, Demirbasoglu S, Mulayim B. The role of inhibin B as a basal determinant of ovarian reserve. *Gynecol Endocrinol* 2003;17:287–93.

26. Seifer DB, Lambert-Messerlian G, Hogan JW, Gardiner AC, Blazar AS, Berk CA. Day 3 serum inhibin-B is predictive of assisted reproductive technologies outcome. *Fertil Steril* 1997;67:110–14.

27. Themmen APN. Anti-Mullerian hormone: Its role in follicular growth initiation and survival and as an ovarian reserve marker. *J Natl Cancer Inst* 2005;34:18–21.

28. de Vet A, Laven JS, de Jong FH, Themmen AP, Fauser BC. Antimullerian hormone serum levels: a putative marker for ovarian ageing. *Fertil Steril* 2002;77:357–62.

29. Seifer DB, MacLaughlin DT, Christian BP, Feng B, Shelden RM. Early follicular serum mullerian-inhibiting substance levels are associated with ovarian response during assisted reproductive technology cycles. *Fertil Steril* 2002;77:468–71.

30. van Rooij IA, Broekmans FJ, te Velde ER, Fauser BC, Bancsi LF, de Jong FH, *et al*. Serum anti-Mullerian hormone levels: a novel measure of ovarian reserve. *Hum Reprod* 2002;17:3065–71.

31. Fanchin R, Schonauer LM, Righini C, Guibourdenche J, Frydman R, Taieb J. Serum anti-Mullerian hormone is more strongly related to ovarian follicular status than serum inhibin B, estradiol, FSH and LH on day 3. *Hum Reprod* 2003;18:323–7.

32. Laven JS, Mulders AG, Visser JA, Themmen AP, De Jong FH, Fauser BC. Anti-Mullerian hormone serum concentrations in normoovulatory and anovulatory women of reproductive age. *J Clin Endocrinol Metab* 2004;89:318–23.

33. Mulders AG, Laven JS, Eijkemans MJ, de Jong FH, Themmen AP, Fauser BC. Changes in anti-Mullerian hormone serum concentrations over time suggest delayed ovarian ageing in normogonadotrophic anovulatory infertility. *Hum Reprod* 2004;19:2036–42.

34. Piltonen T, Morin-Papunen L, Koivunen R, Perheentupa A, Ruokonen A, Tapanainen JS. Serum anti-Mullerian hormone levels remain high until late reproductive age and decrease during metformin therapy in women with polycystic ovary syndrome. *Hum Reprod* 2005;20:1820–6.

35. Nakhuda GS, Sauer MV, Wang JG, Ferin M, Lobo RA. Mullerian inhibiting substance is an accurate marker of ovarian response in women of advanced reproductive age undergoing IVF. *Reprod Biomed Online* 2007;14:450–4.

36. Ficicioglu C, Kutlu T, Baglam E , Bakacak Z. Early follicular antimullerian hormone as an indicator of ovarian reserve. *Fertil Steril* 2006;3:592–6

37. Riggs RM, Duran EH, Baker MW, Kimble TD, Hobeika E, Yin L, *et al*. Assessment of ovarian reserve with anti-Mullerian hormone: a comparison of the predictive value of anti-Mullerian hormone, follicle-stimulating hormone, inhibin B, and age. *Am J Obstet Gynecol* 2008;199:202–8.

38. Gnoth C, Schuring AN, Friol K, Tigges J, Mallmann P, Godehardt E. Relevance of anti-Mullerian hormone measurement in a routine IVF program. *Hum Reprod* 2008;23:1359–65.

39. Shanbhag S, Aucott L, Bhattacharya S, Hamilton MA, McTavish AR. Interventions for 'poor responders' to controlled ovarian hyperstimulation (COH) in in-vitro fertilisation (IVF). *Cochrane Database Syst Rev* 2007;(1):CD004379.

40. Broer SL, Mol BW, Hendriks D, Broekmans FJ. The role of antimullerian hormone in prediction of outcome after IVF: comparison with the antral follicle count. *Fertil Steril* 2009;91:705–14.

41. Fanchin R, Taieb J, Lozano DH, Ducot B, Frydman R , Bouyer J. High reproducibility of serum anti-Mullerian hormone measurements suggests a multi-staged follicular secretion and strengthens its role in the assessment of ovarian follicular status. *Hum Reprod* 2005;4:923–7.

42. Feyereisen E, Mendez Lozano DH, Taieb J, Hesters L, Frydman R , Fanchin R. Anti-Mullerian hormone: clinical insights into a promising biomarker of ovarian follicular status. *Reprod Biomed Online* 2006;6:695–703.

43. Hehenkamp WJ, Looman CW, Themmen AP, de Jong FH, Te Velde ER , Broekmans FJ. Anti-Mullerian hormone levels in the spontaneous menstrual cycle do not show substantial fluctuation. *J Clin Endocrinol Metab* 2006;10:4057–63.

44. Maheshwari A, Gibreel A, Bhattacharya S, Johnson N. Dynamic ovarian reserve tests, a systematic review of diagnostic accuracy. *Reprod Biomedi Online* 2009;18:717–34.

45. Hendriks DJ, Kwee J, Mol BW, te Velde ER, Broekmans FJ. Ultrasonography as a tool for the prediction of outcome in IVF patients: a comparative meta-analysis of ovarian volume and antral follicle count. *Fertil Steril* 2007;87:764–75.

46. Kline J, Kinney A, Kelly A, Reuss ML, Levin B. Predictors of antral follicle count during the reproductive years. *Hum Reprod* 2005;20:2179–89.

47. Muttukrishna S, McGarrigle H, Wakim R, Khadum I, Ranieri DM, Serhal P. Antral follicle count, anti-mullerian hormone and inhibin B: predictors of ovarian response in assisted reproductive technology. *BJOG* 2005;112:1384–90.

48. Verhagen TE, Hendriks DJ, Bancsi LF, Mol BW, Broekmans FJ. The accuracy of multivariate models predicting ovarian reserve and pregnancy after *in vitro* fertilization: a meta-analysis. *Hum Reprod Update* 2008;14:95–100.

49. Sun W, Stegmann BJ, Henne M, Catherino WH, Segars JH. A new approach to ovarian reserve testing. *Fertil Steril* 2008;90:2196–202.

50. Human Fertilisation and Embryology Authority [www.hfea.gov.uk].

51. Wilson JM, Jungner YG. Epidemiology and prevention. In: Beaglehole R, editor. *Basic Epidemiology*. Geneva: World Health Organization; 1993 (2002 reprint). p. 93.

52. Soldevila PN, Carreras O, Tur R, Coroleu B, Barri PN. Sonographic assessment of ovarian reserve. Its correlation with outcome of *in vitro* fertilization cycles. *Gynecol Endocrinol* 2007;23:206–12

53. Lekamge DN, Barry M, Kolo M, Lane M, Gilchrist RB, Tremellen KP. Anti-Mullerian hormone as a predictor of IVF outcome. *Reprod Biomed Online* 2007;14:602–10.

54. Smeenk JM, Sweep FC, Zielhuis GA, Kremer JA, Thomas CM, Braat DD. Antimullerian hormone predicts ovarian responsiveness, but not embryo quality or pregnancy, after *in vitro* fertilization or intracyoplasmic sperm injection. *Fertil Steril* 2007;87:223–6.

Chapter 20
Egg freezing: the reality and practicality

Helen Picton and Emma Chambers

Introduction

In the past three decades, the changing agenda in assisted reproduction, together with the introduction of more restrictive legislation, has increased the interest in oocyte cryopreservation as a means to preserve female fertility. There are many advantages of including oocyte freezing as an adjunct in assisted conception programmes.[1] The indications for oocyte cryopreservation are discussed in Chapter 21.

In summary, when successful, oocyte freezing could be used to improve the efficiency of female fertility treatment in assisted reproduction as it provides an ethically and legally more acceptable long-term storage option for women than embryo freezing. When used as part of an oocyte donation programme, oocyte cryopreservation would remove the need for cycle synchronisation between donor and recipient and it would allow for more effective screening of donors for transmittable diseases such as is currently practised for sperm donors. Oocyte freezing can be used to preserve fertility for women at risk of premature ovarian failure or those with congenital infertility disorders such as Turner syndrome.[2] Finally, oocyte cryopreservation can be used to preserve the germplasm of young women and girls who are likely to lose their fertility as a result or abdominal trauma or ablative cancer treatments.[3-6]

Despite the great potential of oocyte cryopreservation, historically the success rates of oocyte freezing programmes have lagged behind those of embryo and sperm freezing. The low efficiency of initial attempts to freeze oocytes was predominantly due to the use of suboptimal freezing protocols that failed to match the unique biological characteristics of oocytes. However, significant improvements have been made to equilibrium freezing protocols and new tools and devices have been developed to support the ultra-rapid vitrification of oocytes and embryos. This review provides an overview of the principles of cryobiology as applied to oocyte freezing and provides insight into the progress and the clinical practices of oocyte cryopreservation.

Fundamentals of cryopreservation

The consensus among cryobiologists is that freezing protocols must be tailored to the biological characteristics of the cells of interest.[7,8] Furthermore, each cell type has an optimum cooling rate that is dependent of the biological parameters of the cells and their surface area to volume ratio.[8] For example, embryos that have a low surface area to volume ratio and a low water permeability require slow rates of cooling; whereas sperm with a high surface area to volume ratio and a higher value for water permeability can be cooled faster.[8] An in-depth understanding of the principles and practices of cryopreservation is therefore fundamental to the development of strategies for the efficient preservation of oocytes.

Cryopreservation protocols for isolated oocytes and complex ovarian tissues can be broadly classified as equilibrium freezing (slow-freezing protocols) or rapid freezing (vitrification protocols). Fundamentally, oocyte cryopreservation requires that the gametes tolerate three non-physiological conditions:

1. exposure to molar concentrations of cryoprotective agents (CPAs)

2. cooling to subzero temperatures

3. removal of or conversion of almost all of the liquid cell water into the solid state.

Both slow-freezing and vitrification protocols aim to protect the cells from the effects of intracellular ice crystal formation, cellular dehydration and drastic changes in solute concentrations at both high and low temperatures.[7]

When the components of freezing protocols are managed incorrectly, freezing can cause an array of detrimental effects on various aspects of oocyte biology that ultimately result in loss of oocyte function and viability. As cells are cooled to between −5 and −15 °C, ice nucleation is stimulated and ice crystals begin to form.[8] Nucleation initially occurs within the extracellular environment because intact cell membranes restrict the formation of ice within the cytoplasm of the cell.[9] The ice crystals then increase in size as the temperature continues to decline, which concentrates the extracellular solutes and increases the osmolality of the external environment. Consequently, the equilibrium between the extracellular and intracellular compartments is disrupted and an osmotic gradient is created, that leads to the movement of water out of the cell.[10] This considerable efflux of water not only damages the cell membrane[11] but also causes cellular dehydration, shrinkage and an increase in the concentration of intracellular solutes and cytoplasmic osmolality.[12] The presence of a large body of ice within the extracellular environment may also cause deformation of the oocytes and damage to the ultrastructure of the oolemma.[13] The formation of intracellular ice leads to concentration of solutes and an increase in the osmolality of the cytoplasm.[9] Ice formation can lead to the creation of lethal intracellular gas bubbles.[14] The success of cryopreservation is therefore dependent on minimising the impact of these lethal processes and reducing the likelihood of cellular damage.

Cryoprotective agents

Oocytes and reproductive cells are routinely protected from the chilling injuries detailed above by two categories of CPAs:

1. penetrating CPAs, such as glycerol, dimethyl sulphoxide (DMSO), ethylene glycol (EG) and 1,2-propanediol (PrOH), which are all membrane-soluble and can pass into cells

2. non-penetrating CPAs, including sucrose, glucose, trehalose and polymers such as hydroxyethyl starch and polyvinyl pyrrolidone.[15]

The presence of penetrating CPAs in the slow-freezing solution increases the solute concentration in the extracellular compartment and therefore draws water out of the oocytes.[16] In response to this efflux of cellular water, penetrating CPAs diffuse across the cell membrane and enter the intracellular compartment.[15] However, the rate at which CPAs penetrate oocytes is slower than that at which water leaves and consequently cellular volume initially decreases during equilibration (for example, by around 40% in oocytes).[17] The oocyte then returns to normal volume as more of the CPA enters. To limit the osmotic stress caused by these volumetric fluctuations, CPAs are frequently introduced by gradual step-wise increases in concentration in the incubation solutions.[18] Therefore, by the time cooling actually begins in slow-freezing protocols, the amount of intracellular water will have significantly decreased and been replaced by an equivalent amount of CPA. As the external temperature then decreases, ice will form in the extracellular environment, which will lead to a further exchange between water and CPA. The influx of CPAs during the cooling process enables the intracellular volume to be maintained, which limits the overall dehydration and shrinkage of the oocytes.[17] The CPAs within the cell limit the denaturation of cellular proteins[18] and their presence increases the cytoplasmic solute concentration and osmolality. In turn, this leads to an increase in the viscosity of the intracellular compartment, which lowers the temperature at which ice can form[19] and physically hinders ice nucleation and crystal growth. Finally, it has been reported that a number of the penetrating CPAs such as DMSO can stabilise cell membranes at subzero temperatures,[20] which is beneficial with regard to preventing cooling injury.

It is widely recognised that supplementation of the cryopreservation media with low concentrations (0.05–0.3 mol/l) of non-penetrating agents such as sucrose is beneficial during oocyte freezing. The mode of action of non-penetrating CPAs is unclear, although several theories have been proposed. Carpenter et al.,[21] suggested that molecules such as sucrose may preserve the structure and activity of temperature-sensitive enzymes. The constant presence of non-penetrating CPAs in the extracellular environment during cooling will also increase the solute concentration of this compartment and lead to increased viscosity and possible inhibition of extracellular ice nucleation.[18]

Despite the protective effects afforded by CPAs during the process of cooling and warming, the presence of these molecules, in particular the penetrating compounds, can be highly detrimental to cells.[15] Exposure to CPAs has been shown to disrupt the cytoskeleton[22] and trigger calcium release from intracellular stores, which can lead to parthenogenetic activation of the gamete and/or apoptosis.[23] The impact of these problems can be easily managed, as CPA toxicity is strongly temperature dependent with effects increasing above 0 °C.[15] However, the penetrability of the CPAs is also temperature dependent, with the rate of influx occurring more rapidly at higher temperatures.[16] Consequently, oocytes are susceptible to damage during the equilibration, cooling and warming processes. The length of the exposure to CPAs during equilibration also influences the extent of their detrimental impact. Freezing protocols must therefore provide a balance between CPA penetration and minimising CPA exposure and toxicity.

Rate of cooling

The rate at which cells are cooled is fundamental to the success of cryopreservation.[24] There are currently two approaches to this aspect of the procedure: slow freezing and vitrification. The principles and practices of these two methods of oocyte preservation are summarised in Box 20.1.

In slow-freezing protocols, cells are incubated in solutions containing penetrating CPAs at a concentration of 0.1–0.3 mol/l for equilibration before the onset of cooling. Ice nucleation is deliberately induced in the extracellular compartment between −5 and −9 °C, depending on cell type. Following ice seeding, the temperature is

Box 20.1	Summary of principles and practices of equilibrium freezing and vitrification protocols for cryopreservation of tissues and cells
Equilibrium freezing:	**Vitrification:**
• Slow	• Ultra-rapid
• Extracellular ice formed	• Amorphous glass formed
• Risk of cellular dehydration	• No/low risk of cellular dehydration
• Moderate concentration of cryoprotective agents used, low toxicity of cryoprotective agents (CPAs)	• High concentrations of CPAs used, high toxicity of CPAs
• Volume of freezing solution not critical to success	• Volume of vitrification solution critical to success, for example minimal drop freezing
• Ice crystal seeding required	• No seeding required
• Step-wise, slow rate of cooling, approximately 2 °C/minute from room temperature to seeding temperature, then 0.3 °C/minute to −30 or −40 °C	• Very high rate of cooling ranging from 10 000–22 000 °C/minute in devices with larger volumes to approximately 700 000 °C/minute in minimum volume devices.
• Expensive apparatus required	• No expensive apparatus required
• Routinely used for embryos, ovarian cortex and whole ovary freezing	• Used for oocytes and embryos, limited success when applied to ovarian tissue
• Sealed tubes, ampoules and straws most commonly used for gametes and embryos	• Range of devices developed specifically for oocyte and embryo vitrification including solid surface freezing, Cryoloop, Cryotop, Cryo Tip™, Cryoleaf™ systems
• Protocols slow but robust and tolerant to the demands of busy clinical service	• Protocols very quick but intolerant to the demands of busy clinical services
• Protocols require optimisation to improve efficiency for each cell type	• Protocols require further optimisation to improve efficiency for each cell type
• Few safety implications for tissue stored in sealed straws/ampoules in liquid nitrogen	• Safety implications for cells/tissues stored in open systems in direct contact with liquid nitrogen
• Storage and handling relatively easy	• Freeze-fracture of straw/vial contents can occur in storage vessel, storage and handling therefore more difficult

decreased at a controlled rate. In protocols for the preservation of ovarian tissue and oocytes, temperature decreases at a rate of 0.3–0.5 °C/minute are commonly used.[25] The small decreases limit the pace at which extracellular ice crystals can grow and therefore prevent an acute and rapid efflux of cellular water. Instead, water is drawn out in a more regulated manner, ensuring that any fluctuations in cell volume are only minor.[18] The gradual influx of CPAs during slow-freezing protocols also minimises the probability of intracellular ice nucleation. Once the temperature has dropped to −40 °C, the rate of cooling increases as the majority of ice crystals will have been formed,[25] until a temperature of −180 °C is reached, at which point the cell samples are plunged into liquid nitrogen for long-term storage. Although intracellular ice crystal formation is minimised by the CPA exposure during slow-freezing protocols, cellular dehydration is a major cause of damage and loss of cell viability on thawing.

Vitrification systems have been developed as a rapid method for preserving various cell types as this strategy avoids both ice crystal formation and the detrimental effects of cellular dehydration. Vitrification is a vitreous, transparent, ice-free solidification of water-based solutions at subzero temperatures.[26] Vitrification solutions contain far higher concentrations of CPAs than are used in slow-freezing protocols. The high concentrations of CPAs cause a strong osmotic gradient to be set up, resulting in cells rapidly losing water and becoming fully permeated with CPAs before cooling is initiated.[25] Consequently, the concentration of solutes within and the viscosity of the extra- and intracellular environments are both very high. The cells are then preserved by direct immersion in liquid nitrogen at very high cooling rates. The most critical period during vitrification is the initial cooling[27] and the cooling rate required to avoid chilling injury and to lower the CPA concentration used is around 20 000 °C/minute.[28] The rate of cooling and warming are device dependent, with the highest cooling rates of 10 000–20 000 °C/minute[29] and warming rates of 12 000–42 000 °C/minute being recorded for minimal volume vitrification methods. In the absence of solid support and in extremely small volumes (such as is achieved with Cryoloop devices), cooling rates as high as 700 000 °C/minute have been achieved during vitrification.[30] Minimising the volume of the vitrification solutions also helps to reduce the chance of ice crystal nucleation/formation in the cell sample. The high viscosity of the extra- and intracellular compartments prevents ice crystallisation during this rapid cooling. Instead, the solutions vitrify, forming amorphous glass-like solids[19] that maintain the integrity of the cell membrane, minimise damage to intracellular proteins and protect against other deleterious consequences of cytoplasmic ice formation[31] while maintaining the morphology of the oocyte spindle apparatus.[32,33] There are, however, some disadvantages of vitrification that are not encountered during slow freezing. These include increased parthenogenetic activation in oocytes,[34] danger of liquid nitrogen-mediated contamination of cells, freeze-fracture damage of closed storage vessels in nitrogen tanks, the potential toxic impact of exposure to concentrated solutions of CPAs and relative intolerance to minor excursions from the optimised protocol.

Rate of warming

The rate at which the cryopreserved cells are warmed and the subsequent removal of the CPA solution affects the success of all freezing protocols. A slow rate of warming allows small ice crystals to coalesce and recrystallise, which may cause cellular injury.[18] In contrast, rapid warming, which is commonly used in clinical oocyte freezing protocols, enables any ice which has formed to melt and so protects against recrystallisation damage.[24] When the oocytes are placed into an isotonic solution on thawing, there will be an initial influx of water and the cells will swell. These changes can be substantial, for example oocytes have been shown to increase to 140–150% of their normal volume.[17] These large volume changes can lead to cell membrane damage and rupture. A step-wise removal of the CPAs is therefore required on warming both to prevent cell lysis and to regulate the volumetric changes associated with CPA exposure.[17]

Oocyte cryopreservation

The principles of slow freezing and vitrification have been used to develop clinical protocols for oocyte freezing. The success of oocyte freezing and its utility as a clinical strategy to preserve female fertility is dependent on the stage of development at which oocytes are frozen and whether the cells are preserved using slow-freezing or vitrification protocols. Secondary oocytes can be collected and stored at either the mature metaphase II (MII) stage or at the immature germinal vesicle (GV) stage following ultrasound-guided oocyte pick-up. Alternatively, whole ovaries or biopsies of ovarian cortex can be collected laparoscopically[35] and the earliest staged primordial oocytes can be stored *in situ* in slices of ovarian cortex,[36,37] or by whole ovary freezing,[38,39] or primordial follicles can be cryopreserved after isolation. Whichever stage of development is preserved, the freezing strategy used must be matched to the stage of oocyte development and account taken of the characteristics of the cell type(s) being frozen (Table 20.1). While there is no doubt that primordial oocyte/ovarian tissue cryopreservation can be used to preserve the fertility of young cancer patients,[4–6] mature MII oocyte preservation is increasingly being used in clinical practice as an alternative to embryo freezing. The rest of this review will therefore focus on the biological and clinical outcomes associated with MII oocyte freezing.

While there are many advantages of MII oocyte freezing, the published clinical statistics on the efficacy of this treatment are hugely variable and, in many cases, are difficult to interpret as there is no standardisation of women's ages or clinical treatment demographics between clinics or even between studies published by the same clinic. There is a very clear need to objectively evaluate the efficiency of human oocyte freezing methods.[40–43] The problem is further confounded by the inconsistency in the presentation format of the published clinical data. While it is possible to use the characteristics of embryo development *in vitro* as a means to assess the efficacy of oocyte freezing[42] when considered in isolation, data on pregnancy rates following transfer of highly selected embryos are highly misleading as very few of the published trials of oocyte freezing take into account the post-thaw oocyte survival and fertilisation rate, the embryo selection criteria used, endometrial programming or implantation factors.

Table 20.1 Comparison of the characteristics that influence the suitability of human oocytes for cryopreservation

	Immature primordial oocytes	Fully grown secondary oocytes	
Nuclear maturity	Germinal vesicle stage	Germinal vesicle stage	Metaphase II stage
Tissue availability/type	Abundant, harvested from ovarian cortex	Scarce, present in antral folicles, harvested from follicles >4 mm diameter	Scarce, present in antral follicles, harvested from preovulatory follicles of approximate size range 10–20 mm diameter
Ease of collection	Laparoscopic cortex biopsy or ovariectomy	Ultrasound-guided oocyte retrieval	Ultrasound-guided oocyte retrieval
Size	30–40 micrometres	Approximately 110–120 micrometres	Approximately 110–120 micrometres
Support cells	Few, very small pregranulosa cells	Numerous compacted cumulus cells	Numerous expanded cumulus cells
Nuclear status	Resting prophase I, nuclear membrane	Germinal vesicle, has nuclear membrane	On temperature-sensitive spindle, no nuclear membrane
Zona	Absent	Present	Present
Cortical granules	Absent	Present and centrally located	Present and peripherally located
Surface area to volume ratio	High	Low	Low

Overall, the data on embryo development from frozen–thawed oocytes suggest that these embryos exhibit retarded development *in vitro* when compared with fresh tissue.[42] The most important indicator of the success of oocyte freezing regimens is to evaluate the full developmental potential of oocytes (and the resulting embryos) after freeze–thawing in relation to similar parameters measured in fresh oocytes from women with similar demographics.

Cryopreservation of mature MII oocytes has been achieved in a number of animal species and also in clinical practice. The early attempts to freeze MII oocytes using equilibrium freezing methods met with only limited success owing to relatively low post-thaw survival rates, which ranged from 24% to 54%.[44,45] The poor survival of the cells from these early studies was attributed to the use of freezing protocols that did not match the biological requirements of MII oocytes, as detailed in Table 20.1. Mature oocytes have a very low surface area to volume ratio, which hampers adequate cellular dehydration during the cooling process and renders the cells susceptible to intracellular ice formation. At the MII stage of development, oocytes have undergone nuclear maturation and cytoplasmic maturation, which are characterised by the expulsion of the first polar body, chromatin condensation and chromosomal alignment at the equatorial region of the metaphase spindle. The spindle apparatus is highly sensitive to cooling and partial or complete depolymerisation of the spindle occurs following transient or sustained temperature loss of only 2–4 °C.[46] Changes in spindle morphology can also occur after CPA exposure.[46–48] Spindle disassembly will disrupt chromatid separation and lead to a high risk of chromosomal abnormalities in the oocytes,[49] which will be manifest not only by high aneuploidy rates in the embryos so derived but also by high first-trimester miscarriage rates in the fetuses (Table 20.2). Other biological causes of poor oocyte developmental potential after cryopreservation include increased DNA fragmentation,[50] loss of oolemma integrity, ultrastructural modifications to the microvilli, mitochondria and vesicles,[51] alteration of intracellular pH, parthenogenetic activation, irreversible loss of high mitochondrial membrane potential and associated defects on Ca^{2+} signalling after insemination,[52] and zona hardening due to precocious cortical granule exocytosis and breakdown.[53,54]

Recent attempts to improve the success rates of MII oocyte cryopreservation by slow freezing have been centred on the modification of the freezing solutions. The greatest successes have been achieved by increasing the sucrose content of freezing media from 0.1 mol/l to 0.3 mol/l as detailed by Fabbri *et al.*[55] The improvements in the success rates of slow freezing after these modifications have been summarised in Table 20.2. The inclusion of higher sucrose concentrations improves the retention of intact meiotic spindles[56] and reduces the post-thaw osmotic stress of the cells.[57] Using the revised slow-freezing protocols, the survival rates of cryopreserved MII oocyte have been increased to 80–90% in the best clinical programmes.[58,59] Unfortunately, the morphological normality of oocytes after freeze–thawing frequently does not equate to retention of oocyte developmental competence. Consequently, in the series of published results detailed in Table 20.2, only 180 healthy pregnancies/births have been produced from 6161 viable oocytes after slow freezing and, with the exception of the data of Konc *et al.*,[59] the chance of a healthy pregnancy or birth per oocyte thawed appears to have peaked at around 4.5%, which is still significantly lower than the pregnancy rates achieved following the insemination of fresh oocytes[60,61] or the transfer of frozen pronuclear embryos[62] by the same clinics. There are only limited data available on viability of oocytes after long-term storage. The developmental competence of stored MII oocytes has been shown not to be compromised after slow freezing and storage for 5 years.[63]

Table 20.2 Details of the methodology, survival and pregnancy rates obtained after slow freezing of metaphase II human oocytes using 1.5 mol/l 1,2-propanediol and 0.2–0.3 mol/l sucrose

Publication, (no. of women studied; no. of oocytes frozen), source of women	Type of CPA	No. of survived oocytes/ no. of thawed oocytes (% survival)	Fertilisation rate after ICSI (cleavage rate)	CPR/ET, IR/thawed cycle, MR	No. of continuing pregnancies or live births (% per oocyte)
Fabbri et al. (2001)[55] (96; 1769), infertility patients	1.5 mol/l PrOH, 0.2 mol/l sucrose	796/1502 (53%)	58% (91%)	N/A	N/A
Fosas et al. (2003)[58] (4; 88), oocyte donors/recipients	1.5 mol/l PrOH, 0.3 mol/l sucrose	79/88 (90%)	73%	57%/ET	4, (4.5%/thawed oocytes)
Chen et al. (2005)[62] (21; 159), infertility patients	1.5 mol/l PrOH, 0.3 mol/l sucrose	119/159 (75%)	67% (91%)	9.7%/woman, IR 11%, MR 11%	7, (4.4%/frozen oocyte; 7.1%/frozen pronuclear oocytes)
Borini et al. (2006)[80] (146; 2450), infertility patients	1.5 mol/l PrOH, 0.2 mol/l sucrose	687/927 (74%)	76% (68%)	8.9%/ET, IR 5.2%, MR 14.2%	18, (1.9%/thawed oocytes)
Chamayou et al. (2006)[81] (34; 470), infertility patients	1.5 mol/l PrOH, 0.3 mol/l sucrose	263/337 (78%)	70% (77%)	5.4%/ET, IR 2.2%, MR 22%	2 (0.6%/thawed oocytes; 0.3%/fresh oocytes)
Levi Setti et al. (2006)[60] (286; 2900), infertility patients	1.5 mol/l PrOH, 0.3 mol/l sucrose	760/1087 (70%)	68% (54%)	12%/ET, IR 6%, MR 33%	13 (1.6%/thawed oocytes; 5.1%/fresh oocytes)
La Sala et al. (2006)[82] (414; 1647), infertility patients	1.5 mol/l PrOH, 0.3 mol/l sucrose	1200/1647 (73%)	75% (>80%)	4%/ET, IR 6%, MR 47%	10 (0.8%/thawed oocytes) (probability of a live birth is 1:65)
De Santis et al. (2007)[83] (131; 1144), infertility patients	1.5 mol/l PrOH, 0.1 mol/l sucrose, and 1.5 mol/l PrOH, 0.3 mol/l sucrose	123/506 (24%) and 282/396 (71%)	54% (72%) and 80% (91%)	17%/ET, IR 12%, MR 40% and 10%/ET, IR 6%, MR 29%	5 (1.0%/thawed oocytes) and 7 (1.7%/thawed oocytes)
Bianchi et al. (2007)[61] (141; 1083), infertility patients	1.5 mol/l PrOH, 0.3 mol/l sucrose	306/403 (76%)	76% (94%)	21%/ET, IR 17%, MR 12%	17 (4.2%/thawed oocytes; 7.4%/fresh oocytes)
Borini et al. (2007)[84] (749; 5448), infertility patients	1.5 mol/l PrOH, 0.2 mol/l Sscrose	2205/3238 (68%)	76% (92%)	15%/ET, IR 8%, MR 22%	88 (4.2%/thawed oocytes)
Konc et al. (2007)[59] (25; 87)	1.5 mol/l PrOH, 0.3 mol/l sucrose	70/87 (80%)	81% (97%)	24%/ET, IR 14%, MR 16%	5 (7.1%/thawed oocytes)

CPA = cryoprotective agent; CPR = clinical pregnancy rate; DMSO = dimethylsulphoxide; ET = embryo transfer; ICSI = intracytoplasmic sperm injection; IR = implantation rate; MR = miscarriage rate; PrOH = 1,2-propanediol

Other modifications of freezing protocols include substitution of sucrose with sugars such as trehalose[64] or taxol,[65] the use of differential sucrose concentrations during dehydration and rehydration processes,[61] depletion of the sodium content of the freezing medium,[66,67] the use of choline-based media[68] and the inclusion of spindle stabilisers and cytoskeletal relaxants such as cytochalasin B in the freezing solutions.[65] These protocol modifications have improved the post-thaw survival of oocytes by 10–20% with a concomitant improvement in pregnancy rates. However, the number of thawed oocytes producing babies after slow freezing of oocytes still remains low.[41]

The cryopreservation of secondary oocytes at the GV stage[69] has been proposed as a way of avoiding the deleterious effects of chilling on the cytoskeleton of slow-cooled MII oocytes. Fully grown GV oocytes are potentially a more suitable source of gametes for cryopreservation than MII oocytes, as cells at this stage have attributes that render them less susceptible to cooling injury (Table 20.1). For example, the meiotic spindle and peripheral cortical granules are absent, which reduces the chance of acquiring spindle damage and chromosomal abnormalities during cooling or suffering zona hardening.[25] There are however, several problems associated with this approach. Perhaps the greatest disadvantage is that GV oocytes must undergo *in vitro* maturation before they can be fertilised.[48,70,71] To date, few pregnancies and live births have been reported following GV oocyte cryopreservation.[48] Cryopreservation of GV oocytes currently offers little or no advantage over the freeze storage of MII oocytes.

In marked contrast to the unpredictable results of equilibrium freezing of secondary oocytes, improvements to vitrification protocols and the development of a series of new vitrification devices have led to significant improvements in both MII oocyte survival and the clinical outcome of oocyte preservation (Table 20.3). There are many advantages of vitrification over slow freezing in a clinical setting. For example, vitrification protocols are simpler and quicker than conventional slow-freezing methods and they do not require the purchase of expensive controlled rate freezing apparatus (Box 20.1). However, vitrification requires the oocytes to be exposed to very high concentrations of combinations of at least two CPAs; typically ethylene glycol and DMSO are used in combination with 0.5 mol/l sucrose (Table 20.3). Consequently, CPA exposure times and temperatures must be very tightly controlled and there is no tolerance of handling errors or minor protocol deviations during vitrification. Oocyte survival rates have been proven to be significantly higher for MII oocytes after vitrification in a number of species including humans.[2,51,61,65,72] A number of devices have been developed based on the minimum drop method to vitrify oocytes and embryos in a number of species. Vitrification devices include electron microscope grids, solid surface vitrification,[61,70] open pulled straws (OPS),[28,73] Cryoleaf™,[48] Cryoloop,[61] Cryotop,[29,72] and Cryo Tip™, which have been derived from the Cryotop methods to minimise contamination from liquid nitrogen.[74] There are advantages and disadvantages associated with using each of these devices but, to date, the highest rates of cell survival and developmental competence have been obtained with the systems based on the minimum drop method of vitrification as this strategy maximises the rate of cooling of the oocytes. Examples of some of the many recent publications on the success of vitrification of human MII oocytes are shown in Table 20.3. A consistently higher proportion (75–99%) of MII oocytes survived vitrification than slow freezing. Furthermore, in the studies shown in Table 20.3, 69 pregnancies or births resulted from 1051 viable oocytes following MII vitrification and the percentage of pregnancy or birth per thawed oocyte appears equivalent to the success achieved for fresh oocytes (8.0–9.0%), suggesting that vitrification has a far greater potential for the production of a viable pregnancy after MII cryopreservation

Table 20.3 Details of the methodology, survival and pregnancy rates obtained in recent large studies on the clinical efficiency of human metaphase II oocyte vitrification

Publication, (no. of women; no. of oocytes frozen), source of women	Combination of CPA	Vitrification device	No. of oocytes survived/ thawed (% survival)	Fertilisation rate (cleavage rate)	Rates	No. of pregnancies or live births (% per oocyte)
Kuwayama et al. (2005)[74] (67; 64), infertility patients	5 mol/l EG	Cryotop	58/64 (90%)	92% (81%)	N/A	N/A
Okimura et al. (2005)[85] (64 oocytes), infertility patients	Not detailed	Cryotop	58/64 (91%)	90% (50% blastocyst rate)	N/A	10 (17.2%/thawed oocytes)
Lucena et al. (2006)[75] (13; 92), oocyte donors/recipients	15% EG, 15% DMSO, 0.5 mmol/l sucrose	Cryotop	63/78 (80%)	90% (93%)	N/A	7 (9%/thawed oocytes)
Selman et al. (2006)[76] (6; 53), infertility patients	15% EG, 15% DMSO, 0.6 mol/l sucrose	OPS	18/24 (75%)	78%	N/A	2 (8.3%/thawed oocytes)
Antinori et al. (2007)[72] (251; 463), infertility patients	15% EG, 15% DMSO, 0.5 mol/l sucrose	Cryotop	328/330 (99%)	93% (97%)	CPR 32%/ET, IR 13%, MR 21%	28 (8.4%/thawed oocytes; 8.0%/fresh oocytes)
Yoon et al. (2007)[86] (28; 426), infertility patients	5.5 mol/l EG, 1 mol/l sucrose, 10% FBS	EMG	302/364 (85%)	77% (94%)	CPR 43%/ET, IR 14%, MR 15%	11 (3.0%/thawed oocytes)
Cobo et al. (2008)[87] (30; 509), oocyte donors/recipients	15% EG, 15% DMSO, 0.5 mol/l sucrose	Cryotop	224/231 (97%)	76% (94%)	CPR 65%/woman, 41% IR, 7% MR	11 (4.8%/thawed oocytes)

CPAs = cryoprotective agents; CPR = clinical pregnancy rate; DMSO = dimethylsulphoxide; EG = ethylene glycol; EMG = electron microscope grid; ET = embryo transfer; FBS = fetal bovine serum; IR = implantation rate; MR = miscarriage rate; N/A = data not available; OPS = open pulled straws

than slow freezing.[72,75,76] Further review of the literature indicates that, to date, the highest success rates for the vitrification of human oocytes have been achieved using the minimum drop method and Cryotop and Cryoleaf™ devices. A follow-up study of 200 babies born from 165 pregnancies from MII oocytes vitrified using these two devices in three fertility centres in Canada, Mexico and Colombia showed that the mean birth weight (± SEM) was 2920 ± 37 g for singletons and 2231 ± 55 g for multiples.[77] Furthermore, the incidence of congenital abnormalities reported for this cohort of newborns was 2.5% (two ventricular septal defects, one biliary atresia, one club foot and one skin haemangioma),[77] which is comparable to that of spontaneous conceptions in fertile or infertile women from the same clinics.[78]

It should be noted that not all of the vitrification devices detailed above are compatible with the stringent quality management systems used in clinical laboratories as many are founded on open systems in which direct cellular contact with liquid nitrogen is used to maximise the speed of cellular cooling. Direct contact with nitrogen is ill advised in a clinical setting because of the known risks of viral transmission in nitrogen storage tanks.[79] An alternative strategy is to seal the vitrification device in a sterile pre-cooled straw for hermetic isolation at the time of storage. The impact of this approach on cooling and warming rates has yet to be evaluated.

Conclusion

Modifications to the slow-freezing and vitrification protocols used for mature oocyte cryopreservation have led to improved survival, fertilisation and developmental competence of mature oocytes after freeze–thawing. These protocol improvements have helped to reduce the extreme chemical and physical stresses associated with cooling oocytes to liquid nitrogen temperatures for long-term storage. However, despite these advances, the pregnancy rates occurring in assisted conception cycles using frozen–thawed oocytes remain unacceptably low. Until the clinical efficacy of oocyte cryopreservation has been fully explored and it has been proven to be reliable, the full potential of MII and GV oocyte banking cannot be realised as a good treatment option for the preservation of female fertility. The recent data on oocyte vitrification are encouraging and suggest that this approach might be a good strategy for oocyte preservation. In general, the improvements in the post-warming survival rates of cryopreserved oocytes, especially those preserved by slow freezing, remain to be translated into increased developmental competence. Consequently, at the time of writing, mature MII oocyte cryopreservation remains a potential solution rather than a practical remedy for infertile women and large-scale, properly controlled trials are required to compare and contrast the efficiency of oocyte preservation by slow-freezing and vitrification protocols.

Acknowledgement

The authors would like to acknowledge that Emma Chambers is supported by a research grant from The Candlelighters, a children's cancer charity.

References

1. Campbell BK, Picton HM. Oocyte storage. *Curr Obstet Gynaecol* 1999;9:203–9.
2. Huang JYJ, Tulandi T, Holzer H, Lau NM, MacDonald S, Tan SL, *et al.* Cryopreservation of ovarian tissue and *in vitro* matured oocytes in a female with mosaic Turner syndrome: case report. *Hum Reprod* 2008;23:336–9.

3. Yang D, Brown SE, Nguygen, Reddy V, Brubaker C, Winslow KL. Live birth after transfer of human embryos developed from cryopreserved oocytes harvested before cancer. *Fertil Steril* 2007;87:1469.e1–4.
4. Picton HM, Kim SS, Gosden RG. Cryopreservation of gonadal tissue and cells. *Br Med Bull* 2000;56:603–15.
5. Meirow D, Baum M, Yaron R, Levron J, Hardan, I, Schill E, *et al*. Ovarian tissue cryopreservation in haematalogic malignancies: ten years' experience. *Leuk Lymphoma* 2007;48:1569–76.
6. Donnez, J, Martinez-Madrid B, Jadoul P, Van Langendonckt A, Demyll D, Dolmans MM. Ovarian tissue cryopreservation and transplantation: a review. *Hum Reprod Update* 2006;12:19–535.
7. Pegg DE. The history and principles of cryopreservation. *Semin Reprod Med* 2002;20:5–14.
8. Mazur, P. Freezing of living cells: mechanisms and implications. *Am J Physiol* 1984;247:c125–42.
9. Paynter SJ, Cooper A, Thomas N, Fuller BJ. Cryopreservation of multicellular embryos and reproductive tissues. In: Karow AM, Critser JK, editors. *Reproductive Tissue Banking: Scientific Principles*. San Diego: Academic Press; 1997. p. 359–97.
10. Mazur P. Kinetics of water loss from cells at subzero temperatures and the likelihood of intracellular freezing. *J Gen Physiol* 1963;47:347–69.
11. Muldrew K, McGann LE. The osmotic rupture hypothesis of intracellular freezing injury. *Biophys J* 1994;66:532–41.
12. Karlsson JOM, Toner M. Long-term storage of tissues by cryopreservation: critical issues. *Biomaterials* 1996;17:243–56.
13. Ashwood-Smith MJ, Morris GM, Fowler R, Appleton TC, Ashorn R. Physical factors are involved in the destruction of embryos and oocytes during freezing and thawing procedures. *Hum Reprod* 1988;3:795–802.
14. Fujikawa S, Miura K. Plasma membrane ultrastructural changes caused by mechanical stress in the formation of extracellular ice as a primary cause of slow freezing injury in fruit-bodies of basidiomycetes (*Lyophyllum ulmarium* (Fr.) Kühner). *Cryobiology* 1986;23:371–82.
15. Meryman HT. Cryoprotective agents. *Cryobiology* 1971;8:173–83.
16. Newton H, Fisher J, Arnold JRP, Pegg DE, Faddy MJ, Gosden RG. Permeation of human ovarian tissue with cryoprotective agents in preparation for cryopreservation. *Hum Reprod* 1998;13:376–80.
17. Newton H, Pegg DE, Barrass R, Gosden RG. Osmotically inactive volume, hydraulic conductivity, and permeability to dimethylsulphoxide of human mature oocytes. *J Reprod Fertil* 1999;117:27–33.
18. Karlsson JOM, Toner M. Long-term storage of tissues by cryopreservation: critical issues. *Biomaterials* 1996;17:243–56.
19. Wolfe J, Bryant G. Cellular cryobiology: thermodynamic and mechanical effects. *Int J Refrigeration* 2001;24:438–50.
20. Yu ZW, Quinn PJ. The modulation of membrane structure and stability by dimethylsulphoxide (review). *Mol Membr Biol* 1998;15:59–68.
21. Carpenter JF, Crowe JH, Arakawa T. Comparison of solute-induced protein stabilization in aqueous solution and in the frozen and dried states. *J Dairy Sci* 1990;73:3627–36.
22. Vincent C, Johnson MH. Cooling, cryoprotectants and the cytoskeleton of the mammalian oocyte. *Oxf Rev Reprod Biol* 1992;14:73–100.
23. Litkouhi B, Winlow W, Gosden RG. Impact of cryoprotective agent exposure on intracellular calcium in mouse oocytes at metaphase II. *Cryo Letters* 1999;20:353–62.
24. Pegg DE. Cryobiology: Life in the deep freeze. *Biologist* 1994;41:53–6.
25. Shaw JM, Oranratnachai A, Trounson AO. Fundamental cryobiology of mammalian oocytes and ovarian tissue. *Theriogenology* 2000;53:59–72.
26. Luyet BJ, Hodapp R. Revival of frog spermatozoa vitrified in liquid air. *Proc Soc Exp Biol NY* 1938;39:433–4.
27. Arav A, Yavin S, Zeron Y, Natan D, Dekel I, Gacitua H. New trends in gamate's cryopreservation. *Mol Cell Endocrinol* 2002;187:77–81.
28. Vajta G, Holm P, Kuwayama M, Booth PJ, Jacobsen H, Greve T, *et al*. Open pulled straw (OPS) vitrification: a new way to reduce cryoinjuries of bovine ova and embryos. *Mol Reprod Dev* 1998;51:53–8.

29. Kuwayama M, Vajta G, Leda S, Kato O. Comparison of open and closed methods for vitrification of human embryos and the elimination of potential contamination. *Reprod Biomed Online* 2005;11:608–14.

30. Isachenko E, Isachenko V, Katkov II, Dessole S, Nawroth F. Vitrification of mammalian spermatazoa in the absence of cryoprotectants: from past partial difficulties to present success. *Reprod Biomed Online* 2003;6:191–200.

31. Ledda S, Leoni G, Bogliolo L, Naitana S. Oocyte cryopreservation and ovarian tissue banking. *Theriogenology* 2001;55:1359–71.

32. Ko CS, Ding DC, Chu TW, Chu YN, Chen IC, Chen WH, *et al.* Changes to the meiotic spindle and zona pellucida of mature mouse oocytes following different cryopreservation methods. *Anim Reprod Sci* 2008;105:272–82.

33. Larman MG, Minasi MG, Rienzi L, Gardner DK. Maintenance of the meiotic spindle during vitrification in human and mouse oocytes. *Reprod Biomed Online* 2007;15:692–700.

34. Somfai T, Ozawa M, Noguchi J, Kaneko H, Karja NWK, Farhudin M, *et al.* Developmental competence of *in vitro*-fertilised porcine oocytes after *in vitro* maturation and solid surface vitrification: effect of cryopreservation on oocyte antioxidative system and cell cycle stage *Cryobiology* 2007;55:115–26.

35. Jadoul P, Donnez J, Dolmans MM, Squifflet J, Lengele B, Martinez-Madrid B. Laparascopic ovariectomy for whole human ovary cryopreservation. *Fertil Steril* 2007;87:971–5.

36. Newton H, Aubard Y, Rutherford AJ, Sharma V, Gosden RG. Low temperature storage and grafting of human ovarian tissue. *Hum Reprod* 1996;11:1487–91.

37. Meirow D, Levron J, Eldar-Geva T, Hardan T, Fridman E, Yemini Z, *et al.* Monitoring the ovaries after autotransplantation of cryopreserved ovarian tissue: endocrine studies, *in vitro* fertilization cycles and live birth. *Fertil Steril* 2007;87:418e7–15.

38. Onions VJ, Mitchell MR, Campbell BK, Webb R. Ovarian tissue viability following whole ovine ovary cryopreservation: assessing the affects of spingosin-1-phosphate. *Hum Reprod* 2008;23:606–18.

39. Martinez-Madrid B, Donnez J. Cryopreservation of intact human ovary and its vascular pedicle- or cryopreservation of hemiovaries? *Hum Reprod* 2007;22:1795–6.

40. Gook DA, Edgar DH. Human oocyte cryopreservation. *Hum Reprod Update* 2007;13:591–605.

41. Oktay K, Cil AP, Bang H. The efficiency of oocyte cryopreservation: a meta-analysis. *Fertil Steril* 2006;86:70–80.

42. Edgar AH, Gook DA. How should the clinical efficiency of oocyte cryopreservation be measured? *Reprod Biomed Online* 2007;14:430–5.

43. De Santis L, Cino I, Coticchio G, Fusi FM, Papaleo E, Rabellotti E, *et al.* Objective evaluation of the viability of cryopreserved oocytes. *Reprod Biomed Online* 2007;15:338–45.

44. Tucker MJ. Clinical applications of human egg cryopreservation. *Hum Reprod* 1998;13:3156–9.

45. Porcu E, Fabbri R, Marsella T, Balicchia B, De Cesare D, Giunchi S, *et al.* Clinical experiences and applications of oocyte cryopreservation. *Mol Cell Endocrinol* 2000;169:33–7.

46. Pickering SJ, Braude PR, Johnson MH, Cant A, Currie J. Transient cooling to room temperature can cause irreversible disruption of the meiotic spindle in the human oocyte. *Fertil Steril* 1990;54:102–8.

47. Mullen SF, Agca Y, Broerman DC, Jenkins CL, Johnson CA, Crister JK. The effects of osmotic stress on the metaphase I spindle of human oocytes, and the relevance to cryopreservation. *Hum Reprod* 2004;19:1148–54.

48. Albarracín JL, Motató R, Rojas C, Mogas T. Effects of vitrification in open pulled straws on the cytology of *in vitro* matured prepubertal and adult bovine oocytes. *Theriogenology* 2005;63:890–901.

49. Gomes CM, Silva CA, Silva MS, Acevedo N, Baracat E, Serafini P, *et al.* Influence of vitrification on mouse metaphase II oocyte spindle dynamics and chromatin alignment. *Fertil Steril* 2008;90:1396–1404.

50. Huang JYJ, Chen HY, Park JYS, Tan SL, Chian RC. Comparison of spindle and chromosome configuration in *in vitro*- and *in vivo*-matured mouse oocytes after vitrification. *Fertil Steril* 2008;90:1424–32.

51. Boonkusolet D, Faisaikarm T, Dinnyes A, Kitiyanant Y. Effects of vitrification procedures on subsequent development and ultrastructure of *in vitro*-matured swamp buffalo (*Bubalus bubalis*) oocytes . *Reprod Fertil Dev* 2007;19:383–91.

52. Jones A, Van Blerkom J, Davis P, Toledo A. Cryopreservation of metaphase II human oocytes effects mitochondrial membrane potential: implications for developmental competence. *Hum Reprod* 2004;19:1861–6.

53. Vincent C, Pickering SJ, Johnson MH. The hardening effect of dimethylsulphoxide on the mouse zona pellucida requires the presence of an oocyte and is associated with a reduction in the number of cortical granules present. *J Reprod Fertil* 1990;89:253–9.

54. Ghetler Y, Skutelsky E, Nin IB, Dor LB, Amihai D, Shalgi R. Human oocyte cryopreservation and the fate of cortical granules. *Fertil Steril* 2006;86:210–6.

55. Fabbri R, Porcu E, Marsella T, Rocchetta G, Venturoli S, Flamigni C. Human oocyte cryopreservation: new perspectives regarding oocyte survival. *Hum Reprod* 2001;16:411–16.

56. Coticchio G, De Santis L, Rossi G, Borini A, Albertini A, Scaravelli G, *et al.* Sucrose concentration influences the rate of human oocytes with normal spindle and chromosome configurations after slow-cooling cryopreservation. *Hum Reprod* 2006;21:1771–6.

57. Boldt J, Tidswell N, Sayer A, Kilani R, Cline D. Human oocyte cryopreservation: 5-year experience with a sodium-depleted medium slow freezing method. *Reprod Biomed Online* 2006;13:96–100.

58. Fosas N, Marina F, Torres PJ, Jove I, Martin P, Perez N, *et al.* The births of five babies from cryopreserved donated oocytes. *Hum Reprod* 2003;18:1417–21.

59. Konc J, Kanyo K, Cseh S. . Does oocyte cryopreservation have a future in Hungary? *Reprod Biomed Online* 2007;14:11–13.

60. Levi Setti PE, Albani E, Novara PV, Cesana A, Morreale G. Cryopreservation of supernumerary oocytes in IVF/ICSI cycles. *Hum Reprod* 2006;21:370–5.

61. Bianchi V, Coticchio G, Distratis V, Di Giusto N, Flamigni C, Borini A. Differential sucrose concentration during dehydration (0.2mol/l) and rehydration (0.3 mol/l) increases the implantation rates of frozen human oocytes. *Reprod Biomed Online* 2007;14:64–71.

62. Chen SU, Lien YR, Chen HF, Chang LJ, Tsai YY, Yang YS. Observational clinical follow-up of oocyte cryopreservation using a slow-freezing method with 1,2-propanediol plus sucrose followed by ICSI. *Hum Reprod* 2005;20:1975–80.

63. Parmegiani L, Fabbri R, Cognigni GE, Bernadi S, Pocognoli P, Filicori M. Blastocyst formation, pregnancy, and birth derived from human oocytes cryopreserved for 5 years. *Fertil Steril* 2008;90:2014.e7–10.

64. Gasparrini B, Attanasio L, De Rosa A, Monaco E, Di Palo R, Campanile G. Cryopreservation of *in vitro* matured buffalo (*Bubalus bubalis*) oocytes by minimum volumes vitrification methods. *Anim Reprod Sci* 2007;98:335–42.

65. Zang J, Nedambale TL, Yang M, Li J. Improved development of ovine matured oocytes following solid surface vitrification (SSV), effect of cumulus cells and cytoskeletal stabilizer. *Anim Reprod Sci* 2009;110:46–55.

66. Boldt J, Cline D, McLaughlin D. Human oocyte cryopreservation as an adjunct to IVF-embryo transfer cycles. *Hum Reprod* 2003;18:1250–5.

67. Boldt J, Tidswell N, Sayer A, Kilani R, Cline D. Human oocyte cryopreservation: 5-year experience with a sodium-depleted medium slow freezing method. *Reprod Biomed Online* 2006;13:96–100.

68. Stachecki J, Cohen J, Garrisi J, Munné S, Burgess C, Willadsen SM. Cryopreservation of unfertilised human oocytes. *Reprod Biomed Online* 2006;13:222–7.

69. Isachenko V, Montag M, Isachenko E, Dessole S, Nawroth F, van der Ven H. Aseptic vitrification of human germinal vesicle oocytes using dimethylsulphoxide as a cryoprotectant. *Fertil Steril* 2006;85:741–7.

70. Picton HM. Oocyte maturation *in vitro*. *Curr Opin Obstet Gynecol* 2002;14:295–302.

71. Chian RC, Kuwayama M, Tan L, Tan J, Kato O, Nagai T. High survival rate of bovine oocytes matured *in vitro* following vitrification. *J Reprod Dev* 2004;50:685–96.

72. Antinori M, Licata E, Dani G, Cerusico F, Versaci C, Antinori S. Cryotop vitrification of human oocytes results in high survival rate and healthy deliveries. *Reprod Biomed Online* 2007;14:72–9.

73. Tucker MJ, Wright G, Morton PC, Massey JB. Birth after cryopreservation of immature oocytes with subsequent *in vitro* maturation. *Fertil Steril* 1998;70:578–9.

74. Kuwayama M, Vajta G, Leda S, Kato O. Comparison of open and closed methods for vitrification of human embryos and the elimination of potential contamination. *Reprod Biomed Online* 2005;11:608–14.

75. Lucena E, Bernal DP, Lucena C, Rojas AJ, Moran A, Lucena A. Successful ongoing pregnancies after vitrification of oocytes. *Fertil Steril* 2006;85:108–111.

76. Selman H, Angelini A, Barnocchi N, Brusco GF, Pacchiarotti A, Aragona C. Ongoing pregnancies after vitrification using a combined solution of ethylene glycol and dimethyl sulphoxide. *Fertil Steril* 2006;86:997–1000.

77. Chian R-C, Huang YJ, Tan SL, Lucena E, Saa A, Rojas A, *et al*. Obstetric and perinatal outcome in 200 infants conceived from vitrified oocytes. *Reprod Biomed Online* 2008;16:608–10.

78. Tan SL, Doyle P, Campbell S, Beral V, Rizk B, Brinsden P, *et al*. Obstetric outcomes of *in-vitro* fertilisation pregnancies compared with normally conceived pregnancies. *Am J Obstet Gynecol* 1992;167:778–84.

79. Tredder RS, Zukerman MA, Goldstone AH, Hawkins AE, Fielding A, Briggs EM, *et al*. Hepatitis B transmission from contaminated cryopreservation tank. *Lancet* 1995;346:137–40.

80. Borini A, Sciajno R, Bianchi V, Sereni E, Flamigni C, Coticchio G. Clinical outcome of oocyte cryopreservation after slow freezing with a protocol utilizing a high sucrose concentration. *Hum Reprod* 2006;21:512–17.

81. Chamayou S, Alecci C, Ragolia C, Storaci G, Maglia E, Russo E, *et al*. Comparison of *in vitro* outcomes from cryopreserved oocytes and fresh sibling oocytes. *Reprod Biomed Online* 2006;12:730–6.

82. La Sala G, Nicoli A, Villani MT, Pescarini M, Gallinelli A, Blickstein I. Outcome of 518 salvage oocyte cryopreservation cycles performed as a routine procedure in an *in vitro* fertilisation program. *Fertil Steril* 2006;86:1423–7.

83. De Santis L, Rabellotti E, Papaleo E, Calzi F, Fusi FM, Brigante C, *et al*. Oocyte cryopreservation: clinical outcomes of slow-cooling protocols differing in sucrose concentration. *Reprod Biomed Online* 2007;14:57–63.

84. Borini A, Bianchi V, Bonu MA, Sciajna R, Sereni E, Cattoli M, *et al*. Evidence-based clinical outcome of oocyte slow cooling. *Reprod Biomed Online* 2007;15:175–81.

85. Okimura T, Kato K, Zhan Q, Kuwayama M, Zhang J, Kato O. Update on clinical efficiency of the vitrification method for human oocytes in an in vitro fertilization program. *Fertil Steril* 2005;84 Suppl 1:S174.

86. Yoon TK, Lee DR, Cha SK, Chung MH, Lee WS, Cha KY. Survival rate of human oocytes and pregnancy outcome after vitrification using slush nitrogen in assisted reproductive technologies. *Fertil Steril* 2007;88:952–6.

87. Cobo A, Kuwayama M, Pérez S, Ruiz A, Pellicer A, Remohí J. Comparison of concomitant outcome achieved with fresh and cryopreserved donor oocytes vitrified by the Cryotop method. *Fertil Steril.* 2008;89:1657–64.

Chapter 21
Assisted conception: uses and abuses

Melanie Davies

Background

The demographic changes in childbearing in Western societies over recent decades have been detailed in previous chapters. More and more women are postponing pregnancy and thus experiencing infertility and pregnancy loss.

Fertility reduces with advancing age: this reduction becomes significant after the age of 35 years and fertility ceases several years before menopause. Observational studies among communities that do not practise contraception show similar results across different times and countries, summarised in Figure 21.1. The famous study by Tietze[1] among the Hutterite community that was published in 1957 showed that 87% of couples were infertile by the age of 45 years. The rate is probably higher in modern Western societies owing to acquired causes of infertility such as chlamydial tubal damage, smoking and obesity.

Pregnancy loss becomes more common with advancing maternal age; indeed, the majority of conceptions to women in their 40s do not lead to a live birth. The rise in the rate of miscarriage is paralleled by the rise in chromosomal disorders in offspring of older mothers. The underlying factor is the increasing risk of genetic abnormality in the eggs of older women.

The evidence supports the Faddy–Gosden model of oocyte depletion.[2] Whereas spermatogenesis is a continuous process in men, there is no genesis of eggs in women; the number of eggs is maximal in fetal life and there is a continuous decline thereafter. Egg loss becomes more rapid in the 40s and leads to complete loss of eggs and menopause around the age of 50 years. It is the reduction in egg quantity and quality that leads to age-related infertility and miscarriage.

What can assisted conception offer to avert this?

In vitro fertilisation

It is a common misconception that *in vitro* fertilisation (IVF) can treat all types of infertility and couples may rely on the false security that 'we can always have IVF'. Unfortunately, IVF cannot compensate for delay in childbearing. The likelihood of success with IVF depends on the number and quality of eggs collected and thus upon ovarian reserve at the time of collection. Indeed, female age is the best single predictor of success (Figure 21.2): livebirth rates of 30% per cycle for women aged under 35 years decrease to 15% for those aged 40 years and to below 5% for those aged 43 years.[3]

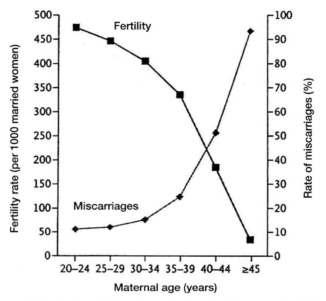

Figure 21.1 Fertility and miscarriage rates by maternal age; reproduced with permission from Heffner[36] (© 2004 Massachusetts Medical Society, all rights reserved) and based on data in Menken *et al.*[37] and in Nybo Andersen *et al.*[38]

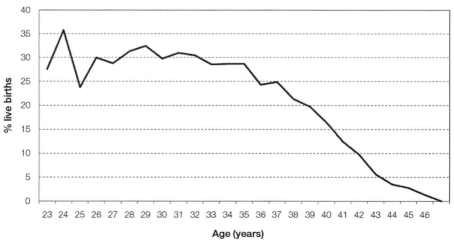

Figure 21.2 IVF livebirth rates by age (fresh embryos, own eggs); 2005 UK data from the Human Fertilisation and Embryology Authority[3]

Leridon[4] developed a mathematical model of the combined monthly probabilities of conceiving spontaneously, of miscarriage and of age-related infertility (Table 21.1). The proportion of women conceiving a successful pregnancy (that is, one leading to a live birth) within 1 year was estimated as 75% for women aged 30 years, decreasing to 66 % for those aged 35 years and 44% for those aged 40 years. By extending this model to 4 years, the success rates rose to 91%, 84% and 64%, respectively. Making the assumption that all unsuccessful women went on to have IVF and received treatment more quickly in the older age groups, Leridon superimposed the effect of assisted reproduction. This achieved more pregnancies than waiting for spontaneous conception for women aged 35 years but had minimal benefit for those aged 40 years. Assisted reproduction did not close the gap: treatment made up for only one-half of the births lost by postponing childbearing from the age of 30 years to the age of 35 years and less than one-third of those lost by postponing from the age of 35 years to the age of 40 years.

Preimplantation genetic screening

Cytogenetic abnormalities of the human oocyte, as described by Pellestor et al.,[5] are remarkably common and there appears to be a multifactorial effect of maternal ageing. Aneuploid embryos are common following IVF, even in unstimulated cycles.[6] The increasing proportion of abnormal embryos with increasing maternal age underlies the increasing risk of miscarriage in older women: by far the most common cause of first-trimester miscarriage is aneuploidy. This is paralleled by the rising incidence of Down syndrome with increasing maternal age.

A widely used diagnostic technique for prenatal diagnosis of Down syndrome is fluorescence in situ hybridisation (FISH), which is applied to fetal cells following amniocentesis. This rapid method of genetic analysis can be applied to single cells derived from embryonic biopsy and thus allow embryo selection. This is an attractive proposition: screening embryos for chromosomal abnormalities might identify the best embryos for transfer back to the uterus and allow older women to have better success rates and fewer miscarriages.

Sadly, preimplantation genetic screening (PGS) has not lived up to these expectations. No benefit has been demonstrated in randomised controlled trials (RCTs), although observational studies with matched controls have shown an improved implantation rate after PGS for 'advanced maternal age'.[7,8] There are several randomised trials, none of which have shown a significant improvement in implantation or clinical pregnancy

Table 21.1 Mathematical probability of pregnancy at various ages; data from Leridon[4]

Spontaneous pregnancy			
Age when starting to conceive	30 years	35 years	40 years
Successful within 1 year (%)	75	66	44
Successful within 4 years (%)	91	84	64
Using assisted reproduction			
Age when starting ART	34 years	38 years	42 years
Successful before ART (%)	91	82	57
Successful with ART (%)	30.1	23.6	16.5
Total % successful	94	86	64

ART = assisted reproductive technology; 'successful' = conception leading to live birth

rates.[9-13] Indeed, the largest showed a significant reduction (continuing pregnancy rate ratio 0.69; 95% CI 0.51–0.93; n = 408).[11] This study has been criticised for poor patient selection and failings of technique[14] but John Collins,[15] in an editorial in the *New England Journal of Medicine*, considered that the RCT results were sufficiently strong to rule out genetic screening for chromosomal abnormalities 'solely because of advanced maternal age'.

Nevertheless, despite the current lack of supportive evidence, PGS is growing in popularity. The PGD Consortium of the European Society of Human Reproduction and Embryology (ESHRE) collects self-reported data from up to 50 centres, almost all in Europe, and reports annually. The number of PGS cycles has risen from 1211 cycles in the calendar year 2002[16] to 2275 cycles in the latest report from 2005,[17] plus an unknown number of cycles in the USA and the rest of the world. The technique is widely advertised by IVF clinics.

While many scientists feel that genetic screening remains a plausible method of embryo selection, the current limitations of PGS mean that it cannot be used by older women to circumvent the problems of IVF failure and miscarriage. The process of embryo biopsy is technically demanding and expensive. It is an invasive procedure and there are no long-term follow-up data for human babies born from biopsied embryos. Moreover, to undertake PGS, the laboratory needs a good number of cleaving embryos so this actually excludes many older women who are 'poor responders' to ovarian stimulation. Braude and Flinter,[18] writing in the *BMJ*, reviewed the application of PGS 'in patients who are desperate for a successful pregnancy' and reached a robust conclusion: 'A technique that only works in certain enthusiasts' hands may have little to recommend it ... The widespread use of this expensive technology ... is arguably unethical.'

Fertility insurance – cryopreservation

Since IVF and PGS do not improve the reproductive performance of older women, what alternative approaches can be considered? Preservation of fertility by storing embryos, eggs or ovarian tissue is now widely offered to young women facing cancer treatment that will induce premature menopause. Why not extend this to offer cryopreservation to all women who face ovarian ageing? Cryopreserved gametes will remain genetically young, at the age of the woman at the time of storage. Indeed, as storage takes place at extremely low temperatures in liquid nitrogen, gametes can be preserved indefinitely and retain eternal youth.

Embryo freezing

Embryo freezing has been an extremely valuable adjunct to IVF over the past 20 years; the storage of spare embryos saves women from undergoing repeated ovarian stimulation and oocyte retrieval procedures. However, livebirth rates from frozen–thawed embryos are generally half that of fresh embryos (and less than natural conception in fertile couples). Thus couples are best advised to proceed with pregnancy rather than store embryos and postpone their family. Furthermore, the consent of both parties is required in UK law before stored embryos can later be used in treatment, and there have been high-profile cases where a relationship has broken down and one partner is unwilling to become a parent.[19] Women who are not in a relationship could theoretically use donor sperm, but their future partner may have reservations about having a donor family. Moreover, the clinics and regulator may consider the storage and disposal of donor embryos that have been created 'just in case' to be ethically contentious.

Egg freezing

Egg freezing has proved to be technically much more difficult than embryo freezing. Using conventional slow freezing, success was elusive until fertilisation rates were improved with the use of intracytoplasmic sperm injection in the mid-1990s.[20] However, with conventional freezing techniques, livebirth rates are around 2% per oocyte thawed[21] and only a few hundred births have been reported worldwide. This number is expected to increase rapidly with the recent development of vitrification techniques resulting in better freeze–thaw survival.[22] Initial safety data are reassuring as the children born show no increase in abnormalities.[23] Oocyte freezing is now becoming established as a method of fertility preservation.

Ovary/tissue freezing

Storage of immature eggs in ovarian tissue is still an experimental technique, with less than ten reported pregnancies from regrafted tissue biopsies. The loss of follicles during freeze–thawing means that the graft's lifespan is short and thus removal of a whole ovary may be necessary. This is acceptable for women with cancer facing ablative treatment but not justifiable for healthy women who are hoping for natural conception. Laboratory isolation and maturation of immature eggs from the stored samples for IVF has not been achieved.

Extending reproductive choice

Women who are concerned that their fertility is slipping away are turning to oocyte freezing for hope. In most IVF clinics, requests for oocyte storage from healthy fertile women outnumber those from cancer patients. Although the American Society for Reproductive Medicine strongly warns women against relying on egg freezing to postpone motherhood, US clinics are marketing this aggressively, with statements along the lines of 'Egg freezing is an incredible breakthrough for women' and 'Egg freezing allows women to take control of their fertility'. Some clinics link this service to ovarian reserve screening with a message equivalent to 'If the result is poor, hurry to freeze your eggs'. More than one cycle of stimulation may be needed to store a sufficient number of eggs. Information on clinic websites minimises the potential risks of ovarian stimulation: 'the process is … quite routine. At the appropriate time we will use a simple procedure to collect the eggs'.[24] The costs of egg freezing are typically £3,000 per cycle. Certain clinics will waive the fee in exchange for 'egg-sharing' or for donating half the number of eggs collected. Whether this 'exchange of services' is ethically justifiable can be debated. The clinics have long waiting lists of women requiring donor eggs, the egg recipient is paying for the donor's cycle and this recruitment exercise will attract fertile young donors. These young women – perhaps students who cannot otherwise pay for egg freezing – need to be counselled carefully about the implications of donation. Egg donation is highly successful and recipients of fresh donor eggs have a likelihood of pregnancy that is probably twice as good as their own chance of pregnancy with their own thawed eggs in the future. Thus donors may well have genetic offspring whom they will not know. In the UK, they must also be made aware that children born from their donation have the right to trace them when they reach the age of 18 years.

Perhaps we should look at egg freezing as a great advance in reproductive choice but it is difficult for women to obtain a balanced perspective and accurate information from the current media coverage. The media have inflated the situation with sensationalist articles: scientists will 'create a generation of ice babies'.[25] Personal stories of women who have frozen eggs for social reasons are paraphrased: 'How career women will put motherhood on ice'.[26] Even *New Scientist* has used the headline 'Egg freezing: a reproductive revolution'.[27]

Egg donation

Ovarian failure is an untreatable condition but the opportunity for pregnancy can be restored by egg donation. Success rates are high and are maintained with increasing age (Figure 21.3). It is the age of the donor that matters and uterine ageing has very little impact, even beyond the normal reproductive lifespan, as long as hormone replacement therapy is used.

There is a severe shortage of egg donors in the UK. Egg donation is regulated by the Human Fertilisation and Embryology Authority (HFEA), is unpaid and is not anonymous (children born from donation have the right to trace their genetic parent from the age of 18 years). The donor must go through a stimulated cycle with daily subcutaneous injections of follicle-stimulating hormone (FSH), monitoring with ultrasound and blood tests that lead, after 2 weeks, to an admission for egg harvest as a day-case procedure under anaesthesia. There are risks to the donor: the most common complication is ovarian hyperstimulation, which hospitalises at least one in 100 women having IVF and is more likely to affect young fertile women. The risks of egg collection – bleeding, infection, anaesthesia – are small, but the donors also have the discomfort of injections and inconvenience of travelling and scheduling appointments.

As a result of the donor shortage, there are long waiting lists for treatment in many UK clinics. Some centres restrict treatment to couples that are able to bring a donor. To increase the numbers donating, 'egg sharing' was accepted by the HFEA in 1998.[28] This means that infertile women undergoing IVF can donate a proportion (usually

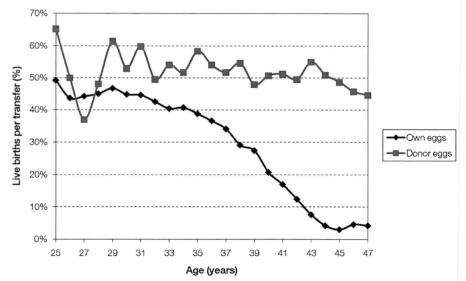

Figure 21.3 Livebirth rates per transfer for ART cycles using fresh embyos from own and donor eggs, 2003; data from US Centers for Disease Control and Prevention[39]

half) of their eggs in exchange for free treatment. Their costs are paid by the recipient couple. This has been described as a win–win situation but it is an indirect payment and can also be viewed as coercion of vulnerable women who are forced to consider donation as they cannot afford to have IVF in any other way. The infertile donor has to understand that she may not achieve pregnancy herself but could still have a genetic child whom she cannot contact but who might seek her out in the future.

Desperate couples go to great lengths to obtain treatment: many advertise for donors in UK newspapers and one couple put an advertisement on the side of a London bus (which attracted several enquiries and led to successful donation).[29] Increasingly, couples go abroad for treatment. Donors are paid in most countries and the UK emphasis on informed consent and independent counselling is lacking. Anonymity is protected in many countries so that children will be unable to trace their donor and donors may be unidentifiable even if genetic information is medically important.

Financial inducement can be overt. In the USA, the American Society for Reproductive Medicine recommends that the upper limit for 'compensation' paid to donors should be US$5,000 but larger sums are frequently involved – this is payment rather than compensation.[30] A frozen egg bank in California advertises a 'basic package' of six eggs for US$15,000 and 'premium package' of 12 eggs for US$25,000.

Reproductive tourism is thriving. Couples from the UK are travelling to Spain, Cyprus, India and the Ukraine. There are now British clinics sending women overseas to have embryos implanted and setting up links to Spain and Eastern Europe. Many women go 'freelance', using internet chat rooms to locate clinics across Eastern Europe and elsewhere that promise to find them donors quickly and cheaply. The exact numbers are not known as embryos implanted overseas are not covered by UK regulations and treatment cycles are not reported to the HFEA. Multiple pregnancies are relatively common: there has been a nine-fold rise in multiple births in women aged 45 years or over in the UK[31] and a substantial number of fetal reduction procedures in London are undertaken on women who had had IVF overseas.[32]

Trading eggs is big business. A report in *The Observer* on the 'Cruel cost of the human egg trade' visited Cyprus and stated that some women viewed egg donation as their main source of income, going through the process of being injected with hormones at least five times a year.[33] The rate of payment was 350 Cyprus pounds (£420) for a cycle in which a woman produced 12 eggs, 500 Cyprus pounds if she produced more: 'They just give their eggs and get the money, it's a pure transaction.' The HFEA website has a new section on fertility tourism – the message must be '*caveat emptor*'.[34]

Egg donation pregnancy may not be straightforward as there are higher rates of hypertension, pre-eclampsia, gestational diabetes and assisted delivery in older mothers. The oldest British mother was aged 62 years when she was delivered by caesarean section in 2006; she could not be treated in the UK but went to Eastern Europe. The dangers of multiple pregnancy are illustrated by Adriana Iliescu, a Romanian woman aged 67 years who had a twin pregnancy but suffered a stillbirth and caesarean section for the surviving twin at 34 weeks. The world's oldest mother, Omkari Panwar, underwent IVF in a last-ditch attempt to produce a male heir to take over the family's smallholdings and was aged 70 years when she delivered preterm twins in India in 2008.

Surrogacy

Reproductive ageing has little effect on uterine function as long as hormone support is maintained. Postmenopausal women undergoing egg donation require hormone replacement therapy to promote uterine growth and endometrial thickening. If the uterus cannot support a pregnancy, for example because of fibroids, or if the potential mother is too unfit for pregnancy, surrogacy will be required. It is possible for the surrogate to be the genetic mother and conception can take place by insemination using sperm from the recipient's husband. However, the surrogate mother is then 'giving away' her genetic child and the psychological and ethical problems are obvious. A third party can act as an egg donor so that the embryos are genetically unrelated to the surrogate. The recipient couple usually take over the care of the baby shortly after delivery but need to go through legal proceedings (parental order or adoption) to become the legal parents.

Again, the regulations in the UK are stringent.[35] Commercial surrogacy is illegal in the UK but the commissioning couple may still be liable for considerable expenses. Couples may only apply for a 'parental order' if they are married and domiciled in the UK and if the child is genetically related to at least one partner. Surrogacy is an uncommon and expensive procedure. Couples are seeking alternative treatment overseas and India is the main destination for surrogacy tourism. In a country with widespread poverty, the potential for exploitation is obvious.

Conclusion

This chapter has examined the ways in which assisted reproductive technologies can be used to improve reproductive outcome in older women. IVF is ineffective and the addition of PGS of embryos has not boosted success rates. Egg freezing offers considerable hope of preserving fertility although it cannot match natural conception rates; this makes it an appropriate technology for young women with cancer but not a panacea for healthy women wishing to postpone childbearing. Egg donation overcomes age-related infertility; the success rates (and the genetic child) relate to the donor not the recipient.

In reviewing the 'uses' of assisted reproduction, some 'abuses' have been revealed. The infertile couples seeking help can be desperate for treatment and therefore be vulnerable to suggestion. The media have an interest in selling copy and thus in promoting dramatic or sensationalist stories and announcing 'breakthroughs' in reproductive technology. IVF clinics may find that the pressure of competition drives them to advertise, to offer new techniques before they are supported by hard scientific evidence and to accede to women's requests for treatment even if it is ineffective or potentially risky. Reproductive tourism is burgeoning, driven by women's needs for treatment but also by commercial interests. Payment for egg donors may distort the profile of the pool of donors compared with altruistic volunteers and change the motivation of donors. In economically deprived areas, women paid for donation might not disclose an unfavourable medical history, may donate repeatedly and ignore risks of overstimulation, and may have more regrets. Egg sharers who obtain free treatment in exchange for donation, which they could not otherwise afford, may be donating under coercion. Overseas surrogacy treatment in developing countries – 'rent a womb' – is an extreme example of economic coercion that many people would consider an abuse, yet to the organisers of such programmes it is a sound commercial proposition.

References

1.   Tietze C. Reproductive span and rate of conception among Hutterite women. *Fertil Steril* 1957;8:89–97.

2. Faddy MJ, Gosden RG. A model conforming the decline in follicle numbers to the age of menopause in women. *Hum Reprod* 1996;11:1484–6.

3. Human Fertilisation and Embryology Authority. *A Long-Term Analysis of the HFEA Register Data (1991–2006).* London: HFEA; 2008 [www.hfea.gov.uk/en/1540.html].

4. Leridon H. Can assisted reproduction technology compensate for the natural decline in fertility with age? A model assessment. *Hum Reprod* 2004;19:1548–53.

5. Pellestor F, Anahory T, Hamamah S. The chromosomal analysis of human oocytes: an overview of established procedures. *Hum Reprod Update* 2005;11:15–32.

6. Verpoest W, Fauser BC, Papanikolaou E, Staessen C, Van Landuyt L, Donoso P, et al. Chromosomal aneuploidy in embryos conceived with unstimulated cycle IVF. *Hum Reprod* 2008;23:2368–71.

7. Gianaroli L, Magli C, Ferraretti AP, Munné S. Preimplantation diagnosis for aneuploidies in patients undergoing *in vitro* fertilization with a poor prognosis: identification of the categories for which it should be proposed. *Fertil Steril* 1999;72:837–44.

8. Munné S, Garrisi J, Barnes F, Werlin L, Schoolcraft W, Kaplan B. Reduced spontaneous abortion and increased live birth rate after PGD for advanced maternal age. *Fertil Steril* 2007;88:S85–6.

9. Staessen C, Platteau P, Van Assche E, Michiels A, Tournaye H, Camus M, et al. Comparison of blastocyst transfer with or without preimplantation genetic diagnosis for aneuploidy screening in couples with advanced maternal age: a prospective randomized controlled trial. *Hum Reprod* 2004;19:2849–58.

10. Stevens J, Wale P, Surrey ES, Schoolcraft WB, Gardner DK. Is aneuploidy screening for patients aged 35 or over beneficial? A prospective randomized trial. *Fertil Steril* 2004;82:S249.

11. Mastenbroek S, Twisk M, van Echten-Arends J, Sikkema-Raddatz B, Korevaar JC, Verhoeve HR, et al. *In vitro* fertilization with preimplantation genetic screening. *New Engl J Med* 2007;357:9–17.

12. Hardarson T, Hanson C, Lundin K, Hillensjo T, Nilsson L, Stevic J, et al. Preimplantation genetic screening in women of advanced maternal age caused a decrease in clinical pregnancy rate: a randomized controlled trial. *Hum Reprod* 2008;23:2806–12.

13. Schoolcraft WB, Katz-Jaffe MG, Stevens J, Rawlins M, Munné S. Preimplantation aneuploidy testing for infertile patients of advanced maternal age: a randomized prospective trial. *Fertil Steril* 2008 Aug 8 [E-pub ahead of print].

14. Cohen J, Grifo JA. Multicentre trial of preimplantation genetic screening reported in the New England Journal of Medicine: an in-depth look at the findings. *Reprod Biomed Online* 2007;15:365–6.

15. Collins JA. Preimplantation genetic screening in older mothers. *N Engl J Med* 2007;357:61–3.

16. Harper JC, Boelaert K, Geraedts J, Harton G, Kearns WG, Moutou C, et al. ESHRE PGD Consortium data collection V: cycles from January to December 2002 with pregnancy follow-up to October 2003. *Hum Reprod* 2006;21:3–21.

17. Goossens V, Harton G, Moutou C, Scriven PN, Traeger-Synodinos J, Sermon K, et al. ESHRE PGD Consortium data collection VIII: cycles from January to December 2005 with pregnancy follow-up to October 2006. *Hum Reprod* 2008; 23:2629–45.

18. Braude P, Flinter F. Use and misuse of preimplantation genetic testing. *BMJ* 2007; 335:752–4.

19. European Court of Human Rights, Council of Europe. *Evans vs The United Kingdom (Application no. 6339/05): Judgment. Strasbourg 7 March 2006* [www.echr.coe.int/ECHR].

20. Fabbri R, Porcu E, Marsella T, Rocchetta G, Venturoli S, Flamigni C. Human oocyte cryopreservation: new perspectives regarding oocyte survival. *Hum Reprod* 2001;16:411–16.

21. Oktay K, Cil AP, Bang H. Efficiency of oocyte cryopreservation: a meta-analysis. *Fertil Steril* 2006; 86:70–80.

22. Kuwayama M, Vajta G, Kato O, Leibo SP. Highly efficient vitrification method for cryopreservation of human oocytes. *Reprod Biomed Online* 2005;11:300–8.

23. Tur-Kaspa I, Gal M, Horwitz A. Genetics and health of children born from cryopreserved oocytes. *Fertil Steril* 2007;88:S14.

24. Quotation from patient information leaflet produced by commercial UK IVF unit, 2008.

25. Marsh B. Egg freezing breakthrough will create generation of 'ice babies'. *The Telegraph* 11 October 2005 [www.telegraph.co.uk/scienceandtechnology/science/sciencenews/3343416/Egg-freezing-breakthrough-will-create-generation-of-ice-babies.html].

26. Fleming N. How career women will put motherhood on ice. *The Telegraph* 6 January 2006 [www.telegraph.co.uk/news/uknews/1507109/How-career-women-will-put-motherhood-on-ice.html].

27. Nowak R. Egg freezing: a reproductive revolution. *New Scientist* 21 March 2007 [www.newscientist.com/article/mg19325964.400-egg-freezing-a-reproductive-revolution.html].

28. Human Fertilisation and Embryology Authority. Chair's letter CH(98)05. London: HFEA; 1998 [www.hfea.gov.uk/en/522.html].

29. BBC News. Baby girl born after bus adverts. BBC News website 30 June 2008 [news.bbc.co.uk/1/hi/england/kent/7480748.stm].

30. The Ethics Committee of the American Society for Reproductive Medicine. *Financial Compensation of Oocyte Donors*. Birmingham, Alabama: ASRM; 2007 [www.asrm.org/Media/Ethics/financial_incentives.pdf].

31. Office for National Statistics. *Birth Statistics: Review of the National Statistician on Birth and Patterns of Family Building in England and Wales, 2007*. Series FM1 No. 36. Newport: ONS; 2007. Table 6.1 [www.statistics.gov.uk/downloads/theme_population/FM1_36/FM1-No36.pdf].

32. McKelvey A, Shenfield F, David A, Jauniaux E. Unpublished data presented at The Royal College of Obstetricians and Gynaecologists 7th International Scientific Meeting, Montreal, 2008.

33. Barnett A, Smith H. Cruel cost of the human egg trade. *The Guardian* 30 April 2006 [www.guardian.co.uk/uk/2006/apr/30/health.healthandwellbeing].

34. Human Fertilisation and Embryology Authority. *Fertility Treatment Abroad*. London: HFEA; 2008 [www.hfea.gov.uk/en/981.html].

35. Office of Public Sector Information. Surrogacy Arrangements Act 1985 (c.49). London: Office of Public Sector Information; [www.opsi.gov.uk/RevisedStatutes/Acts/ukpga/1985/cukpga_19850049_en_1].

36. Heffner LJ. Advanced maternal age – how old is too old? *N Engl J Med* 2004;351:1927–9.

37. Menken J, Trussell J, Larsen U. Age and infertility. *Science* 1986;233:1389–94.

38. Nybo Andersen AM, Wohlfahrt J, Christens P, Olsen J, Melbye M. Maternal age and fetal loss: population based register linkage study. *Brit Med J* 2000;320:1708–12.

39. Centers for Disease Control and Prevention. Assisted Reproductive Technology (ART) Report: Section 4 – ART Cycles Using Donor Eggs. Atlanta, GA: CDC, 2003 [www.cdc.gov/ART/ART2003/section4.htm].

Chapter 22
Future fertility insurance

Discussion

William Ledger: Thanks very much for three very good talks. While the other speakers are returning, perhaps I could ask Professor Dickenson to comment as you have a professional and personal interest in this topic.

Donna Dickenson: Thank you very much. I have in fact written a book on this.[1] I think the situation is actually even grimmer than Melanie portrayed it – and it is quite grim as she portrayed it. The American Society of Reproductive Medicine (ASRM) does set a maximum, or recommends there is a maximum, of US$5,000 but surveys indicate that currently only half of its members obey it.[2] There have been substantiated reports of up to US$100,000.[1] There have also been substantiated evidence-based reports of up to 70 eggs being taken in only one cycle.[3] The other thing which is quite worrying is that although we say that it is an American phenomenon, even in America you cannot buy and sell organs. However, there is an ambivalence in the relevant 1987 Act,[4] which actually makes an exception to the general principle, because gametes, as it puts it, are renewable tissue. So gametes are exempted. So, it is all based on a massive legislative mistake! It is worrying, as you quite rightly point out, that the trade is developing in Eastern Europe, Spain and Cyprus. There is very strong evidence, not just in the *Observer* report,[5] but further reports since,[6,7] of a massive element of trafficking also involved. So, I think the situation is bad. There are a few favourable signs such as the European Union directive[8] barring the sale of eggs for IVF, but not for stem cell research.

Peter Braude: What concerns me is the amount of egg sharing that occurs. It is extraordinary that we ever agreed to it. We know that there are clinics in this country that have secondary enterprises, working either in Middle Eastern countries and certainly through Cyprus and Russia. They will often accompany their patients through IVF for free. Is there no opportunity for professional bodies to do something about it? Even if it is not exactly direct flouting of the law, it is a clear skirting of the law.

William Ledger: One area we do not have represented around the table is an international lawyer who might have answered that point. I know the HFEA [Human Fertilisation and Embryology Authority] have grappled with this but struggled to regulate outside our own shores. And, as we were discussing yesterday, the European Union has kept a very 'arm's length' approach.

Herman Tournaye: Helen, two years ago I was saying the same thing, but I do not share your scepticism against oocyte freezing anymore. If you look at the published data, it is my feeling that vitrification will completely change the clinical approach that we have now. Look, for example, at the published data with poor responders, which many of us are reproducing. These women can do two cycles of ovarian stimulation, where there is a collection of only two eggs each time, which are frozen. In the end they are fertilised using ICSI with very good results. So, I think egg freezing can revolutionise the way we work.

Helen Picton: I agree with you. That wasn't the impression I intended to give. The results from vitrification are extremely encouraging. That is really my 'take-home' message. Slow-freezing has not been very successful and has probably peaked. We cannot do very much more without completely changing our approach. You can only tinker with the sugar concentrations so much and we have not seen a continuous stepwise increase in success rates. Vitrification is a different matter altogether. I was very sceptical when I saw some results 2 years ago about survival rates of 100% after vitrification. We did it ourselves and we are getting 100% so I am confident that reports for vitrification are real. That is beginning to be translated into success rates, and you can see the data from a number of clinics, all of which are consistently showing the same sort of thing. The summaries of the studies (Table 20.3) had, I think, nine or ten published studies on vitrification – not an awful lot of large-scale studies, but all of them consistently showing the same sort of results. It is improving. The bottom line, or caveat, is that, even with vitrification, you have to have good eggs to vitrify. If the tissue is not really good from our stimulation protocols, or if it is compromised, for example if it is a young cancer patient who is quite sick at the time that she has her eggs collected, we can only do what we can with vitrification if we have really good starting material. My money for MII [metaphase II] freezing is definitely on vitrification as the way forward. There are practical issues to be resolved such as the ovum contact with nitrogen. If we can get the quality of the egg right, vitrification of MII's is what we will see being used in clinical practice, and successfully. I do not think slow freezing will match it any way, shape or form.

Stephen Hillier: All three speakers were absolutely fantastic, thank you very much. Melanie, you made the point that there is no insurance: nothing really works in an objective sense. Helen made a point, subject to the sub-qualification you just gave, that freezing does not work, at least not yet. But clearly there are individual situations where it has worked. Bhatty [Professor Bhattacharya] went over all the ovarian reserve tests, diagnostic and prognostic. Clearly they do work, more or less, in terms of predicting numbers of oocytes and numbers of embryos, but they do not predict pregnancy. You can say this is really pessimistic. Or, you could go the other way and argue, as I did yesterday, that the real problem is that every single one of these correlates is an individual personal event that is exclusive to that woman. Until you (or we) as gynaecologists, embryologists, endocrinologists and everybody else get together and try to do everyone's management properly, and optimally for each individual, there is no point doing meta-analyses and comparisons as they are all different cohorts, different ages, different techniques, etc. We still have not completely saturated the potential that exists in one-to-one management on the basis of best practice – best physiological and clinical practice.

Siladitya Bhattacharya: I completely agree with the joined-up thinking approach, but condensed to individualised management. But there is a message: it is managing to convey the right amount of information in the right perspective and not over-sell what we can do. Part of the problem is the mismatch between expectation and reality.

Susan Bewley: Some comments about language and my concerns about hidden concepts. Firstly, the term 'egg sharing' is a misnomer. Sharing usually means you and I split something in half and we both benefit. You can't split an egg! Clearly, if I give you my egg and you give me money – that is not 'sharing', it is 'selling'. I think we should not use the term. 'Sharing' is a cosy way of covering up the discounted IVF that women get when they have no other choice after remortgaging their house. I would rather see free unlimited IVF, particularly when it's most effective below the age of 35, than so-called 'egg sharing'. The second is about the language of 'choice' which seems to dominate all discourse nowadays. Consider the 18-year-old who, to get through her long education, may feel she has no choice but by earning money in one way or another, selling parts of her body in a traditional female way. [laughter] There are other 'choices' that are not encouraged (and I'm looking for Alastair here) such as choosing to know your genetic inheritance. When your parents conceal that, which happens in most donor insemination and conception cases, it's a false or illusory 'choice'. Choice for some, but not others? Lastly, I accept everything Steve said about how we must do better – that is the medical and technological imperative. Nevertheless, for the woman who is being told today that there might be a test, the advertisements say 'Is there a way I can test the fertility in the privacy of my own home?' We should tell her that the best test for fertility is unprotected sex which ends in pregnancy – which has always been the case. Laboratory tests do not look as though they can tell you 'Will I be all right later down the line?'. Yes, freeze your eggs, by all means, but do not let that put you off getting on with it. Those would seem to be simple messages nowadays. I find the language, the selling, the choice and consumerisation very muddling.

Melanie Davies: Quick feedback: ESHRE [European Society for Human Reproduction and Embryology] has a task force on ethics and law and their approach to egg sharing talks about 'exchange of services'.[9] And they say this is morally or ethically more acceptable than frank payment, although I cannot see the difference myself.

Roger Gosden: Regarding the reserve test, I think we are measuring the wrong cell type. We are measuring granulosa cells directly or indirectly. We need to estimate the number of follicles or eggs, and these are a great problem. Maybe we can discuss that later. Melanie, I do not think there is any doubt around the table that we should offer embryo freezing where possible. Egg vitrification: I completely disagree with you about having ovarian tissue off the table. Although you presented the first two papers,[10,11] those were very unsatisfactory in many respects. The problems are with the grafting, as you say, not the cryopreservation, which works very well. The studies published by Silber on the monozygotic twins, which were mainly fresh grafts, show extraordinary success. In the first seven in that series (and this is sister-to-sister donation), all seven had a return to cycles.[12,13] There are five ongoing pregnancies. Just to give an example: the very first case was a 25-year-old woman who started cycling, as they all did, 3–4 months after the graft. She conceived an ongoing and successful pregnancy on the second cycle. She then had a miscarriage, and her first graft failed after 3 years. Then she had a bit of the frozen tissue grafted back and she conceived again and at the very first ovulation. She delivered a child and that graft is still ovulating. I believe there is a place for this procedure, particularly for very young women and for children for whom there is no other option.

Melanie Davies: I am very sorry if I appeared so dismissive, because I do think that ovarian tissue has a place for the young prepubertal cancer patient. But addressing what to do for a 30-year-old woman who comes for fertility preservation – it has got to be egg freezing, does it not?

Kate Brian: I want to return to reproductive tourism. We highlighted the problems for donors but we need to know as well about the problems for recipients when travelling for treatment. We did a survey recently at the Infertility Network UK, about people's experiences.[14] What came across very clearly was that an awful lot of people, about 40%, had absolutely no counselling at all before going ahead. They were not completely thinking through all the issues such as anonymity or multiple-embryo transfers. There are a lot of problems we need to be aware of.

Dimitrios Nikolaou: Just a comment about the so called 'ovarian reserve' tests. I think these tests should be called 'ovarian response' tests rather than 'ovarian reserve' tests. The reason is that they primarily reflect oocyte quantity, rather than quality.[15] Therefore, they cannot assess an individual's current fertility unless they are extremely abnormal. The only way we currently have to make an (indirect) assessment of the qualitative aspects of the ovarian reserve is the performance during an IVF cycle, where we can look at the quality of the embryos, blastocysts, etc. When discussing 'screening' for 'early ovarian ageing',[16] and 'fertility insurance', the question, of course, is whether any of these tests could be transferred from the field of assisted reproduction to the general population to be used in asymptomatic young women to predict their future fertility? We know that poor ovarian response to stimulation with gonadotrophins is associated with an earlier menopause[17,18] and we know that the existing ovarian reserve tests can predict poor response.[19] For 'screening' to be possible we would need to collect data from a large number of healthy women in the general population and create normal charts for all ages.[20-22] A project such as this would require international collaboration and many years to complete. But what can be done for now I think, is this: we know that one in ten women out there are at risk of early ovarian ageing, but how many women actually realise that? This, I think, is very important. We need to raise awareness of the possibility of 'early ovarian ageing', not only among women but also in the medical profession. Which women? Not the women who are 38 years old and come to the infertility clinic, because then it is too late. The message needs to be delivered to women who are young, still in their 20s, by their GP, or at school or university. Also, there are environmental factors that can increase the risk of early ovarian decline, such as smoking, and women should also be made aware of this.

Siladitya Bhattacharya: I agree. There is a sense of *déjà vu* about this returning to where we were this morning. I do not want to go back over ground we covered earlier. The only note of caution is this: any attempt to go into schools to tell young women to have their babies early would probably not be welcomed by many in the society. So we have to find another mechanism.

William Ledger: The optimal age, biologically, for women to have children is between 20 and 35. We heard that from several speakers. Thinking about the end of this meeting, that is not a sociological recommendation. It is not, I think, a sexist comment in any way. It merely emphasises the biology.

Maya Unnithan: Are we fair in thinking of the social implications of authorities' advances in reproductive medicine? They are actually generating different ways for women to relate to their reproductive bodies. It used to be just through motherhood. But now, having your egg which you can then use leads to reproduction in another line of context. This is really interesting in terms of the ways this feeds back. The thinking of yourself as reproductive. So women who are 18 who are not married can be able to think of themselves as reproductive.

Herman Tournaye: This is a point about the insurance. What I hear from the rumours is that women are interested in being able to have children in the future but also want to avoid the symptoms of menopause. That is why we often combine treatments: we stimulate their ovaries and take the eggs for vitrification but we also store ovarian tissue. Because, apparently, according to many people who work in the field of ovarian tissue transplantation, one small chip of ovarian tissue is good for 4 years of cycling with normal menstrual cycles, so the idea would be that …

Melanie Davies: … it's an alternative implant really …

Herman Tournaye: Not just to get children.

William Ledger: OK. With that interesting and provocative thought, thank you very much to our speakers.

References

1. Dickenson D. *Body Shopping: the Economy fuelled by Flesh and Blood*. Oxford: Oneworld; 2008.
2. De Sutter P. Ethical aspects of modern reproductive medicine and research. Women and Bioethics Conference, Austrian National Bioethics Committee, 2 June 2008, Vienna, Austria.
3. Jacobs A, Dwyer J, Lee, P. Seventy ova. *Hastings Cent Rep* 2001;31:12–14.
4. National Conference of Commissioners on Uniform State Laws. *Uniform Anatomical Gift Act* [www.anatomicalgiftact.org/DesktopDefault.aspx].
5. Barnett A, Smith H. Cruel cost of the human egg trade. *The Observer* 30 April 2006 [www.guardian.co.uk/uk/2006/apr/30/health.healthandwellbeing].
6. Alkorta Idiakez I. Egg donation, a new case of gender exploitation? Women and Bioethics Conference, Austrian Naitonal Bioethics Committee. 2 June 2008, Vienna, Austria.
7. Waldby C. Oocyte markets: women's reproductive work in stem cell research. *New Genet Soc* 2008;27:19–31.
8. Directive 2004/23/EC of the European Parliament and of the Council of 31 March 2004 on Setting Standards of Quality and Safety for the Donation, Procurement, Testing, Processing, Preservation, Storage and Distribution of Human Tissues and Cells. *Official J Eur Union* 7 April 2004 [www.who.int/ethics/en/ETH_EU_Directive_2004_23_EC.pdf].
9. ESHRE Task Force on Ethics and Law. III. Gamete and embryo donation. *Hum Reprod* 2002;17:1407–8.
10. Donnez J, Dolmans MM, Demylle D, Jadoul P, Pirard C, Squifflet J, et al. Livebirth after orthotopic transplantation of cryopreserved ovarian tissue. *Lancet* 2004;364:1405–10. Erratum in: *Lancet* 2004;364:2020.
11. Meirow D, Levron J, Eldar-Geva T, Hardan I, Fridman E, Yemini Z, et al. Monitoring the ovaries after autotransplantation of cryopreserved ovarian tissue: endocrine studies, *in vitro* fertilization cycles, and live birth. *Fertil Steril* 2007;87:418.e7-418.e15.
12. Silber SJ, Lenahan KM, Levine DJ, Pineda JA, Gorman KS, Friez MJ, et al. Ovarian transplantation between monozygotic twins discordant for premature ovarian failure. *N Engl J Med* 2005;353:58–63.
13. Silber SJ, DeRosa M, Pineda J, Lenahan K, Grenia D, Gorman K, et al. A series of monozygotic twins discordant for ovarian failure: ovary transplantation (cortical versus microvascular) and cryopreservation. *Hum Reprod* 2008;23:1531–7.

14.   Brian K. Trying times. *The Guardian* 3 June 2006 [www.guardian.co.uk/money/2006/jun/03/careers.work7].

15.   Nikolaou D. How old are your eggs? *Curr Opin Obstet Gynecol* 2008;20:540–4.

16.   Nikolaou D, Templeton A. Early ovarian ageing: a hypothesis. Detection and clinical relevance. *Hum Reprod* 2003;18:1137–9.

17.   Nikolaou D, Lavery S, Turner C, Margara R, Trew G. Is there a link between an extremely poor response to ovarian hyperstimulation and early ovarian failure? *Hum Reprod* 2002;17:1106–11.

18.   de Boer EJ, den Tonkelaar I, te Velde ER, Burger CW, Klip H, van Leeuwen FE; OMEGA-project group. A low number of retrieved oocytes at *in vitro* fertilization treatment is predictive of early menopause. *Fertil Steril* 2002;77:978–85.

19.   Broekmans FJ, Kwee J, Hendriks DJ, Mol BW, Lambalk CB. A systematic review of tests predicting ovarian reserve and IVF outcome. *Hum Reprod Update* 2006;12:685–718.

20.   Nikolaou D, Templeton A. Early ovarian ageing. *Eur J Obstet Gynecol Reprod Biol* 2004;113:126–33.

21.   Wallace WH, Kelsey TW. Ovarian reserve and reproductive age may be determined from measurement of ovarian volume by transvaginal sonography. *Hum Reprod* 2004;19:1612–17.

22.   van Rooij IA, Broekmans FJ, Scheffer GJ, Looman CW, Habbema JD, de Jong FH, *et al.* Serum antimullerian hormone levels best reflect the reproductive decline with age in normal women with proven fertility: a longitudinal study. *Fertil Steril* 2005;83:979–87.

Section 6

Sex beyond and after fertility

Chapter 23
Contraception for older couples

Diana Mansour

Introduction

An unplanned pregnancy at any age can be devastating but is particularly so for women aged 40 years or over. At this age, women are thought to be in control of their lives, with contraception organised and effectively used. Unfortunately, the facts do not support this statement and the number of abortions in this age group continue to rise. In England and Wales in 2007, 8644 women aged 40 years or over had an abortion, with 710 women being aged 45 years or over and 19 aged 50 years or over.[1] In the UK, over 50% of pregnancies in women approaching their 50s are unplanned.

So, are contraceptive choices reduced for the older woman? The answer should be 'no', yet in practice older couples are far more reliant on permanent, surgical methods and are less likely to use pills and condoms. The Omnibus Survey for 2006/07 asked just over 5000 people in Great Britain aged 16–49 years about their contraceptive usage.[2] The most popular methods were oral contraceptives (35%), male and female sterilisation (27%) and condoms (30%). In people aged 40–44 years, male and female sterilisation was the most common choice of contraception (48%), with 20% using condoms, 17% using oral contraceptives and 7% using intrauterine contraception.[2]

There are now 13 family planning methods available to couples in the UK. These methods can be used by people of all ages after identifying any contraindications. Of these, 11 provide a reversible option, which is very important for those delaying starting or completing their family. Women may be unhappy about making such a permanent decision, with those sterilised under the age of 31 years being twice as likely to express regret compared with older women.[3] They are also 3.5–18 times more likely to request information about reversal and about eight times more likely to undergo reversal or evaluation for *in vitro* fertilisation (IVF).[3]

Many women now plan their first child in their 30s. In 2006, the average age of first birth in the UK was 29.1 years, with women in their early 30s more likely to have a baby than those in their early 20s.[4]

Are there additional problems for the older mother? Data suggest that fecundity decreases as one grows older and the incidence of clinically recognised miscarriage increases.[5] For women receiving optimal health care, maternal mortality is not affected by age, although women in their 40s are at a significantly higher risk of pre-eclampsia, gestational diabetes, induction of labour, operative deliveries (including caesarean section), perinatal mortality, intrauterine fetal death and neonatal death compared with women in their 20s.[6,7]

Contraceptive methods for the older woman

Female and male sterilisation

Male or female sterilisation is chosen by almost 50% of British couples in their 40s as their main method of contraception. Of these, 15% of men and 12% of women choose either vasectomy or tubal occlusion.[2] Couples seeking advice about these birth control methods need to be made aware of the permanency of this surgery and the very small failure rates with each procedure.

Vasectomy is the most effective contraceptive method available, with failures now quoted as having a life-time risk of one in 2000 after two azoospermic samples taken 2–4 weeks apart at least 8 weeks after the procedure.[8] Men requesting vasectomy can be reassured that there is no substantial long-term health risk associated with the procedure, although there is a possibility of chronic testicular pain.[8] Male sterilisation has the advantage of being a minor surgical procedure involving the division of both vas deferens and is normally performed under local anaesthetic with few adverse effects. It is a permanent contraceptive method and although it may be reversed, success rates decrease with the time elapsing from the initial surgery.[8]

Female sterilisation, involving surgical division or mechanical tubal occlusion, was always thought to be the most effective method of contraception. However, following publication of the US Collaborative Review of Sterilization (CREST) study in the late 1990s, which was a multicentre, prospective, cohort study involving 10 685 women for between 8 and 14 years, concern was voiced about long-term efficacy. Cumulative 10 year failure rates of between 0.75 and 3.65 per 100 procedures were reported with the highest rate after Hulka-Clemens clip sterilisation and lowest after unipolar coagulation.[9] The cumulative risk of pregnancy was highest in those sterilised at a young age, with failures for bipolar coagulation quoted as 5.43 per 100 procedures and 5.21 per 100 procedures for Hulka-Clemens clip sterilisation.[9]

The Filshie clip is the most commonly used occlusive method in the UK and is considered to be one of the most effective, with a reported risk of failure over a 10-year period of 2–3 pregnancies per 1000 procedures. Its silastic jaws ensure tight apposition across the fallopian tube but with little risk of bisection, thereby reducing the chances of recanalisation.[8] The life-time failure rate for other female sterilisation methods are quoted as one pregnancy in every 200 procedures performed.[8]

Female sterilisation is often perceived to be the ideal contraceptive method for the older woman as it is effective, does not involve hormones and does not 'mask' symptoms of the menopause. Hormone replacement therapy (HRT) is easily commenced, if required. Female sterilisation has not been shown to increase menstrual blood loss or cause dysmenorrhoea but these problems may present when hormonal contraceptives are discontinued following surgery. Women may also be less tolerant of these complaints post-sterilisation as their childbearing days are over. Requests for treatment of menstrual problems are high, with a 17% cumulative probability of women undergoing hysterectomy 14 years after tubal occlusion.[10]

There are now a number of equally effective yet reversible contraceptive methods available that rival female sterilisation, including the newer copper intrauterine devices (IUDs), the levonorgestrel-releasing intrauterine system (LNG-IUS), progestogen-only injectables and contraceptive implants. These should be considered when female sterilisation is discussed.

Copper intrauterine devices

Intrauterine contraceptives are not a popular contraceptive choice for couples in the UK, with only 7% of women aged 40 years or over choosing this method.[2] About 10% of contraceptive users in Europe and more than 100 million women worldwide decide upon the IUD for spacing their families.[11] Copper-bearing IUDs tend to be used by parous women but can safely be used in the nulliparous who wish to avoid hormonal methods but still have effective contraception. IUDs are highly suitable for older women with medical conditions such as hypertension and cardiovascular disease.

Modern copper IUDs such as the TCu-380A provide highly effective contraception with 1–2% failure rates at 5 years.[12] Increasing the surface area of copper in third-generation IUDs and placing copper bands on the transverse arms of the TCu-380A has markedly improved efficacy when compared with those containing less than 250 mm^2 of copper or older inactive devices.

Research has shown that, in long-term users, copper IUDs work mainly by preventing fertilisation rather than implantation.[13] The copper is both toxic to sperm and the ovum and a local 'sterile' endometrial inflammatory reaction prevents implantation.[14] There is no evidence suggesting that IUDs cause or increase the incidence of pelvic infection, even in immunocompromised women.[14] Pelvic inflammatory disease is more closely associated with the presence of or exposure to a sexually transmitted infection and fitting of an IUD without prior screening for infection.

Modern copper IUDs are licensed for 5–10 years of use, with recent data indicating that the TCu-380A is effective for up to 20 years – it is a very cost-effective method of contraception.[15] Increasing the intervals between IUD changes also reduces the insertion-related risks of pelvic infection, uterine perforation and expulsion.

For older women, the type of copper IUD inserted may not be so important. In 1990, the Family Planning Association suggested that first-, second- or third-generation copper IUDs (re)inserted in women aged 40 years or over may remain until contraception is no longer needed, for example 1 year after the last menstrual period in women aged 50 years or over. This is acceptable practice because, with diminishing fertility, the IUD rarely fails.[16]

Two of the most common reasons for early IUD removal are increased menstrual loss and pain. Framed devices can increase menstrual loss by 20–30%. As women in their 40s often report an increase in menstrual loss together with dysmenorrhoea,[17] these menstrual changes must be emphasised when counselling about this method. However, many women requesting a very effective, reversible and hormone-free contraceptive are prepared to balance the advantages against these disadvantages.

Most experts would recommend IUD removal after the menopause because of the theoretical risk of pyometra or pelvic actinomycosis. Giving a short course of local vaginal estrogen may aid removal if the device has been in place for a number of years. If removal proves difficult, particularly if the IUD threads are missing, then, after thorough counselling, the user may elect to avoid further surgery. This decision needs to be documented and she should be advised to seek help if symptoms such as pelvic pain, vaginal bleeding or abnormal discharge occur.

Hormonal intrauterine systems

Mirenai® (Schering), the LNG-IUS, is an ideal contraceptive method for the older woman. Since it was first licensed in Finland in 1990, there have been more than

10 million cumulative users worldwide (unpublished data). However, in the UK in 2006, only 24% of women surveyed had ever heard of this method.[18]

The LNG-IUS is licensed to provide highly effective contraception for a 5-year period, with fewer than 10 in 1000 women becoming pregnant over 5 years.[12] Women aged 45 years or over at the time of insertion and who are amenorrhoeic may keep the LNG-IUS until after the menopause, even if this is beyond the duration of the UK marketing authorisation.[12]

The LNG-IUS is a T-shaped device with the vertical stem containing 52 mg levonorgestrel surrounded by a silastic capsule releasing 20 micrograms of hormone each day in year 1, decreasing to 11 micrograms in year 5. This gives few systemic adverse effects.[19] It exerts its contraceptive action by altering the cervical mucus and uterotubal fluid, inhibiting sperm migration, inducing endometrial atrophy and altering sperm function and motility.[19] The LNG-IUS can suppress ovulation in some women during year 1 by possibly reducing the preovulatory luteinising hormone (LH) surge. Most cycles from year 2 onwards are ovulatory.[19]

Women in their 30s and 40s choose the LNG-IUS not only because it is a highly effective contraceptive method but because women from the general population report a decrease in dysmenorrhoea and lighter menstrual loss. Those complaining of heavy menstrual bleeding with or without fibroids also benefit, with objective blood loss reduced by 86% after 3 months and 97% after 12 months.[20] Irregular bleeding may be an issue in the first 3–6 months of LNG-IUS use, with prolonged spotting more common in women with menorrhagia with or without fibroids.[21]

The LNG-IUS may regulate fibroid growth and help prevent fibroid formation.[22] There is now evidence confirming that the LNG-IUS is a useful medical treatment for women suffering from endometriosis-related problems, with users reporting significant improvements in severity and frequency of pain/menstrual symptoms.[23]

Women in their 40s using the LNG-IUS are more likely to report amenorrhoea and this has been confirmed by Swedish data. After using an LNG-IUS for 5 years, 70% of women reported regular scanty bleeding, 26% had amenorrhoea and 4% complained of irregular bleeding. After 10 years with a second LNG-IUS, 60% of women reported amenorrhoea, 28% stated that they had regular scanty bleeding and 12% had irregular bleeding. It is interesting to note that a return to irregular bleeding or spotting did not occur following insertion of the second or third LNG-IUS.[24]

Long-term use of the LNG-IUS prevents endometrial proliferation and may induce regression of endometrial hyperplasia.[25] It also has the flexibility of being used as the progestogen component for HRT; however, in this instance, the LNG-IUS would need changing every 5 years.[26]

Some concerns have been voiced that LNG-IUS users with oligomenorrhoea or amenorrhoea may be at risk of osteoporosis but this is not the case. It has been shown that the incidence of ovulation and mean plasma estradiol levels do not differ between menstruating and amenorrhoeic women using the LNG-IUS.[19] Evidence has also found no association between this system and the development of neoplasia, including breast cancer.[27]

In summary, the LNG-IUS must be the contraceptive method of choice for the older woman – if only they knew of its existence. As healthcare professionals, we are aware of its enormous potential to help prevent gynaecological disease. Increasing the provision of the LNG-IUS as a long-acting reversible method of contraception and offering alternative contraceptive choice at the time of female sterilisation has been shown to reduce gynaecological intervention over the long term. In Newcastle, where primary and secondary care work closely together, the number of hysterectomies has fallen by over 50% and female sterilisation procedures by 75% in the past 10 years. This has been achieved by increasing provision of the long-acting hormonal contraceptive methods, particularly the LNG-IUS.[28]

Combined hormonal contraception, including the pill, patch and vaginal ring

Epidemiological data support the prescribing of combined hormonal contraceptives (CHCs) to non-smoking, normal-weight, low-risk women who do not suffer from migraine until the menopause. When the UK Medical Eligibility Criteria (MEC) consensus group met, it recommended that no contraceptive method – including CHCs – is contraindicated by age alone.[29] The UK's Faculty of Sexual and Reproductive Healthcare advises that CHCs can be used unless there are coexisting diseases or risk factors.[30] For women in their 40s, it is normal practice to prescribe the lowest dose preparation that gives good cycle control.

So often when we discuss CHCs our minds are focused on the adverse effects and potential dangers and we forget about the benefits that may be particularly relevant for women in their late 30s and 40s. Combined oral contraceptive pills (COCs) have been shown to reduce menstrual loss and dysmenorrhoea and to give good cycle control.[31] In one randomised controlled study, women complaining of menorrhagia reported a 43% reduction in blood loss when taking the COC.[32]

The majority of studies also suggest that COC use may increase bone mineral density (BMD) in women aged 40 years or over but does not seem to reduce the overall incidence of fractures in premenopausal women.[31]

A number of studies have suggested that epithelial ovarian tumours are less frequently found in women taking the COC. As ovarian cancer is the most common fatal gynaecological malignancy, with a 5 year survival rate of around 40%, and its incidence increases with age, this benefit should be welcomed by women. Overall, even in women taking modern low-dose formulations, the risk is reduced by about 50%[33] and this reduction is similar to that found with older formulations containing double the amount of hormone.[34] The risk decreases with increasing years of use (a 5% reduction with each additional year of use was found in a study published in 2008)[35] and this protective effect lasts for at least 30 years after pill taking has ceased.[34] The COC also protects against the development of endometrial cancer, halving the risk and providing protection for at least 15 years after discontinuation.[30] The COC may decrease the incidence of large bowel cancer by up to 40%,[30] although there are no data, as yet, to suggest that duration of use influences this protective effect.

What about the risks of taking the COC with particular reference to older women in their reproductive years? In 1996, the Collaborative Group on Hormonal Factors in Breast Cancer reanalysed the worldwide epidemiological evidence on the relationship between breast cancer risk and use of hormonal contraceptives.[36] The overall findings were that current users of the pill or those who had used them in the past 10 years were at a slightly increased risk of having breast cancer diagnosed, although the additional cancers tended to be localised to the breast. However, duration of use, age at first use and the dose and type of hormone within the contraceptives had little additional effect on breast cancer risk. There is still some controversy concerning the association between COCs and breast cancer, with four studies[37–40] published after the reanalysis paper of 1996[36] suggesting that there is no increased risk.

Does the COC increase the risk of cardiovascular disease? This is obviously very relevant for the older woman. However, the incidence of myocardial infarction is low in women of reproductive age. Work from the 1980s suggested that pill takers who did not smoke or have other risk factors for cardiac disease were no more at risk of acute myocardial infarction than non-users.[41] A study published in 1999 confirmed this.[42] Both studies highlighted that cigarette smoking and hypertension are independent risk factors for myocardial infarction.

The relationship between cerebrovascular disease and the COC is also important, particularly as the background incidence of stroke increases with age. Approximately 3 per 100 000 women aged under 35 years suffers an ischaemic stroke each year but this doubles with the use of the pill.[30] Other factors associated with an increased risk include a previous history of myocardial infaction (ten-fold increased risk), heavy alcohol consumption (eight-fold increased risk), previous venous thromboembolism (VTE) (six-fold increased risk), treated diabetes mellitus (four-fold increased risk), hypertension (four-fold increased risk), smoking (three-fold increased risk) and migraine (two-fold increased risk).[43,44] Data suggest that high-dose COCs (50 micrograms or more of ethinyl estradiol) increase the risk of ischaemic stroke by approximately two-fold,[45] with the duration of COC use having little influence on the incidence of cerebrovascular events. Approximately 30% of these women will die from this event and a similar proportion will suffer severe morbidity. There is no association between pill use and haemorrhagic stroke.[30]

The incidence of VTE was reported to be increased about five-fold in users of the older high-dose COCs compared with non-users.[46] Data published in 2007 suggest that the COC increases the risk of VTE by about two-fold in low-risk long-term COC users.[47] Whether third-generation COCs containing desogestrel or gestodene further increase this risk is open to debate and this difference probably has little impact on the health of women taking oral contraception. More importantly, there are other independent risk factors that should be taken into consideration when prescribing the pill to the older woman, including obesity (a body mass index over 30 kg/m^2) and a close family history of VTE. With particular reference to the older woman, the incidence of VTE increases with age and thus all risk factors must be excluded before the COC is prescribed.

In summary, it does appear that VTE is about twice as common as arterial complications for women in their 20s. In older women (aged 30–44 years), however, the number of arterial complications exceeds venous disease by about 50%.[48] It must be remembered that women are far more likely to die following an arterial event or to suffer a significant disability.[48] Therefore, healthcare professionals must ensure that CHCs are prescribed safely and only given to those aged 35 years or over with no venous or arterial risk factors.

Progestogen–only pills

Progestogen-only pills (POPs) have normally been reserved for women who are breastfeeding, who are aged 35 years or over or who have contraindications to taking the COC. In the past, there were concerns that POPs were not as effective as COCs and women had to be really good pill takers for it to be effective, as 'the safety window' was just 3 hours. All this changed with the launch of Cerazette® (Schering-Plough), a POP containing 75 micrograms desogestrel. In the UK by 2008, 12–14% of oral contraceptive users took POPs, but this was just 6% before 2002.

So why has Cerazette had such an impact on POP prescribing? The unusual feature of this POP is that it inhibits ovulation in 97% of women as well as having the normal progestogen effects on cervical mucus and the endometrium.[49] Fewer women have regular menstrual cycles when compared with traditional POPs and reports of nuisance adverse effects are similar. The most important feature of Cerazette is that failure rates are similar to COCs[49] (Pearl index less than 1) and extra contraceptive precautions are only required if a tablet is forgotten for more than 12 hours.[50]

POP safety data are very reassuring for the older woman as it does not increase the risk of venous thrombosis, cardiovascular disease or cerebral thrombosis.[51] Are there concerns that the resultant oligomenorrhoea or amenorrhoea may adversely affect BMD? There are limited data in this area but POPs appear to have little effect on BMD.[52]

Can the POP be continued when HRT is prescribed for menopausal symptoms? Again, there are no published studies but it is felt that if the POP is effective in a woman aged 35 years who is producing physiological levels of estradiol then it should be effective in perimenopausal women taking HRT. A sequential or continuous combined HRT should be prescribed as the progestogen content of one POP will not provide the necessary endometrial protection.

Progestogen–only injectables

One of the first long-acting reversible contraceptive preparations to be used was an intramuscular progestogen-only depot that gave contraceptive cover from between 2 and 3 months. The most commonly used progestogen-only injectable is Depo-Provera® (Pharmacia) (depot medroxyprogesterone acetate; DMPA). Is it suitable for contraceptive use in older women?

World Health Organization data suggest that DMPA use is associated with a marked reduction in risk for endometrial cancer[53] and no long-term increase in the risk of breast, cervical or ovarian cancers.[54–56] Increasing numbers of women in their 30s and 40s complain of menstrual problems, including premenstrual syndrome, menorrhagia and dysmenorrhoea. DMPA is a useful treatment option. More than 55% of users are amenorrhoeic after using DMPA for 12 months and this may increase to 68% by 2 years.[57] The National Institute for Health and Clinical Excellence has also endorsed its use, recommending DMPA as a treatment for heavy menstrual loss.[58]

However, DMPA inhibits ovulation by suppressing LH and, to a certain extent, follicle-stimulating hormone (FSH), and thus DMPA administration creates a relative hypoestrogenic state with serum estradiol levels within the early follicular range. Current evidence suggests that BMD in DMPA users generally decreases over time, particularly within the first few years of use, after which it appears to plateau.[59,60] There are very little data investigating fracture risk and DMPA, with one small study finding no significant association.[61]

There is evidence that BMD starts to recover quickly, especially at the spine, when DMPA is discontinued, with rates generally higher than for non-users.[62] If women discontinue using DMPA before their menopause, evidence suggests that they have a similar BMD as postmenopausal women who have never used this form of contraception.[62]

Caution needs to be exercised, therefore, in those women who have lifestyle and/or medical risk factors that put them at increased risk of low BMD (amenorrhoeic athletes, cigarette smokers, women with anorexia nervosa, perimenopausal women and those on long-term corticosteroid treatment). The Committee on Safety of Medicines supports this advice.[59]

Some units restrict the use of DMPA to women aged under 45 years, thereby giving time for recovery of BMD before the menopause. Others weigh up the risks of an unplanned pregnancy against any potential risks of continuing an effective contraceptive with non-contraceptive benefits.

Finally, progestogen-only injectables do not appear to increase the risk of acute myocardial infarction, venous thrombosis or stroke.[51]

Progestogen–only implants

Implanon® (Schering-Plough), the single-rod etonogestrel contraceptive implant, is becoming a popular contraceptive choice for women of all ages. It was launched in 1999, over 3 million women are fitted with Implanon worldwide and more than 80 000 women in the UK request Implanon each year. Year 1 continuation rates have been impressive, with only 25% of women requesting removal in the first 12 months.[63] This continuation rate compares very favourably with other long-acting reversible contraceptive methods[12] and the most common adverse effects are bleeding problems, mood change and weight gain.

Implanon's contraceptive effect lasts for 3 years, with its main modes of action being ovulation inhibition plus alteration of cervical mucus reducing sperm penetrability.[64]

For the older woman, there are some concerns that the irregular bleeding caused by progestogen–only methods may mask endometrial pathology. This has not been borne out in practice. Again, there is no evidence indicating that progestogen–only implants increase the risk of cardiovascular disease or adversely affect BMD.[65,66]

Barrier and natural methods

The Omnibus Survey for 2006/07 reported that 20% of couples aged between 40 and 44 years used condoms as their main method of contraception.[2] With more than one in three couples experiencing divorce, condom use is advised for those entering new relationships to provide protection against sexually transmitted infection as well as contraceptive cover.

For experienced older users, condoms and diaphragms can be effective. Failure rates of less than 1% per year are quoted in proficient, conscientious users of barrier methods and this nears 100% in those approaching the menopause. Diaphragms should be used with a spermicidal preparation but they may be difficult to fit in women with any significant degree of uterovaginal prolapse and they are contraindicated in those who suffer from recurrent urinary tract infections.

For those who suffer with a true latex allergy, male and female condoms made of polyethylene can be tried. Most allergy complaints, however, are related to the presence of a spermicide (nonoxynol-9) on the condom and condoms lubricated with a non-spermicidal silicone base should be tried.

Extra lubricant may be needed in those suffering with vaginal dryness. Care should be exercised when other vaginal preparations are used, for example antifungal pessaries and estrogen creams, as oil-based products may affect the tensile strength of latex condoms and lead to rupture. Male condoms may also be unacceptable in those with erectile dysfunction. For the perimenopausal woman who is having irregular periods, some experts suggest the use of spermicides alone as the risk of pregnancy is low.

Natural family planning methods incorporating the calendar method, monitoring of the basal body temperature and changes in the cervical mucus can provide effective contraception in women who still have regular cycles but whose natural fertility is waning. As with barrier methods of contraception, motivation and experience are the all-important keys to success.

PERSONA® (Swiss Precision Diagnostics GmbH), the hand-held fertility awareness computer system, may also be used. It builds up, month on month, a record of each individual woman's hormonal cycle using a urinary metabolite of estradiol and detecting the LH surge. It must be remembered that natural family planning methods are unsuitable in perimenopausal women with irregular and unpredictable cycles.

Emergency contraception

Emergency contraception is not contraindicated in older women, although awareness in this age group is poor – women in new relationships may once again be using condoms, which increase their chances of a contraceptive failure.

Use of postcoital contraception has escalated since the launch of progestogen-only emergency contraception (POEC) in the late 1990s, which replaced the Yuzpe method. POEC's success is partly related to its high efficacy (failure rate of 0–2%) and also the low incidence of adverse effects. In October 2003, a single pill containing 1.5 mg levonorgestrel was introduced, which aided compliance.

There is evidence to suggest that hormonal emergency contraception may prevent pregnancies even if it is taken between 72 and 120 hours following the first episode of unprotected intercourse in that cycle. Although a copper IUD would be a more effective emergency contraceptive method, POEC could be considered if this was refused.[67] An IUD is also a suitable option if chosen for long-term contraception. It can be inserted up to 5 days after the earliest estimated time of ovulation or up to 5 days after the first episode of unprotected sexual intercourse in that cycle.

When should contraception be discontinued?

The median age of the menopause in Western women who do not smoke is 51.3 years. Although there are no studies giving clear guidance on when contraception can be discontinued, it is standard practice to advise women aged 50 years or over to use a contraceptive method for 1 year after their last natural menstrual period. Women aged under 50 years are advised to continue using a method for a further 2 years as they are at greater risk of 'breakthrough ovulation'.[31]

There is no accurate biological marker to detect the menopause, although FSH is frequently used. Unfortunately, FSH levels vary depending on the day in the cycle that blood is taken. Ideally, FSH should be measured within the first 3–5 days but ovulation can occur in the last month before the menopause or when FSH levels are elevated.

Discontinuing combined hormonal contraception

Symptoms of the menopause are often masked in women using CHCs but some may complain of vasomotor symptoms in the hormone-free week. One option is to change to another contraceptive method at the age of 50 years and continue this until the age of 55 years, when at least 80% of women are 1 year past their last period.[68]

Some would advise checking FSH levels 6–8 weeks after discontinuing the COC if no menstrual bleed has occurred. Levels over 30 iu/l suggest that the woman is menopausal but a confirmatory FSH should be repeated 2 weeks later. If both levels are over 30 iu/l then the woman is menopausal but contraception is still advised for a further 12 months. If either of these levels is below 30 iu/l then contraception must be continued and FSH repeated in 12 months.[68]

Discontinuing progestogen–only methods

Unfortunately, drug-induced amenorrhoea may cause confusion by mimicking the menopause but progestogen–only methods do not mask menopausal symptoms and neither do they greatly affect gonadotrophin levels. In such cases, FSH can be used and if levels are greater than 30 iu/l on two occasions then the woman is probably menopausal and will need to use contraception for the next year. If she is aged under 50 years, she will need to continue using contraception for a further 2 years.[68]

Discontinuing contraception while taking HRT

There is little evidence to suggest that oral or transdermal HRT preparations suppress gonadotrophin levels. FSH can be measured ideally within the first 5 days of the cycle. If two results are over 30 iu/l, contraception should be continued for 2 years if she is aged under 50 years and 1 year if she is aged 50 years or over. If FSH is within the normal range, contraception should be continued and levels checked again in 12 months.

Conclusion

Women in their late 40s often feel that contraception is not necessary and should be reserved for their daughters. However, the risk of an unplanned pregnancy is still present and results in increased morbidity and mortality for mother and baby together with catastrophic psychosocial consequences. There are now a number of very suitable reversible contraceptive methods available that offer effective contraception and non-contraceptive benefits that help to improve quality of life and the transition into the menopause.

References

1. Department of Health. *Abortion Statistics, England and Wales: 2007*. London: DH; 2007 [www. dh.gov.uk].

2. Lader D. *Contraception and Sexual Health 2006/07*. Omnibus Survey Report No. 33. Newport: ONS; 2007 [www.statistics.gov.uk].

3. Curtis KM, Mohllajee AP, Peterson HB. Regret following female sterilization at a young age: a systematic review. *Contraception* 2006;73:205–10.

4. Office for National Statistics. *Summary of Key Birth Statistics: 1996–2006*. Newport: ONS; 2007 [www.statistics.gov.uk].

5. van Noord-Zaadstra BM, Looman CW, Alsbach H, Habbema JD, te Velde ER, Karbaat J. Delaying childbearing: effect of age on fecundity and outcome of pregnancy. *BMJ* 1991;302:1361–5.

6. Godsen R., Rutherford A. Delaying childbearing. *BMJ* 1995;311:1585–6.

7. Jacobsson B; Ladfors L; Milsom I. Advanced maternal age and adverse perinatal outcome. *Obstet Gynecol* 2004;104:727–33.

8. Royal College of Obstetricians and Gynaecologists. *Male and Female Sterilisation*. Evidence-Based Clinical Guideline No. 4. London: RCOG Press; 2004.

9. Peterson HB, Xia Z, Hughes JM, Wilcox LS, Tylor LR, Trussell J. The risk of pregnancy after tubal sterilization: Findings from the U.S. Collaborative Review of Sterilization. *Am J Obstet Gynecol* 1996;174:1161–70.

10. Hillis SD, Marchbanks PA, Tylor LR, Peterson HB. Tubal sterilization and long-term risk of hysterectomy: findings from the United States collaborative review of sterilization. The U.S. Collaborative Review of Sterilization Working Group. *Obstet Gynecol* 1997;89:609–14.

11. Information & Knowledge for Optimal Health (INFO) Project. *The IUD: an Important Method with Potential*. Population Reports, Series B, Number 7. Baltimore: The INFO Project [www. infoforhealth.org/pr/b7/chap1.shtml].

12. National Collaborating Centre for Women's and Children's Health. *Long-Acting Reversible Contraception*. NICE Clinical Guideline 30. London: RCOG Press; 2005 [http://www.nice.org. uk/nicemedia/pdf/CG030fullguideline.pdf].

13. WHO Scientific Group. *Mechanisms of Action, Safety, and Efficacy of Intrauterine Devices.* Technical Report Series. Geneva: World Health Organization; 1987.

14. Clinical Effectiveness Unit. *Intrauterine Contraception.* Clinical Guidance. London: Faculty of Sexual and Reproductive Healthcare; 2007 [www.ffprhc.or.uk],

15. Sivin I. Utility and drawbacks of continuous use of a copper T IUD for 20 years. *Contraception* 2007;75(6 Suppl):S70–5.

16. Newton J, Tacchi D. Long-term use of copper intrauterine devices. *Lancet* 1990;335:1322–3.

17. Rees M. Menstrual problems. In: McPherson A, Waller D, editors. *Women's Health.* 4th ed. Oxford: Oxford University Press; 1997.

18. Family Planning Association. Women must know more about long-acting reversible contraception, says fpa. London: Family Planning Association; 2006 [www.fpa.org.uk/News/Press/Archive/2006/page222].

19. Schering AG, Leiras Oy. *Mirena: Product Monograph.* Finland: Mirena; 2002.

20. Andersson JK, Rybo G. Levonorgestrel-releasing intrauterine device in the treatment of menorrhagia. *Br J Obstet Gynaecol* 1990;97:690–694.

21. Magalhães J, Aldrighi JM, de Lima GR. Uterine volume and menstrual patterns in users of the levonorgestrel-releasing intrauterine system with idiopathic menorrhagia or menorrhagia due to leiomyomas. *Contraception* 2007;75:193–8.

22. Kaunitz AM. Progestin-releasing intrauterine systems and leiomyoma. *Contraception* 2007;75(6 Suppl):S130–3.

23. Bahamondes L, Petta CA, Fernandes A, Monteiro I. Use of the levonorgestrel-releasing intrauterine system in women with endometriosis, chronic pelvic pain and dysmenorrhea. *Contraception* 2007;75(6 Suppl):S134–9.

24. Rönnerdag M, Odlind V. Health effects of long-term use of the intrauterine levonorgestrel-releasing system. A follow-up study over 12 years of continuous use. *Acta Obstet Gynecol Scand* 1999;78:716–21.

25. Varma R, Soneja H, Bhatia K, Ganesan R, Rollason T, Clark TJ, Gupta JK. The effectiveness of a levonorgestrel-releasing intrauterine system (LNG-IUS) in the treatment of endometrial hyperplasia – a long-term follow-up study. *Eur J Obstet Gynecol Reprod Biol* 2008;139:169–75.

26. Inki P. Long-term use of the levonorgestrel-releasing intrauterine system. *Contraception* 2007;75(6 Suppl):S161–6.

27. Curtis KM, Marchbanks PA, Peterson HB. Neoplasia with use of intrauterine devices. *Contraception* 2007;75(6 Suppl):S60–9.

28. Mansour D. Modern management of abnormal uterine bleeding: the levonorgestrel intra-uterine system. *Best Pract Res Clin Obstet Gynaecol* 2007;21:1007–21.

29. Faculty of Sexual and Reproductive Healthcare. *UK Medical Eligibility Criteria for Contraceptive Use (UKMEC 2005/06).* London: FSHRC; 2006 [www.ffprhc.or.uk].

30. Clinical Effectiveness Unit. *First Prescription of Combined Oral Contraception.* London: Faculty of Sexual and Reproductive Healthcare; 2007 [www.ffprhc.org.uk].

31. Faculty of Family Planning and Reproductive Health Care Clinical Effectiveness Unit. FFPRHC Guidance (January 2005) contraception for women aged over 40 years. *J Fam Plann Reprod Health Care* 2005;31:51–63.

32. Fraser IS, McCarron G. Randomised trial of two hormonal and two prostaglandin-inhibiting agents in women with a complaint of menorrhagia. *Aust N Z J Obstet Gynaecol* 1991;31:66–70.

33. Ness RB, Grisso JA, Klapper J, Schlesselman JJ, Silberzweig S, Vergona R, et al. Risk of ovarian cancer in relation to estrogen and progestin dose and use characteristics of oral contraceptives. SHARE Study Group. Steroid Hormones and Reproductions. *Am J Epidemiol* 2000;152:233–41.

34. Collaborative Group on Epidemiological Studies of Ovarian Cancer. Ovarian cancer and oral contraceptives: collaborative reanalysis of data from 45 epidemiological studies including 23 257 women with ovarian cancer and 87 303 controls. *Lancet* 2008;371:303–14.

35. Lurie G, Wilkens LR, Thompson PJ, McDuffie KE, Carney ME, Terada KY, et al. Combined oral contraceptive use and epithelial ovarian cancer risk: time-related effects. *Epidemiology* 2008;19:237–43.

36. Collaborative Group on Hormonal Factors in Breast Cancer. Breast Cancer and hormonal contraceptives: collaborative reanalysis of individual data on 53,297 women with and 100,239 women without breast cancer from 54 epidemiological studies. *Lancet* 1996;347:1713–27.

37. Marchbanks PA, McDonald JA, Wilson HG, Folger SG, Mandel MG, Daling JR, et al. Oral contraceptives and the risk of breast cancer. *N Engl J Med* 2002;346:2025–32.

38. Hankinson SE, Colditz GA, Manson JE, Willett WC, Hunter DJ, Stampfer MJ, et al. A prospective study of oral contraceptive use and risk of breast cancer (Nurses' Health Study, United States). *Cancer Causes Control* 1997;8:65–72.

39. Vessey M, Painter R. Oral contraceptive use and cancer. Findings in a large cohort study, 1968–2004. *Br J Cancer* 2006;95:385–9.

40. Hannaford PC, Selvaraj S, Elliott AM, Angus V, Iversen L, Lee AJ. Cancer risk among users of oral contraceptives: cohort data from the Royal College of General Practitioners' oral contraception study. *BMJ* 2007;335:651.

41. Croft P, Hannaford PC. Risk factors for acute myocardial infarction in women: evidence from the Royal College of General Practitioners' oral contraception study. *BMJ* 1989;298:165–8.

42. Dunn N, Thorogood M, Faragher B, de Caestecker L, MacDonald TM, McCollum C, et al. Oral contraceptives and myocardial infarction: results of the MICA case–control study. *BMJ* 1999;318:1579–83.

43. Nightingale AL, Farmer RD. Ischemic stroke in young women: a nested case–control study using the UK General Practice Research Database. *Stroke* 2004;35:1574–8.

44. Siritho S, Thrift AG, McNeil JJ, You RX, Davis SM, Donnan GA. Melbourne Risk Factor Study (MERFS) Group. Risk of ischemic stroke among users of the oral contraceptive pill: the Melbourne Risk Factor Study (MERFS) Group. *Stroke* 2003;34:1575–80.

45. Lidegaard Ø, Kreiner S. Contraceptives and cerebral thrombosis: a five-year national case–control study. *Contraception* 2002;65:197–205.

46. Prentice RL, Thomas DB. On the epidemiology of oral contraceptives and disease. *Adv Cancer Res* 1987;49:285–401.

47. Dinger JC, Heinemann LA, Kühl-Habich D. The safety of a drospirenone-containing oral contraceptive: final results from the European Active Surveillance Study on oral contraceptives based on 142,475 women-years of observation. *Contraception* 2007;75:344–54.

48. Lidegaard O, Bygdeman M, Milsom I, Nesheim BI, Skjeldestad FE, Toivonen J. Oral contraceptives and thrombosis. From risk estimates to health impact. *Acta Obstet Gynecol Scand* 1999;78:142–9.

49. Collaborative Study Group on the Desogestrel-containing Progestogen-only Pill. A double-blind study comparing the contraceptive efficacy, acceptability and safety of two progestogen-only pills containing desogestrel 75 micrograms/day or levonorgestrel 30 micrograms/day. *Eur J Contracept Reprod Health Care* 1998;3:169–78.

50. Korver T, Klipping C, Heger-Mahn D, Duijkers I, van Osta G, Dieben T. Maintenance of ovulation inhibition with the 75-microg desogestrel-only contraceptive pill (Cerazette) after scheduled 12-h delays in tablet intake. *Contraception* 2005;71:8–13.

51. World Health Organization Collaborative Study of Cardiovascular Disease and Steroid Hormones. Cardiovascular disease and use of oral and injectable progestogen-only contraceptives and combined injectable contraceptives. Results of an international, multicenter, case–control study. *Contraception* 1998;57:315–24.

52. Curtis KM, Martins SL. Progestogen-only contraception and bone mineral density: a systematic review. *Contraception* 2006;73:470–87.

53. World Health Organization Collaborative Study of Neoplasia and Steroid Contraceptives. Endometrial cancer. *Int J Cancer* 1991;49:186.

54. World Health Organization Collaborative Study of Neoplasia and Steroid Contraceptives. Breast cancer. *Lancet* 1991;338:833–8.

55. World Health Organization Collaborative Study of Neoplasia and Steroid Contraceptives. Epithelial ovarian cancer. *Int J Cancer* 1991;49:191.

56. World Health Organization Collaborative Study of Neoplasia and Steroid Contraceptives. Squamous cervical cancer. *Contraception* 1992;45:229–312.

57. Pharmacia. *Depo-Provera Patient Information Sheet.* Pharmacia Ltd; 2004.

58. National Collaborating Centre for Women's and Children's Health. *Heavy Menstrual Bleeding.* NICE Clinical Guideline 44. London: RCOG Press; 2007 [http://www.nice.org.uk/nicemedia/pdf/CG44FullGuideline.pdf].

59. Committee on Safety of Medicines. *Updated Prescribing Advice on the Effect of Depo-Provera Contraception on Bone.* London: Medicines and Healthcare products Regulatory Agency; 2004 [www.mhra.gov.uk].

60. Curtis KM, Martins SL. Progestogen-only contraception and bone mineral density: a systematic review. *Contraception* 2006;73:470–87.

61. Lappe JM, Stegman MR, Recker RR. The impact of lifestyle factors on stress fractures in female Army recruits. *Osteoporos Int* 2001;12:35–42.

62. Kaunitz AM, Arias R, McClung M. Bone density recovery after depot medroxyprogesterone acetate injectable contraception use. *Contraception* 2008;77:67–76.

63. Lakha F, Glasier AF. Continuation rates of Implanon in the UK: data from an observational study in a clinical setting. *Contraception* 2006;74:287–9.

64. Edwards JE, Moore A. Implanon. A review of clinical studies. *Br J Fam Plann* 1999;24(4 Suppl):3–16.

65. Merki-Feld GS, Imthurn B, Seifert B. Effects of the progestagen-only contraceptive implant Implanon on cardiovascular risk factors. *Clin Endocrinol (Oxf)* 2008;68:355–60.

66. Beerthuizen R, van Beek A, Massai R, Mäkäräinen L, Hout J, Bennink HC. Bone mineral density during long-term use of the progestagen contraceptive implant Implanon compared to a non-hormonal method of contraception. *Hum Reprod* 2000;15:118–22.

67. Penney G, Brechin S, Allerton L. Clinical Effectiveness Unit (CEU) of the Faculty of Family Planning and Reproductive Health Care (FFPRHC), Royal College of Obstetricians and Gynaecologists. FFPRHC Guidance (July 2005): The use of contraception outside the terms of the product licence. *J Fam Plann Reprod Health Care* 2005;31:225–41.

68. McKinlay SM, Bramilla DJ, Posner JG. The normal menopause transition. *Maturitas* 1992;14:103–115.

Chapter 24
Ageing, infertility and gynaecological conditions: how do they affect sexual function?

Catherine Coulson

Introduction

Sexual response is a complex psychological and physiological event. It is truly psychosomatic, involving the body and the mind. It is influenced by hormones, the wholeness of the body and neurological factors. It is influenced by the experience of being held and loved as babies and children, by the sum total of all the experiences, good and bad, in life, by mood, health, stress, the nature of the relationship with the lover, and societal and personal belief systems.

A woman's sexual response changes as she ages. In addition to the effects of ageing itself, other factors in her life will have an impact. Experiences of infertility, conception, delivery, parenting, menopause, gynaecological procedures and cancer are but a few of them. Here, I attempt to look at some of these factors. There is a wealth of literature about some aspects but it is a difficult subject to quantify. When confronted with any patient, I believe it is important to see that person as a unique individual and this is even more important when the person presents a sexual problem. Generalisations are only helpful if we can first focus on the person in front of us.

Evidence

Studies to look at sexual problems are difficult to perform. The response rate is often low, possibly because inhibited people may be less likely to respond. Cross-sectional studies look at a group at a point in time. The groups chosen might be population samples from a clinic population or a general practice, or might be randomly assigned by a computer or from a medical insurance-based population. Such studies may carry a bias in sampling and will not control for cohort changes. For example, octogenarians in 2008 would have had different life experiences and education regarding sex and would have been exposed to different sexual mores than octogenarians in, say, 2050. A recent Swedish study[1] confirms this. People aged 70 years were studied in 1971, 1976, 1992 and 2000. There was an increase in sexual satisfaction and frequency of intercourse and a more positive attitude to sex over the 30-year study period.

Longitudinal studies have been conducted and provide useful data but these can also be criticised for sample bias. Many studies just ask about frequency of intercourse; however, many couples enjoy mutual masturbation as part of sexual intimacy and there are no reliable data on this activity. Embarrassment about self-masturbation makes data about this subject very difficult to collect. Not all questionnaires used have been properly validated. Large population studies use patient-completed questionnaires that are private and anonymous. Small researcher-led interviews are more probing and allow narrative research but have no statistical power.

In this chapter, I look at the evidence for the changing interest in, and capacity for, sexual activity associated with ageing in men and women. The contributory factors are psychosocial, such as relationships and retirement, or physical, related directly to ageing or to changing hormone levels.

Later, I look at whether infertility has any impact, both at the time and later in life, and whether this is related to general mood changes or to the infertility journey itself. Parity, mode of delivery, cancer and gynaecological operations may also have an impact on sexuality.

Societal views on ageing and sex

The ageing population is growing. Just over 20% of the UK population is aged 60 years or over and women aged 80 years or over predominate over men. The sexual needs of this group of people have been ignored by healthcare professionals and policymakers. Their sexual needs, for example, are rarely part of a care plan for the elderly. The negative stereotype of 'a dirty old man' is prevalent. The prevalent social sexual construct is ageist, heterosexualist and phallocentric.[2] It is not surprising that the hidden message is that sex for the elderly is not acceptable, or should at least be discreet, and hence it may be difficult for aged people to ask for help. In a review of the literature, Bouman et al.[3] found there to be a rather negative attitude to later-life sexuality by doctors and nurses and by caregivers but that the elderly themselves had a more positive view of sexuality, while also seeing themselves as less attractive and less entitled to the enjoyment of sexual pleasure. Elderly people who still engage in sexual relations benefit from an important reinforcement of self and pleasure that impacts on general wellbeing and mental health.[4]

Sexual capacity

Sexual capacities of men and women diminish with age. In men, the full erection takes longer to achieve and cannot be maintained as long, the need for ejaculation diminishes and the refractory time is longer. In the 40s, the intense genital pleasure changes to a more diffuse sensual feeling but this does not detract from the overall pleasure. With age, men gain more control over ejaculation, which can make sexual relations more pleasurable for both partners.[5–9] Women take longer to achieve orgasm and the duration and intensity diminishes.[8] During orgasm, contractions are reduced and the resolution phase is quicker. A woman's capacity for multiple orgasm remains unchanged. However, these changes are very variable and women can continue to give and receive sexual pleasure all their lives.

Sexual activity

Research shows that people continue to be sexually active in older age but that frequency diminishes. Two large US studies in the 1980s confirmed that old people are interested in sex. Starr and Weiner[10] reported on 800 adults aged from 60 to 91 years: 68% of men and 36% of women were still having intercourse. Brecher[11] interviewed 4000 people aged 50 years or over. Most reported a satisfying sex life, with 60% of men and 40% of women having intercourse and 50% of those aged 70 years or over being sexually active. A UK-based study[12] of people aged 18 to 75 years showed that self-reported satisfaction and partner-reported satisfaction was independent of age. Pfeiffer[13,14] looked at 250 men and women aged 60–94 years over a 20-year period. People who were interested in sex at the beginning of the survey maintained that interest. A decline in men's sexual activity was noted. At the start of the study, 70% of men were sexually active but only 25% were active 10 years later. The proportion of women who were sexually active was lower and constant at 20%. Men are more sexually active than women and decreasing sexual activity with increasing age is probably attributable to loss of interest by the man.

Sexual frequency

Frequency of sex declines with age. Weizman and Hart[15] looked at 81 Israeli men who were full-time workers aged 60–65 years or retirees aged 66–71 years. Of the men without erectile dysfunction, 54% had had more than four sexual encounters in the previous month (64% of those who were aged 60–65 years and 47% of those who were aged 66–71 years). Only 17% had had less than one sexual encounter in the last month (9% of those aged who were 60–65 years and 23% of those who were aged 66–71 years). The older group had masturbated more than the younger group. It might appear that the sexual interest remained constant but that the expression was different.

Libman,[16] in a study of 144 married men and 71 female partners, found that frequency of sex was the same for those aged under and over 65 years, at between once per week and once per fortnight, and that satisfaction was good in both men and women. However, younger people had more desire and fantasies.

Mulligan and Moss[17] studied 1031 war veterans aged 30–99 years. They found that sexual interest remained with age but diminished and that frequency of intercourse fell from once per week for those aged 30–39 years to once per year for those aged 90–99 years.

Sexual practices

Bretschneider and McCoy[18] studied over 200 men and women aged between 80 and 102 years and found that the majority had an active sex life but the definition was vague. Over the last year, 88% of the men and 71% of the women had felt a need to feel close and intimate with someone of the opposite sex. The most common activity was mutual caressing (82% of the men and 64% of the women), masturbation (72% of the men and 40% of the women) and penetration (63% of the men and 30% of the women) in the last year. Of those who had had intercourse, three-quarters of the men but only one-half of the women had found it pleasurable. In Libman's study,[16] the preferred activity was intercourse and men rarely masturbated.

Psychosocial issues

Lifetime experiences impact on sexual function. Bereavement, divorce, abuse and abusive relationships will impact negatively on a person's ability to enjoy sex. Previous positive experiences will condition a healthy and comfortable sexual response. People have learned different ways to negotiate problems. In older age, the children have left and the common interest of bringing them up disappears, leaving couples thrown in on each other. Failing health can produce physical barriers to sexual activity. Body image and self-esteem may suffer. With severe illness and the threat of death, some may wish for greater intimacy but some may begin to withdraw emotionally to prepare themselves for the ultimate separation. Social taboos surrounding elder sex may be difficult to negotiate.

Relationships

Trudel et al.[4,19] reviewed the literature as well as conducting the Quebec Elder Health Study. The frequency of sex declined rapidly in the early part of marriage and subsequent decline was not as great. Remarriage was associated with an increase in sexual frequency. Sexual satisfaction was associated with higher marital functioning and the quality was associated with passionate or erotic feelings for the partner. Conjugal satisfaction was not related to age itself but varied with time spent together; so it was good initially, worse in the middle and better after 25 years, underlining that couples learned to negotiate a way of being together. The divorce rate in older couples is rising, at a time of life when other stresses such as financial implications are more significant. Common sources of marital dissatisfaction in older couples are sexual relations, communication and the amount of time spent together.

Retirement

Retirement can bring a freedom from work and greater leisure time to relax. It can also signal a loss of friendship and status and can bring economic hardship. Retirement brings problems for some couples whereas for others it might be a second honeymoon. It is stressful as they renegotiate the daily tasks.

Women complain more about husbands being at home and invading their space. Research shows that couples organise their life around the home, their social network shrinks and a lot of time is spent with their spouse and they become interdependent. Pre-existing difficulties become amplified. Husbands of retired women are happier than wives of retired men; higher conflict arises when they retire asynchronously than if they retire together. Women who continue to work after their husbands retire are less satisfied. Satisfaction in retirement is different in men and women. Women value the chance of spending more time with their spouse and men value the ability to let go of the responsibilities associated with work.[19]

The ageing male

General health

Cardiovascular disease, diabetes, prostatic disorders and neurological conditions all impact on sexual function. Medical management, whether surgical or pharmacological, often has an adverse effect and many elderly people take a cocktail of drugs. Chronic diseases, such as arthritis, that impact on mobility can affect either partner. Depression is a common cause of loss of desire at all ages and increases with age. Pelvic operations for prostate or bowel can also affect the capacity for ejaculation. The prevalence of erectile dysfunction is 12.4% for men aged between 40 and 49 years, 29.8% for those between 50 and 59 years and 46% for those aged between 60 and 69 years. Erectile dysfunction increases with age, lower economic status, diabetes, heart disease and hypertension.[20]

Hormonal changes

There is an age-related decline in testosterone but it does not seem to be responsible for the increase in erectile dysfunction. Low androgens may be associated with loss of desire.[21,22] The medications for the treatment of erectile dysfunction have allowed some men the possibility to turn back the clock. However, the continuation rate of all phosphodiesterase inhibitors is low after 1 year.

In a discursive paper, Potts *et al.*[23] suggested that the medicalisation of the normal ageing process is not always welcome as it neglects men's experiences of ageing normally and undermines their understanding of such changes as positive outcomes of ageing, experience and maturity. A total of 33 men were interviewed and their narratives were taped and analysed in depth. A subset of these men talked about their changing experience of sex over their lives and, while acknowledging the loss of vigour, had found more meaning and understanding in the shared experience with their partner.

The ageing female

In women, sexual problems increase with age. As women go through the menopause, there are significant decreases in sexual responsiveness, frequency of sexual activity, libido and tender feelings for partner. There is an increase in vaginal dyspareunia and in their male partner's problems as they both age.[24] Women tend to be less interested in sex as they get older. The decline is most marked during the late menopausal transition. Low estrogens predispose women to dryness and dyspareunia and also to reduced desire. The role of testosterone is unclear in naturally menopausal women.

Menopause and hormonal changes

It is difficult to disentangle the impact of ageing from that of the menopause. Hallstrom,[25] in a cross-sectional study of 800 women, stratified them at 38, 46, 50 and 54 years of age. When age was controlled, the relationship between decreased sexual functioning and menopause was strong for all ages but, when menopausal status was held constant the relationship between age and sexual function was not significant. The same findings were reported by a British group[26] in a longitudinal study of women aged 47–54 years. Women were more likely to report a decline in their sex life as they became older but the major change was seen over the menopausal transition.

The Melbourne Women's Midlife Health Project[24] set out to examine the relationship between age and menopause and sexual function. The original cross-sectional questionnaire asked women about their sexual experience over the previous 12 months. A total of 2001 women aged 45–55 years were polled by telephone. A decrease in sexual interest was reported by 31% and was associated with natural menopause rather than age. Decreased wellbeing, lack of paid employment, lower education and increased menopausal symptoms were all associated with a decline in interest. The longitudinal study that followed, on 438 randomly selected women aged 45–55 years, continued for more than 9 years. Annually, each woman completed a questionnaire on sexual function, kept a menstrual diary and had a blood test for sex hormones. Menopause status was evaluated from the menstrual history and divided into early menopause status (menstruated in the previous 3 months), late menopausal status (3–12 months of amenorrhoea) and postmenopausal status (more than 12 months of amenorrhoea). The maximum change in estradiol, follicle-stimulating hormone and free testosterone index was during the late menopause. No significant change in testosterone or dehydroepiandrosterone occurred with the menopause but ageing had a significant impact on dehydroepiandrostenedione.

The role of these hormones in sexual functioning is not understood. There is evidence that the decline in sexual function during the menopause is related to declining estradiol levels. Hormone change is only one of many possible changes and the woman's pre-morbid level of functioning, her personality, education level,[24] stress and physical health are all important. The complexity may explain why a prescription for hormone replacement therapy is often insufficient clinically.

Distress

The newer classification of sexual problems (Box 24.1)[27] also takes the distress to the woman into account. Not all women with sexual decline are distressed about it. Bancroft et al.[28] found that 25% of women aged 20–65 years were distressed about sexual matters but the younger women were more likely to complain than the older women. In the Melbourne Women's Midlife Health Project,[24] of 48 women with partners, 39 women (81%) had sexual dysfunction but only eight of those were distressed by it.

In another longitudinal study in Australia, Howard et al.[29] found that younger women and those with partners had higher levels of distress. Indifference to sexual frequency rose from 26% in women aged 40–49 years to 72% for those aged 70–79 years. This may be explained by lack of partner, normal ageing or hormonal changes.

Cross-sectional studies[30,31] looking at hypoactive sexual desire disorder (HSDD) confirm the theory that declining estrogen level is significant. In a study of 2050 women in the USA,[30] young women with a surgical menopause were more likely to have HSDD (26%) than their premenopausal counterparts (14%). In older women,

---

Box 24.1   Classification of sexual disorders according to Basson et al.[27]

- Sexual desire disorders are divided into two types. Hypoactive sexual desire disorder is the persistent or recurrent deficiency (or absence) of sexual fantasies/thoughts, and/or desire for or receptivity to sexual activity, which causes personal distress. Sexual aversion disorder is the persistent or recurrent phobic aversion to and avoidance of sexual contact with a sexual partner, which causes personal distress.
- Sexual arousal disorder is the persistent or recurrent inability to attain or maintain sufficient sexual excitement, causing personal distress, which may be expressed as a lack of subjective excitement, or genital (lubrication/swelling) or other somatic responses.
- Orgasmic disorder is the persistent or recurrent difficulty, delay in or absence of attaining orgasm following sufficient sexual stimulation and arousal, which causes personal distress.
- Sexual pain disorders are also divided into three categories:
  - Dyspareunia is the recurrent or persistent genital pain associated with sexual intercourse.
  - Vaginismus is the recurrent or persistent involuntary spasm of the musculature of the outer third of the vagina that interferes with vaginal penetration, which causes personal distress.
  - Non-coital sexual pain disorder is recurrent or persistent genital pain induced by non-coital sexual stimulation.

Disorders are further sub-typed according to medical history, laboratory tests and physical examination as lifelong versus acquired, generalised versus situational, and of organic, psychogenic, mixed or unknown origin.

there was no difference between those with a natural (9%) or surgical menopause (14%). HSDD was associated with a decline in arousal, orgasm and pleasure. Women with HSDD were more likely to express dissatisfaction with their relationship and more likely to have other illnesses. It is a major factor in quality of life. The percentage of women who have a low interest in sex increases with age but the proportion who are distressed about it diminishes so that the prevalence of HSDD remains constant. In European women aged 20–29 years, 11% had low desire compared with 53% in women aged 60–70 years.[31] However, the prevalence of HSDD in Europe was 6% for women aged 20–29 years compared with 13% for those aged 60–70 years and, in the USA, 12% of women aged 20–29 years compared with 19% for those aged 60–70 years.

Sex and experience of infertility

Impact of infertility on sex

Couples presenting with infertility are subjected to detailed questions about their sex life, such as how often it occurs and at what time in the menstrual cycle. A previously private area of life becomes public. They try all ways of targeting the fertile time with consequent loss of spontaneity and focus on vaginal intercourse. Sex may become a chore rather than fun. The creative and playful aspects are not procreative and it becomes fruitless and pointless. Sometimes it is easier not to try and be disappointed again, so avoiding tactics are employed.

A number of studies have attempted to quantify the size of the problem. Monga et al.32 compared infertile couples with couples seeking sterilisation procedures. In women there were no statistically significant differences but trends towards lower relationship satisfaction and greater sexual problems were found in the infertile group. However, Hentschel et al.[33] found that infertile women and women seeking sterilisation had similar sexual satisfaction scores. Tayebi and Ardakani34 found that, in a survey of 300 infertile women, 50% mentioned a decrease in coitus since the diagnosis of infertility.

Men in infertile couples had decreased satisfaction with intercourse and a trend to lower desire than their fertile counterparts. Ramezanzadeh *et al.*[35] found that, in a survey of 200 infertile couples, 41.5% of men reported a reduction in desire and 52.5% reported a reduction in satisfaction compared with recalled sexual satisfaction before the diagnosis of infertility. Shindel *et al.*[36] found that 18% of men in infertile couples had mild erectile dysfunction and 4% had moderate erectile dysfunction and that depression, erectile dysfunction and sexual relationship problems are prevalent among male partners of infertile couples. In a separate paper, Shindel *et al.*[37] found that premature ejaculation was prevalent among infertile couples but men might overestimate the level of partner frustration, and 50% of men said they ejaculated quicker than they wished.

Peterson *et al.*[38] attempted to examine the role of anxiety in generating sexual problems in infertile couples by using a questionnaire sent 2 months before they entered an assisted reproductive technology (ART) cycle. Anxiety scores and sexual infertility stress were measured, among others. Women reported greater anxiety symptoms than men: 24% of women and 7% of men reported scores in the mild-to-moderate anxiety range. However, 21% of men and 17% of women reported high levels of infertility sexual stress. There was a strong relationship between anxiety and sexual stress in men and the authors postulated that perhaps this relates to sexual performance and diminished feelings of masculinity as well as pressures from the spouse to have intercourse at the fertile time.

Impact of infertility on mood

Depression has a negative effect on sex drive and impacts on relationships. It is easy to understand the impact at the time of diagnosis and treatment but what long-term effects can be observed? The psychological consequences of fertility treatment, whether successful or not, have been the subject of research and there are disparate results. A systematic review of 25 years of research by Verhaak et al.[39] found three papers that looked at women after both successful and unsuccessful treatment. The most consistent finding was of depression after one or more unsuccessful cycles. It is unlikely to disappear quickly after treatment cycles. Successful treatment, on the contrary, tends to alleviate negative emotional responses. Three papers[40–42] reported variable levels of clinical depression (10–25%) after unsuccessful treatment. This is likely to be due to the treatment failure as most studies show that women entering treatment are normal in terms of depression, although possibly more anxious.[39]

Impact of an infertility diagnosis on the strength of the relationship

Relationship and sexual expression are intricately linked. Some papers are very positive about the strength of the relationships as couples say that coping with the adversity of infertility testing and treatment has brought them together. However, many studies look at couples undergoing ART and these couples often have to present as particularly stable to qualify for treatment and, indeed, couples in distress may not present for fertility treatment or may drop out from treatment early because of the weaknesses exposed in the relationship. Holter et al.[43] looked at marital relationships during the first in vitro fertilisation (IVF) cycle. More men than women perceived that childlessness had caused problems in the marriage both before and during the treatment but there was no difference in the pregnant or nonpregnant group after treatment. Generally, there was evidence that couples supported each other through the treatment and experienced it as positive. This was only a short-term analysis.

Peterson et al.[44] examined the agreement between couples' infertility-related stress and its effects on depression and marital adjustment in infertile men and women. If couples perceived the stress in a similar manner, there was a higher level of marital concord than when they perceived it at different levels. Incongruence between partners regarding relationship concerns and a need for parenting contributed to depression in women but not in men. High levels of agreement between couples allow them to successfully manage the impact of these stressful life events. The most common reason for not pursuing ART is the impact of stress on the couple.[45]

Sydsjö et al.[46] used the ENRICH (Evaluating and Nurturing Relationship Issues, Communication and Happiness) marital inventory to look at marital dynamics before, during and 18 months after 1–3 unsuccessful IVF cycles. The couples demonstrated a stable relationship throughout the treatment. This is in contrast to the findings of Leiblum et al.,[47] who found that women were less positive about their relationship after failed treatment. Sydsjö et al.[46] reported that 73% of unsuccessful couples had decided to adopt. The only discrepancy between men and women was that, after the treatment had finished, women were more likely than men to say that they would like more treatment. Clearly, women find it harder than men to give up on treatment. The authors of this study pointed out that couples must be in stable relationships to be able to enter treatment and there should be no other adverse social factors such as drug dependency, psychiatric illness or psychosocial problems.

Impact years later of a history of infertility

Leiblum *et al.*[47] looked at the impact of fertility treatment 2–13 years after last treatment. The respondents were classified into those who had never conceived, those with a child from IVF, those who had adopted and two groups who were excluded because they presented with secondary infertility or who conceived spontaneously. Questionnaires were related to sexual functioning, marital satisfaction, symptoms and self-esteem. There were no statistical differences in marital satisfaction or work satisfaction but infertile women expressed less satisfaction overall than those who had conceived. There were no statistically significant differences in sexual satisfaction between the groups. Anxiety was slightly more common in the women who had not conceived but none was clinically ill. A single question asking the women about the overall impact of infertility was revealing. One-third of the unsuccessful women said it had had a very negative effect. Similarly, when asked to rate the importance of a variety of reasons to abandon fertility treatments, 58% pointed to the negative effect it was having on their marital and sexual relationship and 59% of adoptive mothers said this was the reason to terminate fertility treatment. One-third of the unsuccessful women reported that infertility had had a negative impact on their relationship compared with 11% of the women who had adopted and 5% of the successful women. The childless women expressed a greater negative impact on the domains of marriage, self-esteem, feelings of adequacy as a woman and sex life.

Repokari *et al.*[48] studied couples who had conceived through ART and compared them with controls who had conceived without apparent problems. It demonstrated that ART had a neutral or positive effect on marital relationships and would support the hypothesis that couples undergoing ART are strong and less susceptible to adverse life events after having undergone the shared stress, bereavement and disappointments of ART.

Olshansky *et al.*[49] reported a series of taped and analysed interviews of nine menopausal women ranging in age from 48 to 72 years with previous infertility at various stages of the menopause. Three had conceived after treatment, three had adopted and three had remained childless. A core concept was generated of finally feeling normal, having felt abnormal throughout their reproductive lives.

Wirtberg *et al.*[50] reported on life 20 years after unsuccessful fertility treatment. Out of a possible 151 women who had had surgery for tubal disease, 91 could be included and were contacted. Finally, 39 women were interviewed, of which 25 had conceived or adopted and 14 had never entered parenthood. These 14 women were the subject of the paper. The method was of semistructured interviews that were written down and shown back to the women to be sure that that was what they had intended. The mean age was 52 years (range 48–60 years). Half were still with the same man, half were divorced and two had remarried. Six of the seven divorced women related the divorce to the infertility and, in every case, it was the man who had left. All but two women were working, with not working being due to illness that the women related to infertility and stress. Five of the 14 women were menopausal and all five were badly symptomatic. Thirteen of the women reported lack of self-esteem and feeling inferior to other women and feeling socially isolated. Half had recovered their self-esteem although they were feeling isolated again as their peers reached grandparenthood. All women raised the issue of no grandchildren and it was felt to be a loss. Effects on sexuality were all negative and one woman did not want to talk about it at all. Nine women said their sexual life and desire were gone forever. Four women said they had regained their desire, two with a new spouse and two with the previous spouse.

There were two predominant adaptations to being without children. One was to care for surrogate children – children of friends or family – and the other was to care for animals. Many had found a meaning to life in the absence of children. However, three women remained self-identified as infertile and were stuck in a non-resolution of the problem.

Other effects on sexual function

Impact of parity and mode of delivery on sexual function

Most studies concentrate on the short-term effects of parity. A metacontent analysis of 59 studies in 1999[51] showed that the decline in female sexual interest in the first trimester became very variable in the second trimester and declined in the third trimester. Couples tended to not practise intercourse for 2 months around the time of delivery and then frequency increased over the next 6 months but not to the prepregnancy level, and it was reported that sexual problems were common. Papers vary on whether the mode of delivery affects sexual function. Griffiths et al.[52] found that, 2 years after delivery, sexual satisfaction was better in women who had undergone caesarean section compared with vaginal delivery. However, Connolly et al.[53] found no difference relating to delivery. Baksu et al.[54] found that mediolateral episiotomy had an adverse effect on sexual function at 6 months postpartum. Botros et al.[55] used an identical twin study to separate out the effects of parity by using a biological control group that eliminated genetic variance. Women were of all ages and at very different stages of life. Nulliparous women reported superior sexual function when compared with their biologically identical counterparts. Obstetric interventions had no impact on subsequent sexual function. Having a child does have a lasting impact on sexual function and whether this is due to the pressures of parenthood or whether there is a biological change is unclear.

Impact of cancer on sexual function

Another life-changing event of relevance to doctors dealing with women as they age is a diagnosis of cancer, which has devastating effects on women. Treatments are now more effective and women are living longer. Quality of life after treatment is important and sexual function is important for self-esteem, relationships and quality of life. Corney et al.[56] assessed sexual function for 5 years after radical pelvic surgery and radiotherapy in 105 women. Before treatment, 90% of the women in relationships had been sexually active. After surgery, 24% had no problems, 66% had problems at 6 months and 15% never resumed intercourse. In women aged under 50 years, 82% of women who had radiotherapy admitted sexual dysfunction, mainly lack of desire. Although their sex lives had deteriorated, only 16% felt their marriage had deteriorated. Younger women were more likely to attribute their personal and marital problems to sexual dysfunction. The women in Corney's study had undergone mutilating treatment but, at the other end of the spectrum, Hellsten et al.[57] studied the impact of referral for colposcopy. There was no difference in women depending on whether they had actually had loop excision or not but spontaneous interest in sex and frequency of intercourse remained low 2 years after colposcopy.

Impact of other operations on sexual function

Changing sexuality with age may be further influenced by gynaecological procedures such as hysterectomy and urinary incontinence treatments.

There have been a number of well-designed trials in Europe and the USA to look at whether a subtotal or total hysterectomy is preferable in terms of sexual functioning. At 2 years there was no difference, although at 6 months there was some benefit to subtotal hysterectomy.[58-60] Data about bilateral oophorectomy are confounded by methodological problems as women have a higher use of hormone replacement. The TOSH (total or supracervical hysterectomy randomised trials) study[58] showed a slower recovery rate in the women who had undergone bilateral salpingo-oophorectomy but at 2 years there was no difference between the groups for sexual function.[61] Women who have had a hysterectomy for pain generally do better sexually after the operation. Those who were depressed as well as in pain preoperatively do less well but still are generally better.[62]

Urinary incontinence studies report an association between incontinence and sexual dysfunction of between 26% and 43%.[63-65] Barber et al.[66] looked at results of treatment for incontinence. Age was the best predictor for sexual activity and the reasons given for no sexual intimacy were complex and included concurrent medical problems, the partner's medical problems, being too tired, the partner being too tired, or lack of interest by the woman or the partner. Of sexually inactive women, 48% gave more than one reason for the inactivity and 20% indicated that the reason for their sexual inactivity was embarrassment at the thought of incontinence. Before treatment, 83% reported that sexual relations were satisfactory and 22% were worried about incontinence or prolapse during sexual activity. Women improved equally with behavioural therapy, topical estrogen and surgery.

How doctors can help

An awareness of the impact of gynaecological treatments and conditions and the effect on sexuality is the first step. Women wish to be asked about this and would like information on what to expect. The doctor does not need to be expert. Generally speaking, sympathetic listening in a non-judgemental way will enable the woman to voice her concerns. Men and women can talk about their sexual concerns without embarrassment if the doctor is not embarrassed. It is helpful to listen carefully and then reframe the history to make sure the person understands. Older women and men can and should be asked about whether they have any sexual concerns. Physical symptoms may be helped with medication such as topical or systemic hormone replacement therapy. Men with erectile dysfunction will often be helped with phosphodiesterase inhibitors but medication is more effective when combined with psychological help. Covert female problems may surface when the male partner becomes more potent. Sexual and marital therapy, such as that offered by Relate, can help relationship issues. It is possible that retirement preparation programmes may also be of use.

There are two organisations offering training to doctors. The Institute of Psychosexual Medicine (www.ipm.org.uk) offers training to doctors working with people seeking help with sexual difficulties and related psychosomatic problems. Such problems may present overtly or in the guise of other symptoms. The training aims to increase skills rather than knowledge and the method of training is concerned with practice rather than theory. It helps to understand how emotional factors, which are not always experienced at the conscious level, interfere with sexual performance and enjoyment. As with non-directive psychosexual counselling, treatment methods involve active listening and reflection but people present to doctors expecting a physical and psychological examination of their complaints. The underlying causes of the problem may be physical or psychological in varying proportions but are rarely limited to one or the other. The attitudes, anxieties and fantasies revealed during the consultation and the physical examination are particularly relevant to the understanding of the sexual problem. The British Society of Sexual and Relationship Therapists (www.basrt.org.uk) offers comprehensive theoretical and practical training to doctors and other professionals.

Conclusion

Women's sexual response changes with age and generalisations are, by nature, inaccurate. Having said that, there is a generally decline in interest and an increase in sexual problems accelerated by the menopause and made worse by infertility, having children, gynaecological procedures and cancer, among others. Psychosocial factors and mood, however, are just as important as physiological and pathological processes in ageing women.

References

1. Beckman N, Waern M, Gustafson D, Skoog I. Secular trends in self reported sexual activity and satisfaction in Swedish 70 year olds: cross sectional survey of four populations, 1971–2001. *BMJ* 2008;337:a279.
2. Boyle M. Gender, science and sexual dysfunction. In: Sarbin TR, Kitsuse JI, editors. *Constructing the Social.* London: Sage Publications; 1994.
3. Bouman W, Arcelus J, Benbow S. Nottingham study of sexuality and ageing. Attitudes regarding sexuality and older people: a review of the literature. *Sex Relat Ther* 2006;21:149–61.
4. Trudel G, Villeneuve V, Anderson A, Pilon G. Sexual and marital aspects of old age: an update. *Sex Relat Ther* 2008;23:161–9.
5. Kinsey AC, Pomeroy WB, Martin CE. *Sexual Behaviour in the Human Male.* Philadelphia, PA: WB Saunders; 1948.
6. Masters WH, Johnson VE. *Human Sexual Inadequacy.* Boston, MA: Little, Brown; 1966.
7. Masters WH, Johnson VE. *Human Sexual Response.* Boston, MA: Little, Brown; 1970.
8. Masters WH, Johnson VE. Sex and the ageing process, *J Am Geriatr Soc* 1981;29:385–90.
9. Masters WH, Johnson VE. *Human Sexuality.* Boston, MA: Little, Brown; 1982.
10. Starr BD, Weiner MB. *The Starr Weiner Report on Sex and Sexuality in the Mature Years.* New York: McGraw-Hill; 1981.
11. Brecher EM. *Love, Sex and Aging.* Boston, MA: Little, Brown; 1984.
12. Dunn KM, Croft PR, Hackett GI. Satisfaction in the sex life of a general practice sample. *J Sex Marital Ther* 2000;26:141–51.
13. Pfeiffer E, Verwoerdt A, Wang HS. Sexual behaviour in aged men and women. *Arch Gen Psychiatry* 1968;19:753–8.
14. Pfeiffer E. Sexual behaviour in old age. In: Busse E, Pfeiffer E, editors. *Behaviour and Adaptation in Late Life.* Boston, MA: Little, Brown; 1977.
15. Weizman A, Hart J. Sexual behaviour in healthy married elderly men. *Arch Sex Behav* 1987;16:39–44.
16. Libman E. Sociocultural and cognitive factors in aging and sexual expression: conceptual and research issue. *Can Psychol* 1989;30:560–7.
17. Mulligan T, Moss CR. Sexuality and aging in male veterans: a cross sectional study of interest, ability and activity. *Arch Sex Behav* 1991;20:17–25.
18. Bretschneider JG, McCoy NL. Sexual interest and behaviour in healthy 80–102 year olds. *Arch Sex Behav* 1988;17:109–29.
19. Trudel G, Turgeon L, Piche L. Marital and sexual aspects of old age. *Sex Relat Ther* 2000;15:381–406.
20. Johannes C, Araujo A, Feldman H, Derby C, Kleinman K, McKinlay J. Incidence of erectile dysfunction in men 40 to 69 years old: longitudinal results from the Massachusetts male aging study. *J Urol* 2000;163:460–3.

21. Kupelian V, Shabsigh R, Travison T, Page S, Araujo A, McKinlay J. Is there a relationship between sex hormones and erectile dysfunction? Results from the Massachusetts male aging study. *J Urol* 2006;176:2584–8.

22. Corona G, Mannucci E, Mansani R, Petrone L, Bartolini M, Giommi R, *et al.* Aging and pathogenesis of erectile dysfunction. *Int J Impot Res* 2004;16:395–402.

23. Potts A, Grace V, Vares T, Gavey N. 'Sex for life?' Men's counter-stories on 'erectile dysfunction', male sexuality and ageing. *Sociol Health Illn* 2006;28:306–29.

24. Dennerstein L, Alexander JL, Kotz K. The menopause and sexual functioning: a review of the population based studies. *Annu Rev Sex Res* 2003;14:64–82.

25. Hallstrom T. Sexuality in the climacteric. *Clin Obstet Gynaecol* 1977;4:227–39.

26. Mishra G, Kuh D. Sexual functioning throughout the menopause: the perceptions of women in a British cohort. *Menopause* 2006;13:880–90.

27. Basson R, Berman J, Burnett A, Derogatis L, Ferguson D, Fourcroy J, *et al.* Report of the international consensus development conference on female sexual dysfunction: definitions and classifications. *J Urol* 2000;163:888–93.

28. Bancroft J, Loftus J, Long J. Distress about sex: a national survey of women in heterosexual relationships. *Arch Sex Behav* 2003;32:193–208.

29. Howard JR, O'Neil S, Travers C. Factors affecting sexuality in older Australian women: sexual interest, sexual arousal, relationships and sexual distress in older Australian women. *Climacteric* 2006;9:357–67.

30. Leiblum S, Koochai P, Rodenberg C, Barton I, Rosen R. Hypoactive sexual desire disorder in post menopausal women: US results from the Women's International Study of Health and Sexuality (WISHeS). *Menopause* 2006;13:46–56.

31. Hayes R, Dennerstein L, Bennett CM, Koochaki PE, Leiblum SR, Graziottin A. Relationship between hypoactive sexual desire disorder and aging. *Fertil Steril* 2007;87:107–12.

32. Monga M, Alexandrescu B, Katz SE, Stein M, Ganiats T. Impact of infertility on quality of life, marital adjustment and sexual function. *J Urol* 2004;63:126–30.

33. Hentschel H, Albertom DL, Sawdy RJ, Capp E, Goldim JR, Passos EP. Sexual function in women from infertile couples and in women seeking surgical sterilization. *J Sex Marital Ther* 2008;34:107–14.

34. Tayebi N, Ardakani S. The prevalence of sexual dysfunctions in infertile women. *Middle East Fertil Soc J* 2007;12:184–7.

35. Ramezanzadeh F, Aghassa M, Jafarabadi M, Zayeri F. Alterations of sexual desire and satisfaction in male partners on infertile couples. *Fertil Steril* 2006;85:139–43.

36. Shindel AW, Nelson CJ, Naughton CK, Ohebshalom M, Mulhall JP. Sexual function and quality of life in male partner of infertile couples: prevalence and correlates of dysfunction. *J Urol* 2008;179:1056–9.

37. Shindel AW, Nelson CJ, Naughton CK, Mulhall JP. Premature ejaculation in infertile couples: prevalence and correlates. *J Sex Med* 2008;2:485–91.

38. Peterson BD, Newton CR, Feingold T. Anxiety and sexual stress in men and women undergoing infertility treatment. *Fertil Steril* 2007;88:911–14.

39. Verhaak CM, Smeenk JMJ, Evers AWM, Kremer JAM, Kraaimaat FW, Braat DDM. Women's emotional adjustment to IVF: a systematic review of 25 years of research. *Hum Reprod Update* 2007;13:27–36.

40. Lok IH, Dee DT, Cheung LP, Chung WS, Lo WK, Haines CJ. Psychiatric morbidity amongst infertile Chinese women undergoing treatment with assisted reproductive technology and the impact of treatment failure. *Gynecol Obstet Invest* 2002;53:195–9.

41. Verhaak CM, Smeenk JMJ, van Minnen A, Kremer JAM, Kraaimaat FW. A longitudinal prospective study on emotional adjustment before, during and after consecutive fertility treatment cycles. *Hum Reprod* 2005;20:2253–60.

42. Newton CR, Hearn MT, Yuzpe AA. Psychological assessment and follow up after *in vitro* fertilization: assessing the impact of failure. *Fertil Steril* 1990;54:879–86.

43. Holter H, Anderheim L, Bergh C, Moller A. First IVF treatment – short term impact on psychological well-being and the marital relationship. *Hum Reprod* 2006;21:3295–302.

44. Peterson BD, Newton CR, Rosen KH. Examining congruence between partners' perceived infertility related stress and its relationship to marital adjustment and depression in infertile couples. *Fam Process* 2003;42:59–70.

45. Olivus C, Friden B, Borg G, Bergh C. Why do couples discontinue *in vitro* fertilization treatment? A cohort study. *Fertil Steril* 2004;81:258–61.

46. Sydsjo G, Ekholm K, Wadsby M, Kjellberg S, Sydsjo A. Relationships in couples after failed IVF treatment: a prospective follow up study. *Hum Reprod* 2005;20:1952–7.

47. Leiblum SR, Aviv A, Hamer R. Life after infertility treatment: a long-term investigation of marital and sexual function. *Hum Reprod* 1998;13:3569–74.

48. Repokari L, Punamaki R, Unkila-Kallio L, Vilska S, Poikkeus P, Sinkkonen J, *et al*. Infertility treatment and marital relationships: a 1 year prospective study among successfully treated ART couple and their controls. *Hum Reprod* 2007;22:1481–91.

49. Olshansky E. Feeling normal women's experiences of menopause after infertility. *MCN Am J Matern Child Nurs* 2005;30:195–200.

50. Wirtberg I, Moller A, Hogstrom L, Trostad SE, Lalos A. Life 20 years after unsuccessful infertility treatment. *Hum Reprod* 2007;22:598–604.

51. von Sydow K. Sexuality during pregnancy and after childbirth: a metacontent analysis of 59 studies. *J Psychosom Res* 1999;47:27–49.

52. Griffiths A, Watermeyer S, Sidhu K, Amso N, Nix B. Female genital tract morbidity and sexual function following vaginal delivery or lower segment caesarian section. *J Obstet Gynaecol* 2006;26:645–9.

53. Connolly A, Thorp J, Pahel L. Effects of pregnancy and child birth on post partum sexual function: a longitudinal prospective study. *Int Urogynecol J Pelvic Floor Dysfunct* 2005;16:263–7.

54. Baksu B, Dava I, Agar E, Akyol A, Varolan A. The effect of mode of delivery on postpartum sexual functioning in primiparous women. *Int Urogynecol J Pelvic Floor Dysfunct* 2007;18:401–6.

55. Botros S, Abramov Y, Miller JJ, Sand PK, Gandhi S, Nickolov MS, *et al*. Effect of parity on sexual function – an identical twin study. *Obstet Gynecol* 2006;107:765–70.

56. Corney RH, Crowther ME, Everett H, Howells A, Shepherd JH. Psychosexual dysfunction in women with gynaecological cancer following radical pelvic surgery. *Br J Obstet Gynaecol* 1993;100:73–8.

57. Hellsten G, Lindqvist PG, Sjostrom K. A longitudinal study of women referred for colposcopy for the first time subsequent to receiving notification after an abnormal smear and a 6-month and 2-year follow up. *BJOG* 2008;115:205–11.

58. Kupperman M, Summitt R, Varner R, McNeeley S, Goodman Gruen D, Learman L, *et al*. Sexual functioning after total compared with supracervical hysterectomy: a randomized trial. *Obstet Gynecol* 2005;105:1309–18.

59. Thakar R, Ayers S, Clarkson P, Stanton S, Manyonda I. Outcomes after total versus subtotal abdominal hysterectomy. *N Engl J Med* 2002;347:1318–25.

60. Zobbe V, Gimbel H, Andersen BM, Filtenborg T, Jakobsen K, Sorensen HC. Sexuality after total versus subtotal hysterectomy. *Acta Obstet Gynecol Scand* 2004;83:191–6.

61. Teplin V, Vittinghof E, Lin F, Learman L, Richter H, Kupperman M. Oophorectomy in premenopausal women: health related quality of life and sexual functioning. *Obstet Gynecol* 2007;109:347–54.

62. Hartmann K, Cindy MPH, Lamvu G, Langenberg P, Steege J, Kjerulff K. Quality of life and sexual function after hysterectomy in women with preoperative pain and depression. *Obstet Gynecol* 2004;104:701–9.

63. Sutherst J, Brown M. Sexual dysfunction associated with urinary incontinence. *Urol Int* 1980;35:414–16.

64. Walters MD, Taylor S, Schoenfield LS. Psychosexual study of women with detrusor instability. *Obstet Gynecol* 1990;75:22–6.

65. Iosif CS. Sexual function after colpo-urethrocystopexy in middle aged women. *Urol Int* 1988;43:231–3.

66. Barber M, Visco A, Wyman J, Fantl J, Bump R. Continence Program for Women Research Group. Sexual function in women with urinary incontinence and pelvic organ prolapse. *Obstet Gynecol* 2002;99:281–9.

Chapter 25
Sex beyond and after fertility

Discussion

David Barlow: Catherine, you mentioned in your presentation that health carers and health professionals can have difficulty recognising that older people have sexual needs. Do you know whether there is similar evidence among health carers and professionals dealing with younger people in healthcare or who have been in hospital for many, many months. Do their carers recognise that they may also have sexual needs?

Catherine Coulson: I certainly have heard it from both sides: disabled people referred to me in the psychosexual clinic where the subject has come up. But I suspect that, generally speaking, it is more comfortable to ignore it, don't you? I did not look at that specifically.

Mandish Dhanjal: Diana, why do you think the IUS [intrauterine system] uptake rate is so low considering it is such a suitable form of contraception and also has added healthcare benefits? I am sure that if you surveyed female gynaecologists, it would be the number one form of contraception they use themselves. Why do you think community general practitioners aren't suggesting that is a good contraceptive?

Diana Mansour: We did a survey recently looking at one particular general practice that we use for training, as well as our own service, and clearly showed that most primary care general practitioners underprescribe long-acting methods including the IUS.[1] Even though there may be some enhanced service payment, they still say that it is too much of a hassle. Well, that is the first excuse they make. There are also some training issues for GPs and the availability of appropriate training. There is always a concern about failure with fitting the IUS as it is a little broader. Although that is rarely spoken about, when you talk to providers about advantages, they look to a smaller, levonogestrel system which is only about 1 mm smaller, a bit like a Nova-T®. It is welcome because of the ease of fitting. Although there are services where you can get an IUS fitted, it is much more relevant for the prospective user. There is still a general feeling in the UK that it is an invasive procedure, is painful and causes infections. I have a lovely slide of a penis with a discharge and say 'That is what causes infection, the device does not.' [laughter] In a recent survey in the USA,[2] 30% of obstetricians and gynaecologists said that they worry about the use of intrauterine devices because of infection. So we have this myth: that you cannot use the IUS in nulliparous women as it is going to cause infertility and all of those things. I suppose it comes from the 1970s, the Dalkon Shield days and when we were unaware of chlamydia, but mothers can remember this. It is an awareness problem, but also a reticence. We do pretty well in Newcastle because there is a consistent message: we have the health professionals, or their wives, using it, nurses, female doctors and gynaecologists. But it is not the same throughout the country.

Diana Mansour: You may not need contraception, but it is ideal for your other problems.

William Ledger: Would you like to comment about the other concern on the internet, which is about weight gain with IUS?

Diana Mansour: There was a European study in the 1980s,[3] with a prototype IUS releasing 20 micrograms per 24 hours of levonogestrel versus a copper IUD [intrauterine device]. It clearly showed, unfortunately, that both groups gained weight and both gained the same proportion. We have seen, from the obesity work, that we all get bigger, and we get bigger as we get older. But, yes, we will all blame anything else. It is not what goes into the mouth … [laughter]

References

1. Mansour D, Rosales C, Cox M. Women's awareness of long-acting, reversible contraceptive methods (LARCs) in community family planning clinics and general practice. *Eur J Contracept Reprod Health Care* 2008;13:396–9.

2. Harper CC, Blum M, de Bocanegra HT, Darney PD, Speidel JJ, Policar M, *et al.* Challenges in translating evidence to practice: the provision of intrauterine contraception. *Obstet Gynecol* 2008;111:1359–69.

3. Andersson K, Odlind V, Rybo G. Levonorgestrel-releasing and copper-releasing (Nova T) IUDs during five years of use: a randomized comparative trial. *Contraception* 1994;49:56–72.

Section 7

Reproductive ageing
and the RCOG:
an international college

Chapter 26
What should be the RCOG's relationship with older women?

Donna Dickenson

Introduction

A 'should' question normally signals work for an ethicist but this ethicist's task is complicated by the normative dimension of all the chapters in this volume. Each author was asked to come up with three recommendations from their own subject area – 'should' statements deriving from the 'is' analysis that they present. If those prescriptions cover the relevant topics, what more is there for an ethicist to do?

I have had a personal interest in obstetricians' relationship with 'older women' since being classified as an 'elderly primigravida' at the superannuated age of 26 years. Apart from that, however, what original contribution can I make? The convenors of the 56th RCOG Study Group gave me plentiful suggestions – perhaps a little too plentiful:

> How should the RCOG approach its constituencies, medical ethics, regulation and its relationship to government and the rest of the medical profession, i.e. the NHS and the market, vested interests, individuals or consumers, families, the unborn, doctors, drug companies, surrogacy, the unborn, trafficking, global adoption, law, research?

I have to admit this was just too much for me. Instead, I want to argue for what may seem a self-evidently simple point. The RCOG describes its mission as 'setting standards to improve women's health' – presumably all women. In the 6 years that I have served on the RCOG Ethics Committee, however, we have almost always been concerned with that minority of the female population who are of reproductive age. There are two things wrong with that slant: it defines women in terms of their reproductive role alone and it risks allowing women above that age (or, indeed, girls below puberty) to vanish from our scrutiny.

I did say my point was self-evidently simple, perhaps even simplistic. The organisers of the Study Group were clearly fully aware of it, since their brief is to expand our awareness. What I want to do is to elaborate on why the narrower concentration is not only professionally blinkered but also morally wrong – and there my background as an ethicist is indeed relevant, particularly as a feminist ethicist. I also want to make three recommendations of my own, which I hope will contribute towards 'consciousness-raising' – itself a feminist method – about older women.

Feminist ethics and reproduction

In the early days of what has come to be called 'second-wave' feminism – that is, the Women's Liberation movement of the late 1960s – feminist activists and academics had plenty to do in asserting women's autonomy and rights in the reproductive context. The popular starting point was probably the collective volume *Our Bodies, Ourselves*,[1] which reads in retrospect as both familiar and strange – familiar because the assertion that women have the right to control their own bodies seems like a platitude to all but militant anti-abortionists, strange because practice in obstetrics and gynaecology has evolved so far away, in most instances, from the taken-for-granted medical paternalism of the earlier period.

In the area of new reproductive technologies, however, feminists came up against not just medical paternalism but also the technological imperative. The cover of the 1984 collection *Test-Tube Women: What Future for Motherhood?*[2] shows a naked and heavily pregnant woman trapped in what looks like a padded cell, with a ludicrously gaudy collection of wires extruding from her stomach. The villain of the piece is the white-coated male doctor whom she's trying in vain to push away. A great deal of feminist concern, much of it quite prophetic, was raised in that book about areas where ethical debates still rage: 'designer genes', for example, as well as surrogacy, egg harvesting, abortion of female fetuses and disability. Reacting against media descriptions of the new reproductive technologies as enabling all women to fulfil their supposedly deepest desire, motherhood, the writers in *Test-Tube Women* typified second-wave feminism's scepticism about whether these new developments were necessarily liberating for women.

That work of challenging the ethical basis of assisted reproductive technologies was, and continues to be, necessary but, ironically, it risks becoming caught up in a sexist stereotype: that reproductive issues, whether 'natural' or 'artificial', are the only rightful concern of feminist ethics. Some feminist ethicists, such as Francoise Baylis and Susan Sherwin, expanded their concerns to power in the doctor–patient relationship more generally, even though the immediate theatre of their concern was pregnancy. In their 2002 essay 'Judgements of non-compliance in pregnancy',[3] the two Canadian professors use pregnancy as a fulcrum, expanding their ethical concerns to:

> ... understanding what is problematic in the circumstances that elicit judgements of patient non-compliance from the perspectives of both the physician and the patient ... We suggest that a subset of the behaviours and choices that the language of non-compliance now captures are not inherently problematic. They ought not to be construed as non-compliance, but rather as informed or uninformed refusals ... A commitment to provide respectful health care requires that these situations be dealt with in a way that enhances, rather than undermines, autonomy-respecting, integrity-preserving patient–physician interactions.

In other words, Baylis and Sherwin broadened feminist concerns to power in the doctor–patient relationship: the power doctors have to brand women who refuse what they recommend as 'non-compliant'. Pregnant women, in their view, should not be treated any differently from other patients who make an informed refusal to consent to a procedure. By implication, this anti-paternalistic position, which might be a truism in relation to other patients, still has to be fought for where pregnant women are concerned. Here feminist ethicists pursue a patient's rights position that applies across the board, to women past reproductive age, and to men as well, even if their starting point is pregnancy.

Other feminist ethicists have left pregnancy behind completely, concentrating instead on developing feminist approaches to such tried-but-not-necessarily-true concepts in medical ethics as autonomy, freedom and property in the body. The concept of 'relational autonomy', for example, has been developed by a number of authors to make up for obvious deficiencies in the 'knee-jerk' standard view that autonomy equals whatever the patient wants. A concept of 'relational autonomy', in contrast, requires both physician and patient to stand back and consider the wider nexus of relationships, both personal and professional, within which autonomy is exercised.[4–6] Of course, relational autonomy may and should be exercised within the patient–obstetrician relationship as well but it is not exclusive to pregnancy and childbirth, although the relationship with the developing fetus may add a further set of considerations.[7,8]

Rethinking the universal concept of autonomy clearly expands our ethical analysis beyond younger women of reproductive age to include older women and men of all ages. Similarly, in my own recent works, the academic book *Property in the Body*[9] and its popular-science sister *Body Shopping*,[10] I have argued that all bodies are in a sense 'open-access' now, as women's bodies were traditionally construed. To that extent, all bodies are 'feminised'. Here I develop and apply the economic, legal and political concepts of property and 'commodification', the process by which we attribute monetary value to something previously outside the market system. Although women's tissue is particularly prone to commodification – think of the huge US market for human eggs – all human tissue is becoming a commodity like any other, when one in five human genes is the subject of a patent, for example. The ethical, economic and political questions which that development raises certainly do not only concern women of reproductive age, although many of the unexpected commercial developments do – private umbilical cord blood banking for one.

Reproductive rights, then, remain 'one of the most important issues for different kinds and different phases of women's movements'[11] but they do not exhaust the ethical concerns of moral philosophers concerned about women's position, any more than they do the range of concerns proper to the RCOG. What else is there, one might ask? Actually, that would be the wrong question because it still prioritises reproduction by reducing everything else to 'else'. Of course, there are many other concerns involving women past reproductive age, such as menopause, hormone replacement therapy, postmenopausal *in vitro* fertilisation, breast, cervical and ovarian cancer screening, sexual disease transmission in older women, incontinence, cosmetic surgery and osteoporosis. My three specific recommendations at the end of this chapter will touch on some of these areas.

However, I want to argue that the RCOG should not adopt a 'scattergun' or 'pick-and-mix' approach to its relationship with older women. There is one particular point that it should concentrate on: preventing the syndrome I have elsewhere called 'the lady vanishes'. Our primary task should be to make sure that the lady does not vanish from public, political and professional sight when she is no longer able to bear children.

The lady vanishes

I first used the term 'the lady vanishes' (apologies to Alfred Hitchcock) to describe public discussion of the ethical issues in stem cell research, where only the status of the embryo seemed to count. Yet because ova are crucial to the somatic cell nuclear transfer variant of stem cell research, there are also important regulatory issues concerning the protection of women from whom ova are taken.[12–14] In most commentaries and debates, however, the women from whom the ova are taken had virtually disappeared from view.

This phenomenon was most evident at the time of the near-universal jubilation over the supposed success of Hwang Woo Suk in creating tissue-matched stem cell lines.[15,16] We now know that Hwang used over 2200 human eggs, many taken from his junior researchers in breach of the Helsinki Declaration, others bought through an international commercial agency in violation of Korean law. In announcing his 'success', however, Hwang claimed to have used less than one-tenth of that number of eggs to create eleven patient-matched cell lines. The few commentators who picked up on that number – or on the very fact that human eggs were involved at all – expressed a degree of incredulity at Hwang's figures, which were wildly out of line with the figure of 400 sheep eggs required to produce one 'Dolly' in the similar reproductive cloning method. But we were drowned out by the far louder and more numerous voices of congratulation. Where there was ethical debate, it focused almost exclusively on the early-stage embryos from which blastocysts had been extracted to create the alleged stem cell lines.

It took the efforts of a collective grouping of Korean feminists known as Korean Womenlink to bring to light the facts about the unethical methods that Hwang had used to collect his eggs and the sheer number of women who had 'contributed'.* Disquiet at those initial findings led Hwang's US collaborator Gerard Schatten to resign publicly from the team and eventually brought the whole flimsy edifice tumbling down. So by ensuring that the lady did not vanish, Korean feminists performed a valuable service for both ethics and science, unwelcome though it was in certain quarters.

The recent ructions in the UK Parliament over the question of human-admixed embryos, or cybrids, in which an enucleated animal egg is substituted for a human one in somatic cell nuclear transfer research, reflect the success of those voices determined to ensure that the very real risks to women in egg donation do not vanish altogether from public sight. Although some of the scientists pressing for cybrid legalisation have made it clear that they hope to move on to using women's eggs if a reasonable success rate can be achieved with animal ones, at least the availability of women's eggs has become a highly public, practical and ethical issue. It is no longer simply taken for granted.

The egg-donating variety of vanishing lady is of reproductive age, of course, but the point about women's invisibility also applies to research involving both younger and older women. Inappropriate experimentation on women of reproductive age has long been a feminist concern. For example, in one birth control study, women seeking contraception were divided into experimental and placebo arms, with 10 of 76 women receiving the placebo becoming pregnant against their wishes.[17] This study gives a whole new meaning to the phrase 'therapeutic misconception' – the way in which control arm participants wrongly believe that by taking part in the experiment, they are assuring themselves of the right to try the new drug.

However, it is the lack of research trials and data on women of reproductive age that is more germane to our subject here – wrongful exclusion rather than wrongful inclusion. Inappropriate generalisation to women from trials only performed on men has led to mismatched drug regimens as well as inaccurate advice about symptoms of major diseases, such as cardiac disease, where signs of an impending heart attack differ markedly between the sexes. Yet equality is difficult to achieve. Although a 2007 study on myocardial infarction found that women showed lower distrust of medical researchers than men, men demonstrated 15% greater willingness to participate in

* For further details, see chapter 4 in *Body Shopping*.[10]

clinical trials than women.[18] Perhaps the popular perception that women are less at risk of heart attack than men lies behind this phenomenon – another instance of the vanishing lady over a certain age, since that benefit essentially ends at menopause.

The disastrous teratogenic effects of thalidomide impelled the US Food and Drug Administration to ban women of reproductive age from early clinical trials in the 1970s but the practice soon spread to women in older age groups as well. With the exception of sex-specific drugs such as hormone replacement therapy, the practice of recruiting only men for trials became so prevalent that many drugs licensed for use in the USA had never been tested on women.[19] All new drug applications in the USA must now include analysis of differential impact on subjects of varying ages, genders, ethnicity and class. Nevertheless, a 2002 meta-analysis concerning representation of women, elderly men and minority ethnic groups found that clinical trials continue to focus on a relatively small percentage of the population at risk of heart failure. Reviewing MEDLINE studies from as far back as 1989, Helat et al.[20] concluded that patients in randomised clinical trials were younger, whiter and more commonly male. There was no improvement in representation from the period of the late 1980s into the 21st century. The lady was still conspicuous by her absence.

Three recommendations and a preliminary warning

I hope I have demonstrated that there are clinical reasons and arguments from gender justice for the RCOG to make a priority of preventing the lady of a certain age from vanishing. The three recommendations I propose all have that goal. But before I present them, I want to raise and then dispel a preliminary objection. If we are concerned to treat women equally, do we need to make them a special case? Is it not patronising to assume that older women need an organisation to speak for them? Does it not smack of the worst kind of medical paternalism? And if we believe in equal treatment of the sexes, what do we make of the fact that men have no Royal College specifically dedicated to their interests?

These sorts of objections are commonly made in all contexts where positive discrimination is an issue. Even if they are well-intentioned – in some cases I think they are just a front for status quo interests – they make one common mistake. They fail to distinguish the more powerful groups from the less powerful. In creating a situation of equality from a situation where one group has more power than another, or is simply more visible than another, we do need to give 'special treatment' to the weaker group, if only to bring them up to a position where they can then function equally well without any further assistance. That is not an insult to women's autonomy or integrity: merely a realistic assessment of the situation. As Catharine MacKinnon wrote in 1989,[21] demands for change in the distribution of power appear to favoured groups to be demands for special protection, but they are really just demands for no group to be more special than any other.

It is precisely because the lady vanishes all too readily that it is incumbent on those concerned for gender justice to advocate for her. We are extraordinarily lucky that the RCOG already exists, with its motto of 'setting standards to improve women's health' and its particular brief to act for women. The recommendations I am proposing are in concord with that mission and with my analysis thus far. The RCOG should do the following:

1. lobby for a lower breast cancer screening age and for genetic testing enabling a more targeted approach, while opposing the growing commercialisation of genetic testing

2. oppose genetic patents that particularly affect women, for example patents on the *BRCA1*, *BRCA2* and *HER2* genes

3. back a safe sex campaign and more funding for sexual health clinics aimed at women over reproductive age.

1. Breast cancer screening and genetic testing

It might appear that the UK's national breast cancer screening programme for women aged 50–71 years is one of the few instances in which the lady has not vanished. That achievement is certainly considerable but it can be improved, particularly in light of the June 2008 findings published in the *New England Journal of Medicine* by Paul Pharoah *et al.*[22] in a paper entitled 'Polygenes, risk prediction and targeted prevention of breast cancer'. The concept of genetic risk stratification needs to be embedded in public health practice, they argue, replacing the one-size-fits-all approach of a national screening programme directed at all women over any particular age, irrespective of family history. (The National Institute for Health and Clinical Excellence [NICE] guidelines in the UK do recommend mammographic screening for women aged 40 years or over if their 10-year risk is over 3% on the basis of family history.)

Individual genes linked to inherited breast cancer, such as *BRCA1* and *BRCA2*, are relatively rare, with a combined carrier frequency of about 0.003 in the general UK population, where there are no common 'founder mutations'. They account for less than 25% of the inherited component of breast cancer.[23] That might not seem sufficient reason to single out women at familial risk in a national screening programme, given that a screening programme to detect and treat carriers would reduce the disease burden in the population by only 0.7%.[22]

Genome-wide association studies, however, have pinpointed a number of more common alleles increasing breast cancer susceptibility, which seem to act in a multiplicative fashion. Profiling women for combinations of these alleles would enable more useful discrimination between higher- and lower-risk groups in the context of population screening. Women's overall risk of breast cancer can vary approximately six-fold when this multiplicative model is converted into absolute risk over a specified time period.

Although risk profiling based on genetic susceptibility is not productive at the individual clinical level, it would provide enough information at the population level to warrant targeted screening programmes for women at greatest risk according to genotype. Currently the 10-year risk for all women aged 50 years is calculated at around 2.3%. If genetic screening were used to stratify the UK population in this fashion, around 20% of women would be classified as low risk and below this level. However, the top 5% of women at highest risk would hit the 2.3% risk level nearly 10 years earlier, at only 41 years of age.[24]

The study by Pharoah *et al.*[22] was the first to apply individual risk calculations to population screening. It has not yet reached a wider popular audience but, when and if it does, it will almost certainly trigger a rush of personalised genetic screening services offered by commercial companies to women who fear they may be in the high-risk bracket. Although Pharoah and his colleagues were careful to state that they did not view risk profiling at the individual level as useful, commercial gene-profiling services will probably disregard that injunction. Without adequate counselling and follow-up services, these genetic profiling 'products' can be seen as preying on older women's understandable anxiety, as accentuating the popular tendency to believe in genetic determination of disease, and as cashing in on the glamour of 'the new genetics'. They may even result in a rash of elective mastectomies, given the publicity which has been given to the stories of women with the much more lethal *BRCA1* gene who have decided to go down that painful route. In the USA, where ancestry tracing is a popular hobby and genetic profiling already much bigger business, such concerns have provoked at least one state, California, to serve 'cease and desist' orders on a score of gene profile companies as a hazard to public health, and to pass a statute banning any new attempts to offer such 'services'.

The RCOG should consider advocating a national programme of genetically stratified breast cancer susceptibility screening, while simultaneously calling for legislation to bar commercial firms from offering breast cancer susceptibility 'profiles'. Admittedly, the efficacy of breast cancer screening may be less good in premenopausal women and the full range of risk factors for breast cancer is not yet established. These new findings, however, do strengthen the case for a genetically stratified risk screening programme to be undertaken by the NHS – not by the commercial gene testing companies that will doubtless spring up soon in the UK, as they already have in the USA. Prohibiting commercial genetic testing is particularly important for women, not only because they are affected by breast cancer, but also because women are more likely than men to be offered and to undergo genetic testing.[25]

2. Genetic patents

Roughly one in five human genes is now the subject of a patent, with the majority in the hands of commercial firms such as pharmaceutical companies.[26] One company, Sciona, holds patents on 2300 genes. This phenomenon is not just some abstract fact of interest only to pedants: it affects daily clinical care. Although the rationale of patenting is to allow researchers and funders a temporary monopoly as an incentive to make scientific discoveries, misuse of genetic patents impairs medical progress and harms patients, particularly the abuses of 'defensive patenting' and restrictive licensing agreements.

These are strong statements, at first glance: what proof do we have that they are true? Two cases particularly affecting older women prove the relevance of these accusations. One of the most worrying cases of restrictive patenting has involved fees for diagnostic tests on the *BRCA1* and *BRCA2* genes, levied by the biotechnology firm holding US patents on these genes, Myriad Genetics. Although the genes were discovered through publicly funded international collaboration, Myriad patented them in 1994 and has enforced its patent rights 'rather aggressively'.[27] Refusing to license any other laboratories than its own US-based operations, Myriad charged a substantial fee for diagnostic testing (up to US$3,000 in the USA) and pursued its rights in court when a strong opposition grew up in Europe. The European Patent Court granted Myriad patents on *BRCA1* in 2001 but subsequently revoked one patent and severely limited the scope of the other two, later amending its similar judgement on *BRCA2* as well.[28] Myriad is still appealing against the judgement, leaving European laboratories who continue to perform the test living in fear of infringement suits. Myriad also challenged Cancer Research UK when the organisation tried to protect its rights to make the genetic test freely available for public health services.

In the USA, where its patents are still valid, Myriad has launched direct mail shots urging women to ask their doctors for a diagnostic test. This attempt to 'grow the market' plays on patients' understandable confusion about the effect of the genes: although the vast majority of women with the *BRCA1* and *BRCA2* genes will develop breast cancer, most breast cancers are not caused by the genes. Urging older women to undergo an expensive genetic test for their supposed peace of mind raises both false alarm and false hope: false alarm because the gene mutations are comparatively rare, false hope because even if a woman tests negatively for the mutation, she can still develop breast cancer.

When a firm holds a patent not just on the diagnostic test kit or drug but on the gene itself, it is very difficult or even impossible to 'invent around' the patent, as is usually feasible with other inventions. The stifling impact of genetic patents on alternative, cheaper treatments was equally evident in the case of the drug Herceptin® (trastuzumab; Roche), which has innovative therapeutic uses against cancer cell production in women with certain genetic predispositions to breast cancer. Herceptin acts on the human epidermal growth factor receptor-2 gene (*HER2*) and increases survival rates in women who have the version of the gene making them prone to some forms of breast cancer. (About 20–25% of all breast cancers are *HER2* positive.) The patent holder of Herceptin, Genentech, also holds multiple patents related to the *HER2* gene itself. Any researcher or drug company wishing to develop an alternative, cheaper drug must obtain permission from Genentech – which it is unlikely to give, for obvious reasons of commercial competition – or risk being sued for patent infringement. It was this monopoly that drove the price of the drug up to such high levels that NICE initially had to restrict its use on the NHS in England and Wales, until a public outcry forced the authority to rethink the decision in 2006. At that time, the NHS Confederation warned that the £100 million annual cost of providing Herceptin – at a price inflated by the monopoly patent – would mean cutbacks elsewhere.

The RCOG has the expertise and the credibility to expose the abuses caused by monopoly patents. It could and should concentrate its skills and authority on supporting the European Patent Court resistance and on making women more widely aware of the way in which the medications they may need are more expensive than necessary because of restrictive licences and monopoly patenting of the genes themselves. There is a growing popular awareness of the 'great genome grab', making RCOG intervention both timely and potentially very influential.

3. Sexual health

Although male celebrities over a certain age evidently have sex – witness new fathers in their 60s such as Jonathan Dimbleby – the soft-porn MTV-generation media still seem uncomfortable with the fact that older women do too. This is a prime case of the vanishing (older) lady: sexualised female bodies are inevitably young female bodies. Much more could be done to get across the 'safe sex' message for older women, and much more needs to be done, since the incidence of sexual diseases among the over-45s has doubled in the past 8 years, according to a Birmingham study of 4445 cases of sexually transmitted infections.[29] Cases of chlamydia, herpes, genital warts, gonorrhea and syphilis all rose, with the overall infection rate per 100000 people up from 16.7 to 36.3.

Older men and women who are divorced and beginning new relationships may be less likely to use condoms to prevent transmission of sexual diseases, since there is less risk of pregnancy. Other factors include the rise of internet dating and the ready availability of Viagra®. More open mores do mean that older women can now visit sexual health clinics without fear of stigmatisation but the rise in their attendance is still not proportional to the rate of disease incidence increase. This, too, is an area in which the RCOG could take a lead, in line with the call from the Health Protection Agency for a safe sex campaign aimed at the middle-aged.

Conclusion

In these three cases, older women do constitute a group with common interests in safer sex, in more targeted screening for breast cancer and in cheaper drugs for the treatment of that disease. Where they are blocked by lack of awareness of statistically complex scientific studies such as Pharaoh's,[22] for example, it is perfectly right and proper for an organisation dedicated to their health to act on their behalf.

It is neither patronising nor paternalistic for the RCOG to use its specialist knowledge, legitimacy and 'clout' to prevent the lady from vanishing.

References

1. Boston Women's Health Book Collective. *Our Bodies, Ourselves*. Boston: Touchstone; 1973.
2. Arditti R, Klein RD, Minden S, editors. *Test-Tube Women: What Future for Motherhood?* London: Pandora Press, Routledge Kegan Paul; 1984.
3. Baylis F, Sherwin S. Judgements of non-compliance in pregnancy. In: Dickenson DL, editor. *Ethical Issues in Maternal-Fetal Medicine*. Cambridge: Cambridge University Press; 2002. p. 285–301.
4. MacKenzie C. Stoljar N, editors. *Relational Autonomy: Feminist Perspectives on Autonomy, Agency and the Social Self*. Oxford: Oxford University Press; 2000.
5. Sherwin S. A relational autonomy approach to autonomy in health care. In: Sherwin S, co-ordinator. *The Politics of Women's Health: Exploring Agency and Autonomy*. Philadelphia: Temple University Press; 1998. p. 19–47.
6. Verkerk MA. The care perspective and autonomy. *Med Health Care Philos* 2001;4:3:289–94.
7. Daniels C. *At Women's Expense: State Power and the Politics of Fetal Rights*. Cambridge, MA: Harvard University Press; 1993.
8. Bewley S. Restricting the freedom of pregnant women. In: Dickenson DL, editor. *Ethical Issues in Maternal-Fetal Medicine*. Cambridge: Cambridge University Press; 2002. p. 131–46.
9. Dickenson D. *Property in the Body: Feminist Perspectives*. Cambridge: Cambridge University Press; 2007.
10. Dickenson D. *Body Shopping: The Economy Fuelled by Flesh and Blood*. Oxford: Oneworld; 2008.
11. Haker H. Reproductive rights in the twenty-first century. In: Widdows H, Alkorta I, Emaldi A, editors. *Women's Reproductive Rights*. Basingstoke: Palgrave; 2006. p. 167–87.
12. Holm S. Going to the roots of the stem cell controversy. *Bioethics* 2002;16:493–507.
13. Dickenson D. Property and women's alienation from their own reproductive labour. *Bioethics* 2001;15:205–17.
14. Jacobs A, Dwyer J, Lee, P. Seventy ova. *Hastings Cent Rep* 2001;31:12–14.
15. Hwang WS, Ryu YJ, Park JH, Park ES, Lee EG, Koo JM, et al. Evidence of a pluripotent stem cell line derived from a cloned blastocyst. *Science* 2004;303:1669–74. Erratum in: *Science* 2005;310:1769. Retraction in: Kennedy D. *Science* 2006;311:335.
16. Hwang WS, Roh SI, Lee BC, Kang SK, Kwon DK, Kim S, et al. Patient-specific embryonic stem cell lines derived from human SCNT blastocysts. *Science* 2005;308:1777–83. Erratum in: *Science* 2005;310:1769. Retraction in: Kennedy D. *Science* 2006;311:335.
17. Levine R. *Ethics and Regulation of Clinical Research*. Baltimore, MD: Urban and Schwarzenberg; 1981. p. 53.
18. Ding EL, Powe NR, Manson JE, Sherber NS, Braunstein JB. Sex differences in perceived risks, distrust and willingness to participate in clincial trials: a randomized study of cardiovascular prevention trials. *Arch Intern Med* 2007;167:905–912.
19. Jones M. Ethical issues surrounding the use of women as subjects in clinical research. In: Boomgaarden J, Louhala P, Wiesing U, editors. *Issues in Medical Research Ethics*. Oxford: Berghahn Books; 2003. p. 57.
20. Helat A, Gross CP, Krumholz HM. Representation of the elderly, women and minorities in heart failure clincial trials. *Arch Intern Med* 2002;162:1682–8.
21. MacKinnon CA. *Feminism Unmodified: Discourses on Life and Law*. Cambridge, MA: Harvard University Press; 1989.

22. Pharaoh PD, Antoniou AC, Easton DF, Ponder BAJ. Polygenes, risk prediction and targeted prevention of breast cancer. *New Engl J Med* 2008;358:26,2796–803.

23. Easton DF. How many more breast cancer predisposition genes are there? *Breast Cancer Res* 1999;1:14–17.

24. Wright C. Polygenic test for breast cancer has utility for screening. PHG Foundation website [www.phgfoundation.org/news/4255].

25. Andrews LB. How is technology changing the meaning of motherhood? In: Widdows H, Alkorta I, Emaldi A, editors. *Women's Reproductive Rights*. Basingstoke: Palgrave; 2006. p. 124–39.

26. Jensen K, Murray F. International patenting: the landscape of the human genome. *Science* 2005;310:239–40.

27. Soini S. Ayme S, Matthijs G; Public and Professional Policy Committee and Patenting and Licensing Committee. Patenting and licensing in genetic testing: ethical, social and legal issues. *Eur J Hum Genet* 2008;16 Suppl 1:S10–50.

28. Matthijs G. European opposition against the *BRCA* gene patents. *Fam Cancer* 2006;5:95–102.

29. Sample I. Sexual diseases double in eight years among the over-45s. *The Guardian* 30 June 2008.

Chapter 27
Reproductive ageing and the RCOG

Discussion

Sean Kehoe: Thank you very much, Donna. Can I just pick you up on one thing? I am a gynae-oncologist and I remember the first *BRCA1* testing. The company was based in Scotland, presumably for legal reasons, and we got a letter from them. Essentially, what the woman had to do was sign a form, then get her GP to sign the form saying that she was counselled, and then send the blood away. Of course, anybody could sign it: they were not going back to check. That test disappeared. We got rid of them. I do not know how it was done but there was a lot of noise made. They tried once but I am sure they will come back again …

Donna Dickenson: There is a continual need to keep vigilant, because lots of companies can find similar things.

Diana Mansour: This is really more of comment: in Newcastle, when we recently opened a session for sexually transmitted infection screening in mature men, I asked: 'What about the mature women?' They said 'It is different. The men are getting their infections elsewhere.' Well, I am sure they are giving it to their wives …

Donna Dickenson: As in your slide, we could show graphically [laughs].

Diana Mansour: Very much so. I was really pleasantly surprised that you actually included that slide. We often think STIs [sexually transmitted infections] are infections only of the young women … purely because of statistics.

Maya Unnithan: I was really interested to see the difference in society's perceptions between men and women. When we talk about the ageing of men, there is not that sort of clear age limit in the way we look at it. But if we look at the ageing of women, there does seem to be a sort of limit: mid-40s and not further. I think that is an interesting point. It struck me when we were talking about broadening the image, you looked at woman beyond the reproductive years …

Donna Dickenson: Yes. We already accepted that point. I think, in general, our limits have broadened. I showed an example of me being classified as rather elderly at 26. So I am pleading for society's perceptions to be broadened even further. I suppose, yes, that is helpful.

Peter Braude: Can I make a comment, Donna? Just looking at the title of your talk, although I entirely understand you in principle, I can only see that one of your issues deals with women specifically. That is the one about contraception and STIs. The other issues you talked about are issues in society in general and should not be sex-related or related to sexuality. The idea of bad ethics committees is not specifically related to women. When you talk about stem cells, we are working towards bringing in stem cell coordinators, who will help reach an agreement on what kind of things would be reasonable to do – and that is not only about women. It is where the HGC [Human Genetics Commission] should be working. I thought that someone of your stature, on that kind of professional body, could actually make a difference. Rather than the RCOG, which, of course, can be supportive, as you said earlier on. It is not the RCOG's main duty to deal with that although they do have a Scientific Advisory Committee. Some of the topics that you separate about women, I don't think are only about women. They are about the society in general.

Donna Dickenson: I won't deny that many of these issues are about society in general. But I think that is actually a good reason for us to try to use issues which are not seen as being just women's issues in order to defend general principles. Certainly the way in which genes are being commercialised is not just limited to the *HER2* and *BRCA1* and *BRCA2* genes. But, coincidentally or not, those have become two of the highest profile instances which have allowed us to campaign against genetic-testing commercialisation at the whole-society level. Just say 'Look, it is affecting women now. It may affect other people soon. Let us do something about it.' And that is the tone that I would like to see the RCOG take. I do not think that is necessarily contradicted by the idea that the HGC could also be doing that. The more of us who do it, the better. But because the RCOG has specialist knowledge, and a specialist mandate, it could also add its weight. I was not asked to produce recommendations that only the RCOG could undertake. Indeed if the RCOG tries to act in conjunction with others, it is likely to be more successful.

Peter Braude: What you just said is a very good example. The way things like *BRCA* testing came to the forefront demonstrates the sway these groups have. They say they are invisible – they are not invisible. They are actually very powerful.

Donna Dickenson: Well, it did not come to the forefront very readily. If you look at the debate on Herceptin, it was not really very clear for most of the debate. It was simply taken for granted that this was the price of the drug. And you really have to look quite hard to find the evidence. That was because there was a patent. That is not brought out in the public discussion. So you know, I am not entirely convinced.

Susan Bewley: What I find reassuring, and I think many Members and Fellows of the College will also find reassuring, is we do not have to 'throw out the baby with the bath water'. Our care and concern for women (as ourselves, our sisters, mothers, daughters or whatever) is not inherently paternalistic or patronising. Obstetricians and gynaecologists have been 'on the defensive'. For example, if a woman says that such-and-such is what she wants, many feel we just have to do it 'or else', whereas we can try to renegotiate the doctor–patient relationship. Is it one of power? Is it one of partnership? Is it one of service? Or are we just like decorators whose clients choose different coloured wallpaper? I think it is very reassuring to hear that. Also, the idea of applying a lens that other medical specialties cannot do – that of gender relations. We did that here with respect to the trading of ova and sperms. There will be differences. If we then start looking at trade in kidneys or lungs, we may see differences which will be due to class, race, poverty or gender. There is something very powerful that the RCOG can do which is to look with a 'gender lens' – because it will bring up other lenses around social justice. This is not very fashionable but it is something that doctors generally believe in – that through health, we do something about inequality. We try to help people live longer, better, fitter lives. Your book *Body Shopping*[1] powerfully brought out the huge debate we are having about our bodies:

can they be bought and sold? Or the parts that are in them? Can we sell our hearts, for example? Not yet, but why not do this on the internet? I wonder whether you would like to expand on a comment in the book that 'everyone has got a female body now'. What did you mean by that?

Donna Dickenson: Before I do that, I want to say thank you for the discussion about paternalism. I have been on the RCOG Ethics Committee for 5 or 6 years now and before this I was on one of the British Medical Association's committees. I am always very favourably struck, and impressed, by the way in which doctors really try extremely hard not to be paternalistic. We always really worry about this. That is why I was trying to reassure you that I do not think they will be in this case, particularly with an ethicist in the room. OK. Regarding the other idea in the book I wrote, *Body Shopping*,[1] I argued that we have some form of feminisation of the body in phenomena such as the one in five human genes being subject of patent and the massive commercial interest in other tissues, or in umbilical cord blood banking for example, which is somewhat similar. Even though it is not actual 'sale', it is still a commercial interest in a body-product that we are witnessing. This is one phenomenon that has actually been the case for women for a long time. Just thinking philosophically about it, there is a blurring of the boundaries about whether the body is an object, or belongs to a subject. So the argument is that, in a sense, the reason that we are worried about developments like the 'one in five human genes', is because they now apply to both sexes. Some of the other developments, like the eggs in a recent case, were not so readily publicised. I am not saying that it is time men also suffered the objectification and commodification that women's bodies have suffered. I am not saying that at all. I do not think 'equal misery' is a very effective rallying cry! We should oppose body shopping for both sexes. Rather like the question that Peter just asked, I am saying that we can act together and have a stronger chance of success.

References

1.   Dickenson D. *Body Shopping: the Economy Fuelled by Flesh and Blood*. Oxford: Oneworld; 2008.

Section 8

Fertility treatment: science and reality – the NHS and the market

Chapter 28
Evidence-based and cost-effective fertility investigation and treatment of older women: moving beyond NICE

David Barlow

Introduction

The management of infertility has been revolutionised by the development of assisted reproduction technology (ART), especially *in vitro* fertilisation (IVF), over the past 30 years. Many serious barriers to success have been overcome through being bypassed. Important examples include overcoming tubal damage by IVF and severe oligospermia/azoospermia being overcome through intracytoplasmic sperm injection (ICSI) in IVF, possibly in combination with epididymal or testicular sperm retrieval. An area where ART has not had such clear success has been in addressing the negative effect of a woman's age advancing to the stage where there is deterioration in ovarian response and/or egg quality. The consequence is a reduced chance of conception with advancing age.

There is no specific threshold age at which reproductive ageing becomes critical. However, it is possible to draw conclusions about average performance and it is clear that reproductive performance declines noticeably between the ages of 35 and 40 years. This affects outcomes at every level of intervention in infertility management but the effect is most readily measured in the IVF context because of the complete data sets that are available.

In general, where a woman is older and seeking fertility assistance it is important that any delay in initiating treatment is minimised. Similarly, it is important that such a couple would come forward to seek help relatively early in the manifestation of the problem. These points were recognised in the UK in the publication of the National Institute for Health and Clinical Excellence (NICE) full clinical guideline on fertility,[1] which provided an evidence- and cost-effectiveness-based approach to the whole of the subfertility experience, from first suspicion by the couple to tertiary level treatment, where appropriate. The issue of female age was relevant to a number of aspects of the NICE guideline but, on the relevance of female age to the approach to be taken, it stated:[1]

> People who are concerned about their fertility should be informed that female fertility declines with age, but that the effect of age on male fertility is less clear. With regular unprotected sexual intercourse, 94% of fertile women aged 35 years, and 77% of those aged 38 years, will conceive after 3 years of trying.

> People who have not conceived after 1 year of regular unprotected sexual intercourse should be offered further clinical investigation including semen analysis and/or assessment of ovulation.

> Where there is a history of predisposing factors (such as …), or where a woman is aged 35 years or over, earlier investigation should be offered.

The ultimate test of ovarian reproductive potential is in IVF. In general, women of around 35 years can reasonably expect to have IVF success that is, on average, not notably inferior to that of younger women. Although responsiveness and implantation rates may be better in younger women, the overall reproductive performance will be acceptable to most people. When birth rates after IVF are considered, the decline in success is accentuated between ages 35 and 40 years. There is no reason to believe that naturally conceived pregnancy outcomes have a different age profile but comprehensive data are much more difficult to generate.

IVF outcomes in the UK

Summary data from the Human Fertilisation and Embryology Authority (HFEA) give a comprehensive overview of outcomes of IVF in the UK.[2] Livebirth rates for the UK (Figure 28.1) indicate that, while there has been a progressive improvement in IVF livebirth rates for younger women, there has not been the same improvement in rates for those aged 35 years or over since 2000, and for those aged 40 years or over there has been no real improvement when comparing 1996, 2000 and 2005. There is a progressive decline in livebirth rates with increasing impact as women approach or pass the age of 40 years

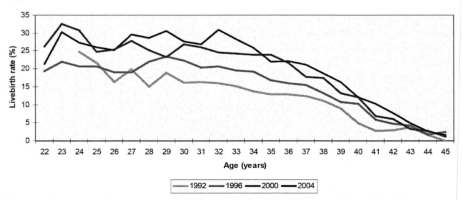

Figure 28.1   Livebirth rates per cycle of IVF or ICSI in the UK for the years 1992, 1996, 2000 and 2005; data from the HFEA[2]

A woman attempting IVF pregnancy at around age 38 years faces an increasing risk of poor response to ovarian stimulation, a reduced chance of pregnancy and live birth and an increased chance of miscarriage. As she approaches around age 43 years, the chance of pregnancy is especially low.

Again, this decline in IVF performance with age was incorporated in the recommendations of the NICE Guideline as follows:[1]

> Women should be informed that the chance of a live birth following *in vitro* fertilisation treatment varies with female age and that the optimal female age range for *in vitro* fertilisation treatment is 23–39 years. Chances of a live birth per treatment cycle are:
> - greater than 20% for women aged 23–35 years
> - 15% for women aged 36–38 years
> - 10% for women aged 39 years
> - 6% for women aged 40 years or older.

The whole process has been regarded as an inevitable reflection of ovarian and reproductive ageing, for which a range of strategies have been proposed. None of these is especially satisfactory. They include:

- estimation of ovarian reserve by a range of techniques that provide some success in predicting ovarian responsiveness but whose use has not been proven to significantly improve birth rates in IVF[3–5]

- oocyte cryopreservation at an age before the start of any decline; this is a theoretical option since birth rates after oocyte cryopreservation are relatively low[6]

- preimplantation genetic screening for aneuploidy aiming to ensure that embryos of the best reproductive potential are used by older women; this has not been shown to improve birth rates[7]

- egg donation, which is an option that bypasses decreased ovarian performance but introduces well-known issues associated with gamete donation about which there are many considerations for those involved.[8]

Implementation of the NICE guideline recommendations by primary care trusts

In February 2004, the NICE clinical guideline on fertility[1] was published under my chairmanship. This large body of work encompassed all aspects of fertility management, from the first querying of whether a couple might have a problem through to all treatment options, although the media attention it received focused on the recommendations concerned with NHS provision of IVF services. This was not surprising, given the importance of this specific aspect of the guideline. One of the recommendations was that couples where the woman is aged below 40 years should be eligible for up to three complete cycles of IVF. The guideline publication was accompanied by a statement issued by the Secretary of State for Health, Dr John Reid, who welcomed the guideline and indicated that he expected primary care trusts (PCTs) to have put in place NHS funding of at least one cycle of IVF by April 2005. The NHS response has been patchy and the politics of this is discussed in Chapter 29. An example of the PCT response to this instruction is provided by a Department of Health-sponsored survey carried out by Infertility Network UK (INUK) that explored PCT funding of fertility services in England in 2006.[9]

The survey addressed the 303 PCTs and 151 (49.8%) of them responded. Some interpretation is required because there was subsequently a reduction of the numbers of PCTs from around 300 to around 150. Of those that responded, 98 (64.9%) indicated that they funded one cycle of NHS IVF, 32 (21.2%) funded two cycles and seven (4.6%) funded three cycles. Finally, 14 (9.3%) either indicated that they did not fund IVF, did not provide details of the number of cycles funded or did not answer that specific question.

In 2007, a PCT survey in England carried out directly by the Department of Health had a 100% response rate. Some provided joint responses and some responses require interpretation in order to classify the provision. My interpretation of the responses can be summarised as follows: 96 (64%) provided one cycle, 40 (27%) provided two cycles and nine (6%) provided three cycles. Five PCTs (3%) either provided no IVF or could not provide data. Forty-nine (34%) of the 145 PCTs that provided some IVF indicated that the provision was 'fresh IVF', which implied that the related frozen embryo replacement cycles were not funded by those PCTs.[10]

The invited title for this chapter includes the statement 'Moving beyond NICE'. In terms of NHS provision of IVF, I would argue that NHS funding has mostly not yet delivered the NICE recommendation, neither in the number of cycles provided nor in the provision of frozen embryo replacement cycles associated with NHS-funded fresh treatment cycles. Another interpretation of 'Moving beyond NICE' in the context of an RCOG Study Group on women in later reproductive life could relate to the fact that the NICE Guideline Development Group recommended that the upper age limit for NHS provision of IVF should be 39 years. It is worthwhile exploring the process involved in reaching this conclusion and, indeed, what the guideline involved more generally since many who have not studied it may believe that it merely outlined the NHS IVF provision.[1]

Cost-effectiveness modelling in the NICE guideline

The NICE guideline took an evidence-based approach to the whole literature on infertility management and encompassed activity across primary, secondary and tertiary care. The tertiary care aspect was largely focused on ART and advanced pelvic surgery. It was noteworthy that a considerable proportion of the infertility literature is not based on the gold standard of the randomised controlled trial (RCT). As a result, only 48 of the 167 recommendations in the guideline were based on level A evidence (RCT based). Many of the sound and sensible recommendations were based on other levels of best available evidence that was assimilated by the multi-faceted Guideline Development Group, and 34 were good practice points where the Group recommended sensible and sound practice advice but without a strong evidence base. Another way of moving beyond NICE will be when the evidence base of infertility management becomes strengthened, particularly by RCTs addressing key questions in clinical practice. The most important and relevant RCTs are likely to be collaborative efforts because of the large scale usually required to produce the statistical power needed to answer the questions. There is a growing trend towards such work being done but the literature remains dominated by relatively small or uncontrolled studies.

The recommendations concerning the older woman who is considering seeking help were that time should be saved as far as possible in deciding to seek help. This pressure applies across management strategies right through to IVF because of the serious decline in the chance of a birth with advanced age. Where the NHS is concerned, this pressure then has to confront the upper age limit threshold for treatment under NHS funding. When the NICE fertility guideline was set up, the scope of the work was defined. This scope determined that the guideline would provide guidance on some key NHS treatment eligibility issues and these are the points that have attracted the greatest interest and are very relevant to the older woman seeking IVF. This scope included the requirement that for advanced fertility interventions the guideline would include clinical eligibility criteria to be met to qualify for NHS treatment, the number of cycles of IVF treatment to be offered by the NHS, the number of embryos to be implanted in any cycle and the optimal lower and upper age ranges for treatment. This type of guidance was unlikely to be able to be based on the outcomes of RCTs but the Guideline Development Group was tasked with providing a best judgement on this.

Where possible, NICE funding advice is based on complex cost-effectiveness modelling designed to provide cost per quality-adjusted life years (QALYs) gained as a result of the intervention under consideration. This is particularly the case for the NICE health Technology Appraisal (TA) programme. This process enables comparisons to be drawn with other health interventions to assist in prioritisation in the provision of health care. In general, interventions that are more expensive than around £20,000 to £30,000 per QALY gained are regarded as not cost-effective. With the NICE fertility guideline, this approach had to be adapted to the circumstances under consideration. There was no underpinning NICE TA; it was appreciated that the modelling would be highly complex because of the layers of costs that would need to be considered when neonatal intensive care costs, and so on, are included but additionally there were valid published arguments (quoted in the guideline) suggesting that:

> QALYs are intended to capture improvements in health among patients. They are not appropriate for placing a value on additional lives. Additional lives are not improvements in health; preventing someone's death is not the same as creating their life and it is not possible to improve the quality of life of someone who has not been conceived by conceiving them.[11]

> Cost–utility analysis has little relevance to the management of infertility where lives are produced and not saved.[12]

In consequence, the approach taken was to use cost-effectiveness where possible and to feed this into cost–impact models. The guideline stated:[1]

> The clinical and cost data that were available were not appropriate for making detailed forecasts of future expenditure on assisted reproduction. ... However, the data did indicate the magnitudes of costs that would be likely to be needed if specific policies were adopted.

The basis for the recommendation that three cycles should be offered was that the evidence base for the effectiveness of IVF in consecutive treatment cycles appeared most convincing for the first three cycles of IVF treatment. Beyond three cycles, the numbers of cases involved in case series were declining such that the reliability that effectiveness is sustained at a level comparable to the first three cycles was not secure. On that basis, the Guideline Development Group recommended three cycles. These were to include the associated frozen–thawed embryo replacements. The cost-effectiveness modelling is detailed in the full guideline and indicates substantially different costs per live birth of £12,931 and £20,056 for women aged 35 and 39 years, respectively (Figure 28.2).[1]

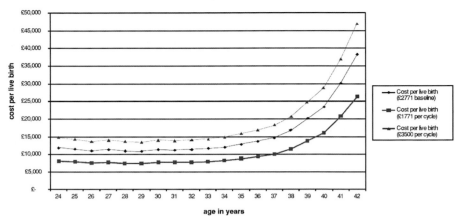

Figure 28.2 Age-specific cost per live birth using three cost estimates for a cycle of IVF treatment; reproduced with permission from the NICE fertility guideline[1]

With the Guideline Development Group having the defined task of advising on the age limits for NHS IVF, the approach was that NHS funding was justified where effectiveness was maintained. The cut-off threshold for NHS funding was set at the age where livebirth rates fell to 50% of the plateau rate observed at younger ages. Based on the HFEA statistics, the livebirth rate fell to 50% of the plateau level for younger women above the age of 39 years and we recommended that NHS IVF was to be offered up to 39 years of age. NICE clinical guidelines carry weight with the NHS but are not mandatory for PCT funding, unlike NICE TAs that do carry a mandatory funding expectation.

What women and doctors need to know

Against this background, I have been asked to outline what women and generalists need to know. In both cases, the need is to have a balanced perspective on the possibilities for achieving pregnancy both without and with some form of ART. Not all women who seek help need think that they will have to become involved in ART but, since it has become the final common pathway for those who are not achieving the desired pregnancy within a reasonable interval, it is important that the couples and their advisers understand what is possible and sensible. Certainly, once a couple has been unsuccessful in trying to achieve a pregnancy for 3 years, we suggested that IVF was justifiable even if the problem is unexplained.

The NICE guideline was published in 2004 and provides comprehensive coverage of the field. I suggest that this remains a good guide to the field, as practised in the UK, for generalists and for those couples who find that the text is accessible.[1] There is also a lay summary of the guideline.[13] Both can be downloaded from the NICE website. For patients looking for guidance on infertility and its management I think that the best source of information is the guide for patients published by the HFEA.[14]

Interpreting published outcome data for IVF clinics

Both the NICE guideline and the HFEA patients' guide provide advice on strategy and on the efficacy of the various treatment options, and describe when they are relevant.

What is especially important for the older woman is understanding how increasing age undermines the effectiveness of options and how this feeds into the advantage of turning to IVF significantly below 40 years if there is to be a reasonable chance of pregnancy. If generalist professionals require information beyond the NICE guideline, I suggest that the most appropriate sources for updating will be the Cochrane Library (www.cochrane.org) for specific fertility topics that are covered by Cochrane and review articles in journals such as *Human Reproduction Update* and *Fertility and Sterility*.

If couples with their clinical advisers decide that referral for IVF at a tertiary centre is appropriate then there may be reference to the published outcome data for the IVF centres that is available on the HFEA website. This information is inevitably used by third parties to construct league tables of IVF success. In some ways, this can be useful to couples since they do wish to have insight into the likely chances of achieving the desired baby at the relevant clinics. Unfortunately, it takes a reasonable degree of insight into the processes of IVF and IVF clinics to be able to interpret meaningfully the multiple outcome measures that are provided. Media-constructed league tables tend to focus on the headline livebirth rate and there is a competition incentive for clinics to aim at achieving a good headline rate, within which there may be important underlying issues. Where a clinic is in the private sector, the importance of having a good headline livebirth rate is accentuated by the business importance of this in attracting couples to the clinic.

Couples looking at clinic data ideally need to understand what may lie behind headline figures. To assist couples, the HFEA published a guide for patients on how to read the clinic data.[15] For the older woman it is important that she looks at the age-specific data that are contained in the HFEA reports on the specific clinics. I have used, as an illustration, the current HFEA website figures for the Oxford Fertility Clinic.[16] I directed this service for 20 years up to 2005 but have no current responsibility for it.

Figure 28.3 shows how the HFEA presents the headline statistics. The HFEA has sought to move away from headline rates and closer to a careful presentation of the data in a meaningful way and a guide on how to interpret the statistics is provided. It can be seen that there is no single headline figure in the HFEA presentation but when external groups make league tables it tends to be the livebirth rate for the main body of patients, which would be the group where the woman is under 35 years old and using fresh embryos.

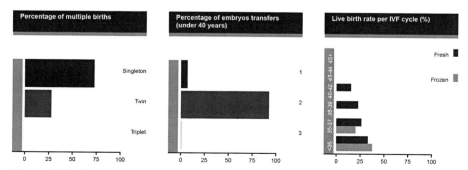

Figure 28.3   HFEA publication of UK IVF clinic data; headline data for the Oxford Fertility Clinic; reproduced with permission from HFEA[16]

The graph of livebirth rate per IVF cycle presents rates stratified by female age. This is appropriate but for most clinics the numbers of older women treated are much smaller than for younger groups so the reliability of the rates can be weakened. The information necessary to better understand this is in the detailed tabulation provided by the HFEA (Table 28.1). Again, this presents livebirth rates stratified by age but it also provides the actual number of cycles of treatment and where the numbers involved are too small to provide reliable percentage rates, no percentage is given. For best interpretation of performance, the eye is drawn to the rows of statistics shown shown in bold text. These are the livebirth rate per cycle started and the singleton livebirth rate per cycle started. The first of these indicates the overall livebirth rate for the indicated age of a woman and is a key guide, but the HFEA provides the important contextual information on the singleton livebirth rate, recognising the importance of singleton birth as the ideal outcome in fertility therapy. As the women approach or pass age 40 years, it can be seen that the singleton livebirth rate gets closer and closer to the overall livebirth rate. However, beyond age 42 years it is a common experience that the number of live births based on the woman's own eggs being used is negligible.

When reviewing clinic-specific data, it is important to realise that pregnancy rates are affected by factors that are not readily obvious to the outsider. These include the case mix of the clinic, with clinics that predominantly treat less complex cases, fewer older women or cases with less extended durations of failure to conceive being likely to have higher success rates. The HFEA has sought to encourage couples who are examining clinic-specific data to consider the likelihood of a multiple pregnancy, which is likely to correlate with the transfer of more than one embryo.

Conclusion

Overall, couples seeking help with a subfertility problem where the woman is older face challenges in addition to the many issues associated with infertility management that all subfertile couples must face. In this context, a 35-year-old woman is merely

Table 28.1 HFEA publication of UK IVF clinic data; detailed performance data for the Oxford Fertility Clinic; data from HFEA[16]

| | Livebirth rates by age for IVF and ICSI embryo transfers using own eggs[a] | | | | | |
	Below 35	35–37	38–39	40–42	43–44	Over 44
Fresh embryos						
Cycles started	**33.1%** (108/326)	**26.2%** (61/233)	**22.5%** (27/120)	**15.0%** (19/127)	(0/9)	N/A
Embryo transfers	35.2% (108/307)	28.0% (61/218)	23.9% (27/113)	16.2% (19/117)	(0/8)	N/A
Implantation rate	26.6% (158/593)	20.9% (88/422)	18.5% (40/216)	10.1% (26/258)	(0/16)	N/A
Singleton live births	**22.4%** (73/326)	**19.3%** (45/233)	**17.5%** (21/120)	**13.4%** (17/127)	0	0
Multiple births	10.7% (35/326)	6.9% (16/233)	5.0% (6/120)	1.6% (2/127)	0	0
Frozen embryos						
Cycles started	**37.6%** (32/85)	**20.0%** (13/65)	(5/31)	(5/35)	(0/3)	N/A
Embryo transfers	37.6% (32/85)	20.0% (13/65)	(5/31)	(5/35)	(0/3)	N/A
Implantation rate	27.2% (47/173)	11.9% (15/126)	8.5% (5/59)	14.1% (11/78)	(0/9)	N/A
Singleton live births	**23.5%** (20/85)	**18.5%** (12/65)	(5/31)	(3/35)	0	0
Multiple births	14.1% (12/85)	1.5% (1/65)	0	(2/35)	0	0

ICSI = intracytoplasmic sperm injection; IVF = *in vitro* fertilisation

[a] Percentage of ICSI = 38% and IVF = 62%

approaching the age where this becomes important whereas a 40-year-old woman is clearly in that situation. One of the important differences for these women compared with younger women is the much greater level of uncertainty around the chance that there will be a baby after treatments have been tried. For women aged below 30 years seeking help with subfertility there can generally be reasonable optimism that, if all appropriate treatment options are explored, the couple are likely to have a baby. For women aged 40 years or over the reverse is the case. For this reason, it is very important that information giving is appropriate, that hopes are tempered by a realistic view of the prospects and that all involved appreciate the importance of achieving a sensible progression through investigation and treatment without delays so that appropriate interventions can be explored before further time-based deterioration of reproductive potential occurs.

References

1. National Collaborating Centre for Women's and Children's Health. *Fertility: Assessment and Treatment for People with Fertility Problems.* London: RCOG Press; 2004 [www.nice.org.uk/nicemedia/pdf/CG011fullguideline.pdf].

2. Human Fertilisation and Embryology Authority. *A Long-Term Analysis of the HFEA Register Data 1991–2006.* London: HFEA; 2008 [www.hfea.gov.uk/docs/Latest_long_term_data_analysis_report_front_cover.pdf].

3. Broekmans FJ, Kwee J, Hendriks DJ, Mol BW, Lambalk CB. A systematic review of tests predicting ovarian reserve and IVF outcome. *Hum Reprod Update* 2006;12:685–718.

4. Smeenk J, Sweep F, Zielhuis G, Kremer J, Thomas C, Braat D. Antimullerian hormone predicts ovarian responsiveness, but not embryo quality or pregnancy, after *in vitro* fertilization or intracytoplasmic sperm injection. *Fert Steril* 2007;87:223–6.

5. Gnoth C, Schuring AN, Friol K, Tigges J, Mallmann P, Godehart E. Relevance of anti-Mullerian hormone measurement in a routine IVF program. *Hum Reprod* 2008;23:1359–65.

6. Tao T, Del Valle A. Human oocyte and ovarian tissue cryopreservation and its application. *J Assist Reprod Genet* 2008; 25,287–96.

7. Anderson RA, Pickering S. The current status of preimplantation genetic screening: British Fertility Society Policy and Practice Guidelines. *Hum Fertil (Camb)* 2008;11:71–5.

8. Sauer M, Kavich SM. Oocyte and embryo donation 2006: reviewing two decades of innovation and controversy. *Reprod Biomed Online* 2006;12:153–62.

9. Infertility Network UK. INUK Survey of PCTs 2006 [www.infertilitynetworkuk.com/uploadedFiles/InfertilityAwareness/DH_079807[1].pdf].

10. Department of Health. *Primary Care Trust Survey – Provision of IVF in England 2007.* London: DH; 2008 [www.dh.gov.uk/en/Publicationsandstatistics/Publications/PublicationsPolicyAndGuidance/DH_085665].

11. Devlin N, Parkin D. Funding fertility: issues in the allocation and distribution of resources to assisted reproductive technologies, *Hum Fertil (Camb)* 2003;6(2 Suppl):S2–6.

12. Collins J. An international survey of the health economics of IVF and ICSI. *Hum Reprod Update* 2002;8,265–77.

13. National Institute for Clinical Excellence. *NICE Fertility Guideline CG11 – Information for the Public* [www.nice.org.uk/nicemedia/pdf/CG011publicinfoenglish.pdf].

14. Human Fertilisation and Embryology Authority. *Infertility: The HFEA Guide.* London: HFEA; 2007 [www.hfea.gov.uk/docs/Guide2.pdf].

15. Human Fertilisation and Embryology Authority. *How to Read the Clinic Pages.* HFEA guide for patients on how to read HFEA clinic data [www.hfea.gov.uk/docs/how-to-read.pdf].

16. Human Fertilisation and Embryology Authority. HFEA clinic data [www.hfea.gov.uk/docs/South_East-2008.pdf].

Chapter 29
Bang for the buck: what purchasers and commissioners think and do

Berkeley Greenwood

Introduction

It is perhaps a little premature to comment in depth on the mindset and motivations of healthcare commissioners in the area of infertility. Department of Health research continues into which assisted reproductive technology (ART) services are being bought by the primary care trusts (PCTs), which problems they are facing and what their longer-term intentions are. This will be coupled with support work to help them to improve commissioning for those who have problems conceiving. This work is being led by Infertility Network UK (INUK), the leading patient voice in infertility, together with a group of other experts guiding the Department of Health on particular aspects of infertility care.

Evidence-based precision on the nature of what goes on in the commissioner's mind is difficult to achieve, partly because there is no such thing as a 'typical' commissioner. The work of the expert group advising ministers on how to improve uptake of the National Institute for Health and Clinical Excellence (NICE) fertility guideline[1] may shed some clear light on this when it reports in the summer of 2009. Meanwhile, everything we can say on the matter is necessarily rather anecdotal and speculative but this chapter is based on a lengthy observation of PCTs' reaction to spending on subfertility. There are some definite trends in commissioning behaviour that are helpful to observe.

But perhaps those who are wedded always to the need for a rigorous evidence base had better look away now.

History

To understand why we are where we are with the funding of ART, it is helpful to review the history of this issue. We will primarily review the situation in England rather than the UK. The first *in vitro* fertilisation (IVF) birth was achieved in 1978. In the years that followed, what had initially been presented by the press and media as a '*Star Wars*'-style technique gradually became a more commonplace and straightforward procedure. It started to become available in limited quantities through the NHS too. As so often has been the case, it was rapidly picked up and more readily embraced in the less conservative healthcare environments elsewhere in Europe.

Being a new area of medicine, there was absolutely no budget in existence for it in the NHS and so creating one meant taking money from elsewhere in what, throughout the past 20 years, has been a continually cash-strapped system. This has been the major challenge for campaigners in this area. It is arguable, too, that the very fact that the 'high-tech' label has been attached to this area of medicine represents a major drawback in gaining funding and that this has been reinforced by the political and funding developments since.

Science has developed on from the now relatively basic and clumsy process of IVF – simply mixing gametes together outside the body and reimplanting them. Now we have even more delicate techniques such as intracytoplasmic sperm injection (ICSI), assisted zona hatching and preimplantation genetic diagnosis, among many others. Each one of these unfolding developments has been lovingly captured in the world press with accompanying 'oohs' and 'ahs'. Indeed, the press coverage that the European Society of Human Reproduction and Embryology (ESHRE) conference attracts each year equals anything that any cancer or cardiac disease congress can gain. The national newspapers in the UK will regularly carry at least two full two pages of stories on the conference for every day that it is on. Public fascination with reproductive health continues unabated. This has helped to reinforce the sense that these treatments are still on the edge of science, with the concomitant feeling that they are associated with limited success rates. In short, it may scare commissioners off.

It is unclear when the first publicly funded cycles of IVF were provided by the NHS but suffice it to say that in the public mind (or more precisely among couples needing treatment) there was a growing expectation by the early 1990s that it was reasonable to expect the NHS to fund ART. One of the main objectives of the first National Fertility Week in 1993 was a desire to raise the profile of fertility treatment's benefits and success rates and the lack of public funding. National Fertility Week became the National Infertility Awareness Campaign (NIAC) and the objective of raising the profile has been prominent in every major NIAC conference.

In the early 1990s, ministers had difficulty in accepting that infertility was a health need at all. They were reflecting wider public opinion (indeed 'smug haves' or 'smug don't wants' can still be found loudly opining against NHS provision of such treatments at dinner tables whenever this topic is discussed). After much campaigning, the Department of Health – in around 1995 – at last began to concede in their correspondence (to NIAC and to patients) that infertility was indeed 'an important health need'. However, the department still was not going to instruct anyone to fund it and the area remained outside the waiting list targets.

The improvements in service that took place in the 1990s from health authority to health authority were largely the result of enterprising groups of patients taking up the cudgels with local commissioners and forcing them to make some provision. This was backed by approaches to Members of Parliament at national level to try to persuade them to take the issue up with directors of public health in their patch. Interestingly, this has always been an area that has commanded genuine cross-party support, among backbenchers at least, and early day motions tabled as early as 1993[2] and as late as 2008[3] bear testimony to this. The arguments that came back were that fertility treatment was not a priority, was not successful and could be categorised alongside wisdom tooth extraction, breast reduction, varicose veins and sterilisation in terms of its value.

In 1997, the Government changed and, despite readily signing up to NIAC's aims in opposition, the new Labour Government found that life was a little different when one actually held the purse strings. Ministers were supportive (see the many questions tabled by the opposition frontbench team in the 1992 Parliament). Frank Dobson,

Labour's first Secretary of State for Health, had commissioned his own survey of provision in 1987 when in opposition and reiterated his support when in office[4] and Tessa Jowell was stout in her desire both for improved quality and quantity of tertiary infertility services. But there was so much else to do and the NHS had large debts.

Enter NICE and a way out of the conundrum. The then Health Minister, Yvette Cooper, after some arm-twisting that was greatly aided by press stories about the gap between provision in the UK compared with everywhere else in Europe, referred the subject of infertility to NICE's clinical guideline process. In 2004, 2 years later, out popped the NICE clinical guideline on fertility[1] in all its 216 page glory. The guideline recommends that three cycles of IVF or ICSI should be provided. It makes no binding recommendations as to the eligibility criteria that define which patients should or should not receive treatment but it does point the way on factors such as age, smoking and body mass index (BMI).

The guideline's publication was accompanied by a statement from the Secretary of State for Health, who at that time was John Reid. He asked PCTs – what the health authorities had now become – to begin to move towards implementing the guideline over time, but initially by providing one cycle of treatment from April 2005.[5] On the same day, the Prime Minister in the House of Commons made it plain that he expected PCTs to implement the whole guideline over time: 'We hope that over the next couple of years we shall see at least very substantial progress towards implementation of the full NICE guidelines … In the longer term, however, we think that we can extend it even further, but we will release details of that when we are ready to do so'.[6] The period that followed was perhaps the most cash-strapped period that the NHS has ever endured. Despite huge resources being poured into the service, budget deficits accelerated. A Treasury-driven desire to balance the books meant that major efforts were needed to clear this debt. Anything that was not nailed down went over the side and, far from implementing one cycle, some PCTs actually began to disinvest.

Infertility was fortunate at this point to have a succession of three Ministers, each of whom strongly believed that those who desired to have a child but could not should be given that chance. Melanie Johnson, Caroline Flint and now Dawn Primarolo (who as a backbencher had introduced a private member's bill calling for better-funded services)[7] have all pressed hard to prompt PCTs to comply (for example, the letters to PCTs from Caroline Flint in June 2006, via the *Chief Executive Bulletin*,[8] and from Dawn Primarolo in July 2007[9]). INUK and the Department of Health have carried out their own surveys of provision, both indirectly through the College of Health reports[10-15] and directly (informally via the Department of Health in the late 1990s, then via INUK and then with its own formal survey in 2006) and will no doubt continue to do so. These show some signs of progress.

It is an uphill battle but one in which there is, at long last, evidence of success. More PCTs than ever before now fund at least one cycle and increasing numbers seem tentatively to be beginning to fund two.[16] What is not clear is whether they are 'cheating' by providing more cycles to a smaller number of people, using widely varying eligibility criteria to narrow down the numbers of people who will qualify for treatment. This is the next phase in the challenge that we face to ensure that ART is properly funded. Encouragingly, though, ministers have now commissioned work to look precisely at eligibility criteria and how these are applied.[17]

International comparators

So how bad is the UK in comparison with the rest of the world? A regular series of data has been published for some years now by ESHRE. This suggests that the gap between the UK and the rest of Europe has traditionally been large and continues to be so, both in terms of overall cycles and of those provided by the state. Although the ESHRE data do not allow a direct comparison of state funding among different countries, they do provide an indicator of attitudes towards ART.

It is clear that the UK undertakes fewer cycles of ART per woman of reproductive age than most major European countries, including all types of funding. The major exception is Germany, which performs about the same and is a country that has seen its state provision slashed in the past few years, leading to a significant fall in total cycles.

It is reasonable also to assume that the UK lags behind other countries in terms of state provision since examining the funding policies of various countries does, as a rule, show a more generous approach to funding ART. ART is indeed regarded in the infertility world as being relatively poorly funded in the UK and, although this is now improving, there is, according to ESHRE's surveys, a long way to go to match the average in Europe.

Improving provision – today, tomorrow, the next day ...

Ministers have repeatedly made plain that they expect decisions to be made in the light of local need. Lord Darzi reiterated this in his recent report.[18] Indeed, no major political party thinks markedly differently and the thrust of NHS reform will continue to take decision making as close to the patient as possible.

From NIAC's conversations with PCT commissioners, it is clear that some commissioners feel that, on the one hand, Ministers tell them to make decisions on priorities for their populations but, on the other, complain when infertility is not made a priority. Equally, some PCTs (and sometimes the same ones) say they want clearer guidance on what they should provide regarding ART. Certainly, in the days of the College of Health surveys, the majority of the health authorities said that they wanted clearer instructions by the Department of Health as to what they were expected to do with regard to infertility. For example, the 1997 Fifth Report[14] showed that 57% wanted guidance on the level of funding, 67% on which services to provide and 69% on eligibility criteria. One could certainly be forgiven for feeling a little surprised that anyone should feel that there is any lack of such guidance. And, oddly enough, when they were given clear indications, they did not rush to implement them. Indeed guidance has been to hand from as early as 1992 with the *Effective Healthcare Bulletin* on the management of subfertility to which Ministers in parliamentary answers regularly suggested that health authorities should attend.[19]

Whatever the truth, Ministers do not feel that they can simply order PCTs to do something that they do not wish to do. Exceptions to this are the central priority areas (coronary heart disease, cancer and mental health), the 'core' standards, which include elements of these three areas among others, the mandated areas such as NICE technology guidance and those areas of public health that are laid down in statute.

The next layer down in terms of national priority were until recently 'developmental standards', which were areas in which the NHS had to demonstrate that it is working towards achieving and these typically include NICE clinical guidelines. But the rules were vague here about what constituted 'reasonable progress'. Decisions on infertility continue to be made locally and ministers have left themselves with limited weaponry with which to cajole reluctant funders into improving services for people with fertility problems. Practice-based commissioning could easily make this situation worse, if GPs were generally more sceptical about ART, as is sometimes claimed.

Whatever weaponry that ministers have has been well used. The process of surveying existing provision is itself helpful in focusing attention within a PCT both on the expectations that are on it and on its progress in delivering them. Ministers have reinforced this by funding INUK to work with PCTs to try to find out why they have not made more progress in this area of medicine and to help them to plan and commission services better. It is early days for this work, the detail of which is being worked on at present, and it will be interesting to see what effect it has.

Ministers also have the ability to seek clarification from PCTs as to why they have not done particular things, even if it cannot order them to. Human nature dictates that such a polite enquiry would be likely to make all but the most hardened PCT wake up a bit!

Again, anecdotally, it is clear from discussions with PCTs that far fewer of them rely now on the argument that infertility is not a health need at all. Most will also accept that a higher degree of priority now applies to this area than in the past. Typically, those that do not fund or who have tried to cut services recent years have cited budget restrictions as their reason for doing so (for example, Hampshire, Northamptonshire, Gloucester and North Lincolnshire). So any process by which funding in PCTs is improved must help in easing this pressure by removing the excuse.

Pressure on NHS finances does appear to have lifted a little. Figures for the final quarter of 2007/08 showed that the NHS was comfortably back in surplus – indeed, this was boasted about rather than being viewed as an embarrassment of riches.[20] There was also media gossip that contracts for the 2008/09 financial year were pulled back into 2007/08 to reduce this surplus, which implied that the NHS might be sitting on an even bigger cash pile. Perhaps it is time to spend a little of it on infertility.

Other factors may also enter the picture. It will presumably not just be around the dinner-party table that opponents of state funding for infertility will be found. Some commissioners – whatever they say publicly to the contrary – must feel instinctively that these are treatments that do not deserve to be funded and this will have an effect on the enthusiasm with which they pursue the commissioning process.

Pressure from patients can be important in tackling this. There is no doubt that a well-organised and determined band of patients (and it does not need to be a large band either) can make a PCT see the error of its ways better than any minister. This is especially effective when it catches the attention of the local press. Pressure from clinicians should not be underestimated either, least of all by clinicians themselves. But the best results have come from a united front of patients, clinicians and local politicians demanding to know when their PCT will implement a NICE guideline which was, after all, produced by a special health authority of the NHS – in other words, a home-grown body.

Age dependency

So are any of the factors surrounding funding dependent on age? Clearly they are. Almost all, if not all, PCTs will apply upper age limits on women receiving treatment and some do so on men. Some also apply a lower age limit, which is 23 years in many cases (in line with the NICE guideline) but can be as high as 30 years or even 35 years.

There is one scarcely believable case with North Yorkshire and York PCT, which allows a window for treatment of just 6 months up to the age of 40 years.[21] This is about as unscientific, cost-ineffective, random and reluctant as it is possible to be. Why not simply offer a treatment to a left-handed, dark-haired woman, born on a Monday in June, and then only if you really have to?

Upper age limits may well be grounded in sensible scientifically based reasoning, namely that the effectiveness of the treatment falls with age.[1] But lower age limits – at least down to 23 years, below which NICE says there is little available evidence – are surely only about budget restraint. What matters on clinical grounds is the duration of the attempt to conceive and the nature of the woman's problem. It hardly makes clinical, cost-effectiveness or social sense to delay treatment in, say, a 26-year-old who is in a stable and longstanding relationship, has tried for 3 years to conceive and has a known cause of infertility.

Other elements of the funding debate around infertility are not related to age in any particular way, although the need for treatment at all may be related, of course, given that women are apparently leaving it later to have families and fertility declines after the age of 38 years or so. This may well raise questions for policy makers as to whether they should do more to raise awareness of the impact of ageing on reproduction but this is a controversial issue and is not one that we shall tackle here.

Is fertility treatment worth the money?

When NICE examined the question of infertility, it used a fairly basic estimate of cost-effectiveness related to the numbers of cycles performed and their cost and likely success rates in various age bands. It did not attempt to perform a more sophisticated cost-effective analysis resulting in a quality-adjusted life year (QALY) estimate, arguing that this methodology was more geared to saving life and gaining quality of life than to creating additional lives.[1] So there is no QALY provided for ART, certainly not through any official process. One would imagine, though, that given the years of high-quality life that ART can create, it would look pretty cost-effective on normal measures. This is discussed further in Chapter 28.

Work has been undertaken, too, to look at the time it takes to 'pay back' the system for funding IVF treatment. This suggests that children born of IVF take only 2 years longer to 'repay' the total cost of their upbringing, including that of actually bringing them into the world, than natural conceptions. These figures did appear to take account of failed cycles by factoring in variations in treatment costs to achieve a successful pregnancy.[22]

This is an area that merits much more detailed study to gain a clearer picture of the real costs and benefits of IVF in 2008. Into this calculation must come not only the life produced as a result of the treatment but the morbidity avoided in terms of depression, failed marriages, underperformance at work and other factors that are reported comorbidities in some who are unable to have children. This is discussed in depth in the NICE guideline.[1] Against this are the costs that arise as a result of ART and particularly from the increased incidence of multiple births and their consequences.[23]

New challenges and opportunities

As mentioned earlier, the thorny issue of eligibility criteria is one with which the infertility world continues to have to wrestle. These vary widely from PCT to PCT and are strongly suspected by patients and some clinicians and politicians of being used primarily to ration services.

NICE partially addressed the issue of eligibility criteria and the British Fertility Society has also taken a view. The main areas of criteria are age (which we have discussed above), BMI, pre-existing children, previous number of cycles, duration of infertility and/or of the couple's relationship, history of sterilisation and whether the couple are the same sex. Most PCTs specify an age range and stipulate a maximum and minimum BMI. In the latter case, if this can be seen to drive clinical success rate or the welfare of mother or child, then it may be seen to be reasonable.

Criteria with regard to secondary infertility are much more contentious and – arguably – inadvertently discriminate against older people, since these are more likely to be in second or third relationships. Denying a couple the chance of treatment if there is a pre-existing child from any previous relationship seems especially harsh but is frequently applied. Other PCTs deny treatment to people only where the child is from the same relationship or from a previous relationship but living with the couple. This is often regarded by people in that situation as very unfair since it ignores the desire for the woman to have her own child or for the couple to have a child that is the fruit of their particular relationship. Some couples also say that the pain from secondary infertility is every bit as bad as that from primary infertility, not least because the couple now know the very real joy that a child brings.

There is also wide variation among PCTs regarding their views on pre-existing relationships, duration of infertility and number of previous cycles received either privately or on the NHS. Only on the question of previous sterilisation does there seem to be agreement, with PCTs either barring treatment to those previously sterilised or (much more rarely) taking no view.

The future

So where does all this take us? There is a chink of a smile appearing on the resolutely poker face that has been infertility funding and some feel that sense is beginning to prevail in the NHS as to the appropriateness of funding ART. Certainly, political endorsement at national level has never been higher, with ministers and other politicians being as one in believing that ART should be routinely funded by the state.

Good evidence exists on the Human Fertilisation and Embryology Authority (HFEA) database as to the value of the treatment and success rates have continued to rise over the past 10 years. We have now found a way of producing broadly acceptable success rates while replacing only one embryo in younger women, which means that we can make a major onslaught on the incidence of multiple births and inroads into the cost that they incur for other parts of the service. Frozen-embryo transfer, too, offers an option – the success rates of which will no doubt improve over time – of squeezing more 'bang for the buck' from a full cycle of treatment. Developments such as embryo vitrification also look interesting in this area.

So all the signals are on green and yet we are still the poor neighbour of much of the rest of Europe in what we provide: 5 years on from the guideline, most PCTs are still only providing one cycle and at least two-thirds of all the cycles undertaken in the UK are private.

What needs to happen now? A combination of different inputs is needed to carry on the work of the past few years and to take it to its final goal. At national level, more of the type of input that we have seen from ministers – gently coaxing and occasionally vaguely threatening commissioners to do what the NHS's own body, NICE, has asked – is vital. This interest from the centre not only lifts morale among campaigners but definitely makes PCTs think twice. Ministers do carry the legitimacy that comes from being part of elected government after all; PCTs do not.

Practical manifestations of this are for the Department of Health to make sure that 18 week waits are applied fully and properly to infertility. It also needs to continue to survey PCTs as to their levels of provision. This will force PCTs each year to face the issue and reveal what they do, with the inevitable local press onslaught if they are falling behind. Such attention does make PCTs sit up.

The move towards single-embryo transfer might also prove to be helpful, since patients are unlikely to accede to this if they believe that they have a reduced chance of success and will not receive, or be able to afford to pay for, further cycles of treatment. Given that the costs of multiple pregnancies (often created in the private sector) are borne by the public purse, it makes economic sense to encourage a move towards single-embryo transfer and to aid this by ensuring that women have their optimal number of cycles with state funding. This point was made by the interim head of the HFEA in a letter to Directors of Public Health.[24,25] We need to make more of this and to force the issue with commissioners in a way that we have not to date.

Clinicians also could do more. A few hardy souls put their heads over the parapet to complain about poor services but they are too often unsupported by colleagues and it happens too rarely to generate real momentum. Policymakers do feel uncomfortable about well-timed criticism from the medical profession: *vide* Lord Winston's criticism about the UK's poor showing versus Europe, which caused quite a flap in Whitehall at the time.[26]

Equally, we would do well to downplay the uniqueness of particular developments in assisted reproductive medicine and to stress instead how commonplace much of ART really is. Commissioners desire as much certainty as possible when planning services and need to be reassured that treatments will work and that success rates are solidly based.

On this theme, we should stress more the concept of packages of treatment to produce a live birth rather than judge each cycle in isolation. No one would measure the results of chemotherapy to treat a cancer on the basis of one dose: it would be judged on the whole course, since that is what would be required to stand a chance of achieving the intended goal. Why should ART be any different? The success rates arising from NICE's recommended three cycles would be, at the very least, 50%. If only the NHS could count on that success rate for all its interventions. We should make more too of the idea of the full cycle of treatment – with any remaining frozen embryos replaced subsequently as part of the same cycle. Ministers accept that this is what should be provided[7] and it offers a cost-effective and potentially increasingly clinically successful option for the future.

Perhaps the biggest boost could come from NICE itself. Its guideline is expected to be reviewed in 2010–11 and any reiteration of its previous advice would carry considerable weight. Would ministers really wish to admit that they had presided over a situation where NICE had provided and reconfirmed its advice but that it still had not been implemented? The guideline should be reviewed quickly and the advice reiterated. Any reaffirmation should be accompanied by a message to PCTs to get on and implement the whole guideline, plus a threat to check for progress in a year. Adding the provision of three cycles to the Care Quality Commission's annual health check would be very helpful too. NICE could help additionally in clarifying aspects of the guideline to make the implementation pathways clearer, so that PCTs did not have any excuse for saying that they did not understand what was required to provide an adequate service.

Most crucial, though, is the united front of patients, clinicians and politicians pressing individual PCTs for the guideline to be implemented. Even a small number of successes would have a wide effect if they had a high profile. This is the single approach which, if maintained over time, stands the greatest chance of delivering success. For various reasons, it does not happen often enough, which lets commissioners off the hook. We must hold the system to account. Consider this the call to arms!

References

1. National Collaborating Centre for Women's and Children's Health. *Fertility: Assessment and Treatment for People with Fertility Problems*. Clinical Guideline 11. London: RCOG Press; 2004.

2. Wigley D. Early Day Motion (EDM 1974): Infertility Treatment. Session 1992–3 [edmi. parliament.uk/EDMi/EDMDetails.aspx?EDMID=5508&SESSION=696].

3. Taylor D. Early Day Motion (EDM 2308) National Infertility Day 2006. Session 2005–6. [edmi. parliament.uk/EDMi/EDMDetails.aspx?EDMID=30855&SESSION=875].

4. BBC. *On the Record* 29 November 1998.

5. Department of Health. Press Notice 25 February 2004 [http://www.dh.gov.uk/en/ Publicationsandstatistics/Pressreleases/DH_4074060].

6. Hansard. Debate, 25 February 2004. col. 278. London: Hansard; 2004. [www.publications. parliament.uk/pa/cm200304/cmhansrd/vo040225/debtext/40225-03.htm#40225-03_spmin10].

7. Hansard. Debate, 8 June 1993. col. 148–9. London: Hansard; 1993. [www.publications.parliament. uk/pa/cm199293/cmhansrd/1993-06-08/Debate-1.html].

8. Flint C, Department of Health. Letter to Primary Care Trusts in England. Facilitating the sharing of good practice in the implementation of the NICE guideline on the assessment and treatment for people with fertility problems, and screening for chlamydia. *Chief Executive Bulletin* Issue 324, 23–29 June 2006 [www.dh.gov.uk/en/Publicationsandstatistics/Lettersandcirculars/ Dearcolleagueletters/DH_4136285].

9. Primarolo D. Letter to All Chief Executives of Primary Care Trusts in England. London: Department of Health; 2007. Gateway ref. 8614 [www.dh.gov.uk/en/Publicationsandstatistics/ Lettersandcirculars/Dearcolleagueletters/DH_077068].

10. College of Health. *Report of the National Survey of the Funding and Provision of Infertility Services*. London: College of Health; 1993.

11. College of Health. *Report of the National Survey of the Funding and Provision of Infertility Services*. London: College of Health; 1994.

12. College of Health. *Report of the Third National Survey of NHS Funding of Infertility Services*. London: College of Health; 1995.

13. College of Health. *Report of the Fourth National Survey of NHS Funding of Infertility Services*. London: College of Health; 1996.

14. College of Health. *Report of the Fifth National Survey of the Funding and Provision of Infertility Services*. London: College of Health; 1997.

15. College of Health. *Report of the Sixth National Survey of the Funding and Provision of Infertility Services*. London: College of Health; 1998.

16. Department of Health. *PCT Survey – Provision of IVF in England in 2007*. London: DH; 2008 [www.dh.gov.uk/en/Publicationsandstatistics/Publications/PublicationsPolicyAndGuidance/ DH_085665].

17. Primarolo D. Interim Report of the Expert Group on Commissioning NHS Infertility Provision: Letter from the Public Health Minister Dawn Primarolo, to Chairs of All Primary Care Trusts. London: DH; 2008 [www.dh.gov.uk/en/Publicationsandstatistics/Lettersandcirculars/ Dearcolleagueletters/DH_087134].

18. Department of Health. *High Quality Care for All: NHS Next Stage Review Final Report*. London: DH: 2008 [www.dh.gov.uk/en/Publicationsandstatistics/Publications/ PublicationsPolicyAndGuidance/DH_085825].

19. Hansard. Debate, 8 July 1994. London: Hansard; 1994. col. 370w amongst others.

20. Department of Health. *The Quarter: quarter 4, 2007–08*. London: DH; 2008 [www.dh.gov.uk/en/ Publicationsandstatistics/Publications/PublicationsStatistics/DH_085244].

21. Brown J; North Yorkshire and York PCT. Letter to patients. January 2009 [northyorkshireivf. blogspot.com/search/label/Funding%20for%20IVF%20treatment%20in%20North%20Yorkshire].

22. Hoorens S, Gallo F, Ledger W, Connolly M. *The Impact of NHS Funding Decisions for in Vitro Fertilisation (IVF) on Treasury Department Revenues: a Simplified Lifetime Net Tax Calculation*. Abstract presented at National Institute for Health and Clinical Excellence (NICE) Annual Conference; December 2006.

23. British Fertility Society. *Multiple Births in the United Kingdom: A Consensus Statement.* Bradley Stoke: British Fertility Society; 2007 [www.britishfertilitysociety.org.uk/news/pressrelease/07_04-MultipleBirths.html].

24. Doran A; Human Fertilisation and Embryology Authority. *The Public Health Challenge of Multiple Births.* Letter to Directors of Public Health. 24 January 2008. Gateway ref. 9375 [www.hfea.gov.uk/docs/1039_001.pdf].

25. All Party Parliamentary Group on Infertility. *Infertility Treatment in the UK: Taking The Next Steps.* London: All Party Parliamentary Group on Infertility; July 2007.

26. BBC Radio 4. *You and Yours.* London: BBC; 6 July 2000.

Chapter 30
Fertility treatment: science and reality – the NHS and the market

Discussion

Diana Mansour: I am a bit frightened to put my name to this because I think in Newcastle we actually have fairly reasonable commissioners. But, having been involved in sexual health around England, I realise we do not have very good commissioning generally, and that is one of the biggest issues. Most commissioners are overworked and do not have a clue of what they are supposed to be commissioning. You are quite right: they probably do not know about the guidelines. But to go back to NICE, obviously that's England. What's happening in Scotland, Wales and Northern Ireland?

Berkeley Greenwood: Wales is probably the worst, because the minister said very recently that she has no intention of funding more than one cycle at the moment. David is probably in a better position to comment on Scotland than I am. Historically, it has been better than England.

David Barlow: There is the report of the Expert Advisory Group on Infertility in Scotland (EAGISS)[1] that sits separately from the NICE guideline. NICE guidelines are advisory in England but they are even more advisory in Scotland [laughter], although it is something to pay attention to. The EAGISS guideline is a bit more liberal.

Siladitya Bhattycharya: The EAGISS report[1] which predated the NICE guideline by a couple of years. It is made somewhat easier by the fact that there are fewer units in Scotland, so they are working together, in dialogue and engagement with the politicians, to see what can be done. There was an initial positive move from the Government, but the pressure is on. The devil is really in the detail, hammering out what exactly is a cycle, whether frozen embryo transfer should be included, etc. But it is looking better. Except, of course, we have not actually got the sort of promises in writing that the East of England, in particular, have seen recently.

Berkeley Greenwood: In terms of the practical effect, there are probably more treatment cycles in Scotland per head of population. However, there are long waiting lists in some areas, very short ones in others, and the eligibility criteria issue rumbles on, as everywhere else. We took our foot off the gas in Scotland at a crucial moment, when we shouldn't have. We made no real, palpable progress in terms of waiting lists in Scotland in the last 2 years, whereas we have made quite good progress in England. Northern Ireland is slightly up in the air at the moment. Essentially, they were only funding one cycle, and not even a full one. That has gone into review again, more quickly than was expected, partly because of good political campaigning, and the recommendations are with the minister. I think what will happen is that they will slacken the eligibility criteria, making it slightly less onerous, and then move to waiting list initiatives to try to shift the enormous waiting lists that exist. Don't expect to see a second cycle in the next stage. That campaign, I think, has a long way to run yet.

Susan Bewley: When NICE used quality-adjusted life years (QALYs), did the costings include the cost of obstetric and neonatal care in relation to the outcomes of IVF pregnancies, particularly taking account of the rate of multiples and the long-term care of babies that might be damaged through prematurity?

David Barlow: It was all done by health economic experts. It attempted to and certainly included neonatal costs – the different proportions for singles and twins and triplets, etc. I cannot remember the calculation of obstetric care. There was so much detail put into these calculations that I cannot believe that we did not include that.

Susan Bewley: I asked because I am very sympathetic to the pain of infertility and am also a taxpayer. Looking at the success rates in 34-year-olds compared with 39-year-olds, surely more women could be relieved of infertility? If the relief of infertility and the costs of pain and stress could be measured in QALYs, do taxpayers not wish to help two couples for their pound, rather than one? Is there not an opportunity in the next round of NICE to say 'This treatment is important and should be unlimited for younger women'? Getting the twin rate down makes the QALY calculation work better. And in terms of bang for the buck, treating under-35-year-olds will relieve more infertility than treating 39-year-olds. I do not think you could do it suddenly, but would that not also have an important symbolic public message about the fertile years? The existence of infertility treatment suggests that the door is open. It encourages women to think: 'Well, maybe I'll get away with it. You even get IVF on the NHS at the age of 39'. So we have more infertility, thanks to treatment existing, than in the days when treatments did not exist. Primary prevention of infertility is also critical. I am sorry to have used a complicated way of saying it. Would it be better to be hard and say 'Unlimited NHS-funded attempts up to 35. Get an insurance plan over this age.' [laughter] Infertility is core treatment. It really matters. It's core, central, integral to heath and wellbeing. And you should get IVF, absolutely everything you need, up to 35. And then, after that, if you happen to meet Mr Right late … well, you will need a savings plan.

David Barlow: For a considerable body of people, the full recommendation of NICE was three cycles, plus all the frozen cycles that go with them, which is a large number of replacements. That would go a considerable way towards unlimited treatment. There are not that few people going for four or fifth fresh attempts. So it is almost what you were saying, but NICE was saying that that can go up to 39.

Berkeley Greenwood: The danger with that argument, from my point of view, is that it gets into the idea that this somehow deserves to be rationed. Whereas, if there is scientific evidence to suggest the treatment is effective, my position would be absolutely hard-line. It should be funded, in line with the NICE guideline, which is clinically based. And the commissioners have a responsibility to get on and develop the implementation of that guideline. As soon as you start deciding between whether you should treat the older or the younger, having accepted that there was a reasonable cost-efficacy argument that is the age-group, etc., you get into the feeling that somehow the area doesn't deserve to be treated like any other healthcare area.

Susan Bewley: I agree with you so long as the treatment is effective. Why has NICE not been fully implemented? Could we say 'Fund all treatments, so long as you have a certain, say 20%, chance of success'? Then age would be just one of many factors in the equation as to whether treatment will work. At least then it would become equitable. You talked about equity, but it is a very inequitable area. You have to have a reading age of about 25 to get through the HFEA literature! We see a lot of inequity issues playing; between different classes, races and economic factors. If treatment was in terms of cost-effectiveness, in which age would feature, would that not be more equitable?

David Barlow: But that is what we did. That is what exactly what we did up to twice as expensive. The cost of a live birth becomes twice as expensive beyond the age of 39, hence the existing NICE guideline recommends funding up to the age of 39.

Berkeley Greenwood: You are always going to get variations of cost-effectiveness. There will always be some patients that are less cost-effective because they respond less well to treatment. So, you are always defining a set of parameters which you compare to provide an element of treatment. My concern is when there is evidence of good clinical effectiveness (and cost-effectiveness comes secondary, where there is good clinical effectiveness), you have got to think hard about why you would not provide the treatment. It is only when it becomes so onerously cost-ineffective to provide that treatment that I think it's reasonable for the health system to start asking questions. My view is that 40 is a reasonable cut-off. I am comfortable with defending that against commissioners.

David Barlow: QALYs do not work because it is new life that you are generating. It only affects the quality of life of the parents.

Kate Brian: In relation to cost-effectiveness, we can be pretty certain that commissioners do not understand this when it comes to IVF. Why on earth would they be funding treatment only for women between the ages of 38 and 38½, if they had the least understanding of cost-effectiveness? I do not think that really comes into play where commissioners are concerned.

Peter Braude: Can we return to the topic of bang for the buck in the fertility market? If we look at the bigger picture of fertility there seems to be extraordinary schizoid thinking. Every Wednesday I do a fertility clinic. At least 10% of the women are sent by their GPs at the age of 40 to 47 with 'Can you do something?' I see them with their partner and am entitled to arrange all the tests, do tubal surgery or myomectomies (which are very common in our area) and yet we know they're never going to make a difference at this age. We do all that with the PCT's money. There is no limit. It is only limited when you start to talk about IVF, which is the most effective treatment we have for many of the age groups. Why has nobody looked at this area? This bothers me enormously – when we look at the pressures for providing NHS treatment. Overall, as you rightly said, probably 65–70% of IVF currently, and fertility in general, is in the private sector. Now, a lot of pressure is not going to come from them – just as turkeys don't vote for Christmas! If we did actually get more funding to do IVF on the NHS, these clinics will lose vast amounts of money. IVF and plastic surgery industry are the two big medical industries we have in this country. IVF will see a reduction in monies if we fund more NHS treatments. I do not know whether there is any real push, or perhaps a reticence, because there is somebody who could lose.

David Barlow: If the cost-effectiveness drive had been taken around the generality of therapies and not just assisted reproduction (such as myomectomy in a 43-year-old simply for fertility indication and not for other reasons)… if modelling had been done, then it is very possible that a range of things that happen over 40 would be judged not to be accessible through the NHS. Two years of work were involved with the modelling for IVF. It was all based on ministerial instruction of what had to be done. If the model included the rest of the fertility work, we might have found a range of thresholds.

Peter Braude: I am simply saying that huge amounts of money are put into so-called fertility treatment, perhaps unnoticed, outwith assisted reproduction. We never ask a 43-year-old if she has got three kids already. I can see her and treat her. It is only when it is IVF that money becomes a barrier.

Berkeley Greenwood: We did recognise that. An All-Party Parliamentary Group on infertility produced a couple of reports.[2,3] In the first report we recognised there were repeated procedures going on both in primary care and specialist settings. There is a lot of wastage. When the Northern Irish guideline was reviewed there was quite a lot of discussion about that. There is some understanding in parts of the system that there is a double standard operating, particularly in terms of where you apply the age cut-off. I have to say, though, Peter, that my attitude is that I don't want to get bogged down in side-arguments. I want to focus on the fact that the NICE guideline is there. It makes the recommendation. Ministers back that recommendation and it should be implemented. Anything that deflects us from that central point is destructive. The key thing for me, for the next year, is to focus on that. Let us keep banging that message.

Catherine Coulson: I want to respond to Peter, because our local PCTs want to find money to fund ICSI which they hadn't funded previously. In conversation with the local consultants who provide the service, it was agreed to set up guidelines on which patients were allowed to be referred to the NHS infertility clinic. It included restrictions on the number of children the couple already have, the age of the woman, the age of the father, coexisting conditions, that sort of thing. Money was clawed back from not doing useless things like investigating women of 46. Remarkably, from the money saved and with more money coming in, our waiting list has gone down to eighteen weeks, over a period of about a year.

Anna Kenyon: It doesn't seem fair to use the NICE fertility guideline to deliver the message of the safest age to have children. I appreciate that, as a group, we may not have control over it but, given the fact that this is already a highly emotive area, when we talk about two or three cycles and frozen cycles, not every woman feels physically able to go through their cycles back-to-back. There would be pressure on them to do that. And it just seems unfair to further penalise this group of women by using them as the means to deliver the message. There should be other ways.

Melanie Davies: I am not a believer in 18-week targets and think they are completely inappropriate for fertility practice. But to use them in another way, they do focus on investigation. We may be giving David an impossible task here, but the amount of money that is wasted in primary care and general gynaecology on fertility investigations is probably substantial. When you think of the large number of patients being referred with inappropriate and unnecessary investigations (for example, poor scans that you just end up repeating). A large number of patients and a few hundred pounds wasted on each might add up to a significant amount of money saved if there were more direct referral patterns to specialist care for appropriate investigation. That should also be a driver for future national guidance.

David Barlow: It is very relevant but you have to then keep that money within the infertility box in order for the money saved to go into other aspects of purchasing.

Berkeley Greenwood: From memory, we reckoned it was £30 to 35 million at the time that your guideline came out, David. And obviously the point was made: should it be used to pump into a primary care service that does not currently exist. Adam Balen had done some work on this so it was observed with pretty accurate data.[2]

David Barlow: Just as I started my presentation, I would like to say to those who are in clinical practice in infertility: Read the NICE guideline – the full guideline document and especially the economic modelling at the back. We are all so busy, we do not read things we don't have to. There is a lot of good meat in that document if you have the time to look at that and it would answer some of these questions.

References

1. Expert Advisory Group on Infertility Services in Scotland (EAGISS). *Evidence & Equity: A National Service Framework for the Care of Infertile Couples in Scotland.* Edinburgh: Scottish Programme For Clinical Effectiveness In Reproductive Health; 1999.
2. All-party Parliamentary Group on Infertility. *Infertility Treatment in the UK: Taking NICE Forward.* London: All-party Parliamentary Group on Infertility; 2004.
3. All-party Parliamentary Group on Infertility. *Infertility Treatment in the UK: Taking the Next Steps.* London: All-party Parliamentary Group on Infertility; 2007.

Section 9

The future: dreams and waking up

Chapter 31

In our wildest dreams: making gametes

Peter Braude

An unfortunate group of women, often in their mid- to late 30s, find themselves in the position of being perimenopausal prematurely. For a few, this may occur because of loss of oocytes due to chemotherapy or autoimmune disease. However, for the majority, the reason for the low ovarian reserve is unclear, perhaps simply having fewer oocytes colonising the gonads *ab initio*. These women often are identified for the first time when they seek help for subfertility and are found to have raised, or sometimes normal, follicle-stimulating hormone levels but are found to be less responsive than expected to follicular induction for *in vitro* fertilisation (IVF).[1]

Currently, little can be offered other than receipt of oocytes from another source or adoption. Oocyte donation in itself brings both practical and ethical problems (see Chapters 21 and 26). Not surprisingly, owing to demand of the desperate, a number of alternatives have been entertained. The use of fetal oocytes from the many therapeutic abortions undertaken annually has been an option considered.[2] Although a source of numerous oocytes, the mere suggestion provoked a furore of correspondence and public and professional condemnation.[3,4] The thought that a resulting child would have no identifiable genetic mother or would have 'a dead fetus as a mother' made it unacceptable. Reproductive cloning where a somatic cell nucleus from the woman could be used as the source for maintaining the genetic link has also been considered.[5,6] However, notwithstanding the legitimate concerns over safety[7] and the worldwide ban, the fetus would contain only DNA from the woman or the man whose somatic cells provided the nucleus. Alternatively, some form of cellular haploidisation might be undertaken to allow somatic nuclei to be used as gametes. Attempts have been made in mice to use the haploidisation potential of the oocyte cytoplasm to redirect somatic nuclei into a meiotic or pronuclear state and thereby provide a vehicle to accept or provide the other available gamete.[8] However, both cell nuclear replacement (CNR) and haploidisation require the availability of oocytes so the argument becomes circular. Clearly, the ability to derive human gametes *in vitro* would be a significant advance provided this could be achieved with sufficient ease, in sufficient numbers and with safety and effectiveness in generating embryos that are competent to develop into normal offspring. One approach has shown promise: the derivation of gametes from human embryonic stem cells *in vitro*.[9] To understand how this might be possible requires an understanding of the way in which gametes develop *in vivo* from primordial germ cells (PGCs) within the embryo.

In insects and amphibia, it has been long appreciated that early developmental decisions are influenced by instructions that are laid down within, or segregated to particular areas within the oocyte itself. Mammals seem to buck this trend, although the extent to which this is the case stimulates considerable argument in the developmental literature.[10-12] However, it is clear that PGCs can be identified in the wall of the yolk sac close to the attachment of the allantois in the human embryo after 3 weeks, and migrate cephalad in the dorsal mesentery of the hindgut into the genital ridges on each side of the midline. Depending on the genetic sex of the embryo, testes or ovaries appear as differentiated by 7 weeks.[13] The central question to be asked is whether these are special cells within the preimplantation embryo that are destined to become PGCs, or whether forces can act upon any embryonic cell and drive it towards a germ cell fate. Although examination of fixed human embryos can reveal the anatomical origins and path of these PGCs, the mechanisms of how they achieve differentiation remain unclear. Inevitably, much of our understanding of the molecular processes underpinning this evolution has been gained from experiments conducted on PGC generation in the mouse.[14]

The stages leading to the production of gametes within the gonad may be divided into four stages: initiation, specification, migration and colonisation (Figure 31.1). Detailed experiments of transcription factors active at around 6 days *post coitum* reveal that PGC specification is induced from the proximal epiblast by extrinsic factors secreted by the extra-embryonic ectoderm cells, mainly BMP4 (bone morphogenetic protein-4, a member of the transforming growth factor-beta [TGFβ] family), which augments expression of a cell surface molecule, *fragilis*. After gastrulation begins, a subset of *fragilis*-positive cells (about six cells initially in the mouse) begin to express *Blimp1* (which codes for B-lymphocyte-induced maturation protein 1) that intiates the germ cell's programme and suppresses the somatic programme. These specified cells (around 40) can be identified at the posterior end of the primitive streak by alkaline phosphatase staining and early on day 7 begin to express another transcription factor *Stella* and, later, *Oct4*, *Sox2* and *Nanog*, which are factors associated with pluripotency in stem cells (see below), as well as other active genes which identify them as maturing germ cells (*Dazl*, *Vasa*). By 8.5 days *post coitum*, the endoderm is invaginating to form the hindgut and the PGCs are carried together with the endoderm cells as well as by active migration. In addition, examination of cells that are in the process of migration reveals that imprinting genes, which are normally identified by their state of methylation, become unmethylated, indicating an erasure of imprints during this time. From this information, it appears that 'germcellness' is induced rather than being pre-segregated in the early embryo and those cells that react to factors at the interface continue along a clear mechanistic path of identifiable molecular change and imprinting that will result in cells that are pluripotent and ready to accept imprints according to the molecular niche in the gonad.[15] This pathway and sequence of gene activation and methylation and sex specification is crucial to the functional development and identification of any putative *in vitro*-derived gametes.

The final stage in the generation of gametes *in vivo* is sex differentiation, whereby the fate of the evolving gamete is determined according to the genetic sex of the other cells within the genital ridge. The mitotic and meiotic fates of male and female gametes are different.[16] Male-derived cells remain in mitotic arrest from birth, resuming mitosis around puberty whereafter, as a germinal epithelium, they periodically enter into rounds of spermatogenic meiosis. Female-differentiated gametes, after rounds of mitosis, enter into the dictyate stage of meiotic prophase within the embryonic gonad where they will remain until they are individually induced to complete meiosis by the action of gonadotrophins in each ovarian cycle. Thus we can envisage a full circle of life: the relationship of fertilised egg, embryo, PGC, gamete, to embryo (Figure 31.1). It is at certain of these points that the opportunity to intervene allows the possibility of *in vitro* gamete generation.

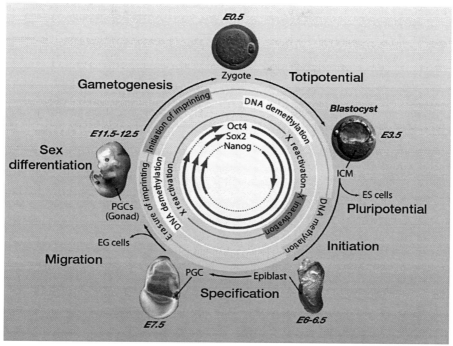

Figure 31.1 Genetic and epigenetic factors regulate the circle of development. The totipotent zygote contains maternally inherited epigenetic modifiers and transcription factors, including Oct4, Sox2 and Nanog. These, together with the embryonic transcripts, regulate development to the blastocyst stage, where the pluripotent cells are established in the inner cell mass (ICM). In the post-implantation embryo, pluripotent epiblast cells are controlled by diverse repressive mechanisms during their differentiation into somatic and germ cell lineages. The primordial germ cells (PGCs) migrate to and populate the developing gonad, where they are induced to form sperm or oocyte precursors by factors controlled by the sex of the surrounding tissues. The ensuing epigenetic reprogramming within this lineage regenerates totipotency in the formation of gametes. Adapted with permission from Surani *et al.*[31]

Stem cells

The possibility of *in vitro* isolation and culture of pluripotent cells from embryos was first demonstrated in the mouse by Martin Evans and Matt Kaufman in 1981.[17] However, it was only following the isolation and culture from human embryos in 1998 that interest increased geometrically with the promising possibilities of use in regenerative medicine.[18] Human embryonic stem (hES) cells can be derived from the inner cell mass of human blastocysts derived by IVF and are defined by their property not only of being able to replicate themselves but also in being pluripotent – they are able to give rise to the entire range of cells and tissues in the body, apart from trophectodermal derivatives. This property can be demonstrated experimentally by their ability to give rise to tissues from all three primary germ layers when injected into immuno-naive 'nude' mice: skin and neural tissue, which are ectodermal derivatives;

bone, cartilage and muscle, which are mesodermal; and gut and glands, which are endodermal (Figure 31.2). Apart from hES cells, pluripotency can also be demonstrated in cells obtained from the gonads of 5- to 9-week-old fetuses; referred to as embryonic germ (EG) cells.[19] It has been shown that somatic cells can be induced to develop into hES cell-like pluripotent cells (induced pluripotent stem cells [iPS cells]) by the use of four transcription factors,[20] two of which are found in hES cells, namely Sox2 and Oct4, although whether these are identical to hES cells is still to be demonstrated.

Deriving gametes *in vitro*

Using mouse embryonic stem (mES) cells transfected with a green fluorescent protein Oct4 construct (*gcOct4-GFP*) containing known germ cell and epiblast enhancers, Schöler and colleagues were able to select clones of cells by fluorescence-activated cell sorting (FACS) that were capable of producing follicle-like structures.[21] These were capable of secreting not only estradiol in culture but also the characteristic zona proteins ZP-1, ZP-2 and ZP-3 and spontaneously underwent a form of cleavage producing morula-like and blastocyst-like structures. It is interesting to note that these 'oocytes' could be isolated from both XX and XY lines, perhaps reflecting an inappropriate or inadequate expression of the male *SRY* or *DAZ* gene needed for differentiation into spermatozoa. In a similar set of experiments in mice, mES cells

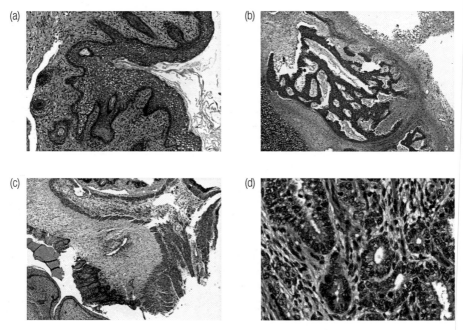

Figure 31.2 Tissues found in teratoma generated by injecting human embryonic stem (hES) cells into nude mice, demonstrating tissues derived from all three germ layers: (a) skin and derivates – ectoderm; (b) bone and cartilage – mesoderm; (c) gastrointestinal tissue and derivates – endoderm; (d) malignancy changes in gastrointestinal tissue – endoderm; images courtesy of Dr Carlos A Castro, University of Pittsburgh

that had been maintained so as to produce three-dimensional balls of cells called embryoid bodies (EB), rather than employing mES cells in sheets, were exposed to retinoic acid from which haploid cells could be isolated.[22] It is noteworthy that not only did these cells show expression of markers for the early stages of male germ cell development (*Oct4*, *fragilis*, *Stella*), but at day 7 of EB development most of the embryonic germ-like cells demonstrated an unmethylated pattern, and by day 10 of EB development all embryonic germ clones had lost imprinting of the maternally derived *Igf2r* gene, as would be expected during normal gamete development. When injected into oocytes, these 'gametes' were able to produce diploid blastocysts, with both XX and XY in equal proportions. In a similar series of experiments, Engel and colleagues demonstrated that, when transplanted into the testes of irradiated mice, these early gametes were able to progress through most of the stages of spermatogenesis, and when these were injected into mouse oocytes they were capable of fertilising and giving rise to preimplantation embryos that gave rise to live pups when transferred to the oviducts of prepared mice. However, the offspring were either smaller or larger than controls and died prematurely (from 5 days to 5 months after birth), perhaps as a result of disturbed methylation patterns of the major imprinting genes.[23]

Implications of the use of *in vitro*-derived gametes

Apart from providing an extraordinary test bed for examination of the morphological, chromosomal and molecular changes that occur during gametogenesis, these experiments have provoked an excitement at the possibility of developing both male and female gametes *in vitro*. However, this excitement needs be tempered by our incomplete understanding of the imprinting requirements during gametogenesis and the potential that, as with reproductive cloning, substantial errors of development might be provoked.[24] In addition, it should be clear that, even if gametes could be derived from stem cells in humans, they are likely to have been derived from embryos with a tissue type that is foreign to the individual in need of replacement gametes and not containing their own DNA. Hence, in effect this would not be different from the use of donated sperm or oocytes, albeit that they may be seen as an easier and more readily available resource. In addition to any biological implications, there would of course be consent implications from the donor of the embryo from which the hES cells had been derived: were they aware and did they consent to gametes being derived from their cells, and were they aware that they might be used to create embryos for therapeutic use? Current consent forms developed in the UK by the Human Embryonic Stem Cell Coordinators (hESCCO) network specifically request permission or refusal for use in therapy but do not address their use in derivation of gametes.[25] Derivation of gametes *in vitro* is allowed under UK law and thus could be licensed by the Human Fertilisation and Embryology Authority, as can the creation of embryos *in vitro* for research provided the experiments are necessary or desirable, but the use of embryos created from such gametes in therapy is disallowed.

Creation of tailor-made gametes, those that would contain the individual's own DNA, would require the process of 'therapeutic cloning' or CNR, whereby a nucleus from one of their somatic cells would be transferred to a donated oocyte and a stem cell line created therefrom. Besides the circular argument that many donated oocytes would be needed for CNR for the creation of oocytes where there is a need or lack, CNR has an extraordinarily low success, making this a non-viable alternative currently.

However, the field of stem cell research has progressed so rapidly in the past few years that new technology may have the capacity to provide additional hope. In addition, it has forced us to readdress the whole concept of cellular differentiation and dedifferentiation and whether gametes are indeed the special cells that they have always been deemed to be. For example, it has been demonstrated that cultures of fetal porcine fibroblasts *in vitro* can be coaxed to form oocytes and then blastocyst-like structures simply by the addition of 5% porcine follicular fluid and gonadotrophins for 10 days.[26] Furthermore, another group was able to derive spermatogonial-like cells from bone marrow in mice that, when transplanted to the testes in chemotherapeutically sterilised animals, repopulated the testes with spermatozoa.[27] Most extraordinarily, Yamanaka's group have demonstrated that the addition of only four transcription factors associated with pluripotency (Oct4, Sox2, Klf4) and tumorogenicity (c-myc) can turn a proportion of fibroblasts into hES cell-like cells.[20] The iPS cells seem to behave like hES cells in forming teratomas, being able to generate embryoid bodies and also be incorporated into chimaeras to give live young. Other experiments suggest that induction may not even require all four factors;[28] indeed, unpublished work suggests that a simple chemically derived mixture may be able to achieve the same effect. It was totally unexpected that reversal of differentiation would yield to so few factors or such a simple cocktail.

The field is progressing exponentially and its ramifications are likely to be profound. If stem cells can be induced simply from somatic cells, previous technology suggests that gametes will be derived from them in humans in a timescale that was never anticipated as being so rapid. It is also likely that, whatever the potential hazards, there will be a rapid and urgent demand from both men and women for their use in overcoming sperm or oocyte deficiency.

So where do we go from here?

How do we test effectiveness and safety? This would require attempted fertilisation of oocytes donated for research with *in vitro*-derived sperm, or vice versa, which may be easier to acquire. However, what would be the criteria of safety? How would we estimate veracity of imprints and likely long-term effects? The fact that such embryos could, and indeed would be likely to, develop into blastocysts and perhaps even outgrow into stem cells themselves, gives little reassurance of long-term safety after implantation and of normal fetal development. Would animal experiments on transfer be sufficient from which to extrapolate? When human IVF was first attempted therapeutically, it was some 10 years after the first human fertilisation[29] and followed an extensive literature of *in vitro* culture, development and transfer in both laboratory and domestic species. The first cloning of sheep only resulted in a successful offspring after many attempts[30] and, in all species, there have been quite bizarre and unexpected abnormalities that could be associated with imprinting abnormalities.[7] Although these are reluctantly tolerated in animal husbandry, the safety demands in human reproduction are naturally much higher. The difficulty will be tempering demand from patients desperate to reproduce using their own genes. The concern is that the potential for fame and profit may drive some less scrupulous individuals to try it.

Acknowledgement

The author would like to thank Dr Azim Surani for his help in providing illustrative material and in perusing the manuscript.

References

1. Sunkara SK, Tuthill J, Khairy M, El-Toukhy T, Coomarasamy A, Khalaf Y, *et al.* Pituitary suppression regimens in poor responders undergoing IVF treatment: a systematic review and meta-analysis. *Reprod Biomed Online* 2007;15:539–46.
2. Shushan A, Schenker JG. The use of oocytes obtained from aborted fetuses in egg donation programs. *Fertil Steril* 1994;62:449–51.
3. Dillner L. Use of fetal eggs for infertility treatment is banned. *BMJ* 1994;6950:289–90.
4. ASRM. Use of fetal oocytes in assisted reproduction. *Fertil Steril* 2004;82(Suppl 1):258–9.
5. Elsner D. Just another reproductive technology? The ethics of human reproductive cloning as an experimental medical procedure. *J Med Ethics* 2006;32:596–600.
6. Prainsack B, Cherkas LF, Spector TD. Attitudes towards human reproductive cloning, assisted reproduction and gene selection: a survey of 4600 British twins. *Hum Reprod* 2007;22:2302–8.
7. Cibelli JB, Campbell KH, Seidel GE, West MD, Lanza RP. The health profile of cloned animals. *Nat Biotechnol* 2002;20:13–4.
8. Nagy ZP, Chang CC. Current advances in artificial gametes. *Reprod Biomed Online* 2005;11:332–9.
9. Nagy ZP, Kerkis I, Chang CC. Development of artificial gametes. *Reprod Biomed Online* 2008;16:539–44.
10. Gardner RL. The case for prepatterning in the mouse. *Birth Defects Res C Embryo Today* 2005;75:142–50.
11. Hiiragi T, Solter D. Fatal flaws in the case for prepatterning in the mouse egg. *Reprod Biomed Online* 2006;12:150–2.
12. Zernicka-Goetz M. The first cell-fate decisions in the mouse embryo: destiny is a matter of both chance and choice. *Curr Opin Genet Dev* 2006;16:406–12.
13. Hua J, Sidhu K. Recent advances in the derivation of germ cells from the embryonic stem cells. *Stem Cells Dev* 2008;17:399–411.
14. Hayashi K, de Sousa Lopes SM, Surani MA. Germ cell specification in mice. *Science* 2007;316:394–6.
15. McLaren A. Primordial germ cells in the mouse. *Dev Biol* 2003;262:1–15.
16. Kimble J, Page DC. The mysteries of sexual identity. The germ cell's perspective. *Science* 2007;316:400–1.
17. Evans MJ, Kaufman MH. Establishment in culture of pluripotential cells from mouse embryos. *Nature* 1981;292:154–6.
18. Thomson JA, Itskovitz-Eldor J, Shapiro SS, Waknitz MA, Swiergiel JJ, Marshall VS, *et al.* Embryonic stem cell lines derived from human blastocysts. *Science* 1998;282:1145–7.
19. Shamblott MJ, Axelman J, Wang S, Bugg EM, Littlefield JW, Donovan PJ, *et al.* Derivation of pluripotent stem cells from cultured human primordial germ cells. *Proc Natl Acad Sci U S A* 1998;95:13726–31.
20. Takahashi K, Yamanaka S. Induction of pluripotent stem cells from mouse embryonic and adult fibroblast cultures by defined factors. *Cell* 2006;126:663–76.
21. Hubner K, Fuhrmann G, Christenson LK, Kehler J, Reinbold R, De La Fuente R, *et al.* Derivation of oocytes from mouse embryonic stem cells. *Science* 2003;300:1251–6.
22. Geijsen N, Horoschak M, Kim K, Gribnau J, Eggan K, Daley GQ. Derivation of embryonic germ cells and male gametes from embryonic stem cells. *Nature* 2004;427:148–54.
23. Nayernia K, Nolte J, Michelmann HW, Lee JH, Rathsack K, Drusenheimer N, *et al. In vitro*-differentiated embryonic stem cells give rise to male gametes that can generate offspring mice. *Dev Cell* 2006;11:125–32.
24. The Hinxton Group. *Science, Ethics and Policy Challenges of Pluripotent Stem Cell-Derived Gametes. Meeting Overview.* Baltimore, MD: The Hinxton Group: 2008 [www.hinxtongroup.org/au_pscdg_ovw.html].
25. Franklin SB, Hunt C, Cornwell G, Peddie V, Desousa P, Livie M, *et al.* hESCCO: development of good practice models for hES cell derivation. *Regen Med* 2008;3:105–16.
26. Dyce PW, Wen L, Li J. *In vitro* germline potential of stem cells derived from fetal porcine skin. *Nat Cell Biol* 2006;8:384–90.

27. Drusenheimer N, Wulf G, Nolte J, Lee JH, Dev A, Dressel R, *et al.* Putative human male germ cells from bone marrow stem cells. *Soc Reprod Fertil Suppl* 2007;63:69–76.

28. Nakagawa M, Koyanagi M, Tanabe K, Takahashi K, Ichisaka T, Aoi T, *et al.* Generation of induced pluripotent stem cells without Myc from mouse and human fibroblasts. *Nat Biotechnol* 2008;26:101–6.

29. Edwards RG, Bavister BD, Steptoe PC. Early stages of fertilization *in vitro* of human oocytes matured *in vitro*. *Nature* 1969;221:632–5.

30. Campbell KH, McWhir J, Ritchie WA, Wilmut I. Sheep cloned by nuclear transfer from a cultured cell line. *Nature* 1996;380:64–6.

31. Surani MA, Hayashi K, Hajkova P. Genetic and epigenetic regulators of pluripotency. *Cell* 2007;128:747–62.

Chapter 32
The future: dreams

Discussion

Siladitya Bhattacharya: The development of inducible pluripotent stem [iPS] cells is terribly exciting. Is there a timescale to this?

Peter Braude: There is a film called *The NeverEnding Story* [laughter]. I don't know the timescale but I can say that even 2 years ago the idea of an iPS cell line was outrageous. Then we got to this point and it now looks as if not very many transcriptional factors are going to be needed. The development was jumped on by the anti-abortion lobby who immediately claimed that this is the future and we can stop all ongoing embryo stem cell research. I imagine President Bush would like this very much. I do not think there is a short timescale. Therapeutic use is still a long way off, but every time we said that in the past, something happened very fast.

Susan Bewley: Can I ask a question about the 20–30 years of these amazing breakthroughs. What is the relationship with use in veterinary science? Has that been a predictor of what could happen in the human, or is it an entirely separate field?

Peter Braude: Generally, veterinary science has been helpful, barring one anomaly, that is that no one got ICSI to work in animals. Is that correct?

Roger Gosden: In horses ICSI is extremely difficult.

Peter Braude: ICSI did not work when they tried it in mice. Then it worked in humans by accident in Brussels and they were able to take advantage of it.[1] They were trying to do SUZI [subzonal insertion of sperm] and injected the sperm into the cytoplasm of the egg, and the next day had the good sense to look at it and see whether it had divided. However, all the other developments such as egg and embryo freezing, were started in mice and then moved to larger animals. If I remember correctly, sperm freezing was used in pigs. Certainly cloning has been trialled in animal species with production of huge numbers of defective animals, but now it is being perfected and used in animal husbandry.

Stephen Hillier: That was a brilliant exposition of the fantasy and reality of iPS cells. I would counsel extreme caution in terms of how you, as clinicians, raise the expectations of patients in this area. I have seen this happen time and time again, that clinical colleagues have opened this vista of wonderful potential and encouraged patients to clamour for a new treatment before it is ready. Clinical application of iPS cell science does seem likely in the fullness of time but we do not know what timescale we are talking about. We will at some point have enough knowledge to apply this type of technology to create gametes and embryos that may possibly be useful for therapeutic purposes. But to allow patients to believe that in the near future we will be able to overcome reproductive ageing is, perhaps, irresponsible at the moment. Clinicians, scientists and ethicists have to be extremely cautious about how we advertise this potential.

Peter Braude: You are 100% right. What is important is to realise why people do this work. The majority of scientists are asking questions such as 'Where do the germ cells come from? How did they get induced? How do they produce different kinds of transcription factors? What actually happens during imprinting?'

Roger Gosden: Thank you for a lovely presentation. I agree with everything that was said. I do believe that the immediate benefits of this work are both conceptual and also experimental. Who knows about the clinical timescale? From a conceptual point of view, I think it fits in with an awful lot what we have learned about cell biology over the last 20–30 years. How much more flexible biology has turned out than we were ever taught in our embryology class. Cloning is one example, and the biology of iPS cells another. I think we will eventually produce germ-cell-like cells from human embryonic stem cells but there are only one or two papers at the moment and not very convincing.[2] I do agree that timescales are extraordinarily difficult to predict. Some things that we thought were going to be relatively easy some 20 years ago have turned out to be much more difficult. We would probably have said 20 years ago that by 2008 we will be able to pick the best embryo to transfer but it is still beyond our grasp. Other things leapfrog forward unexpectedly and ICSI is an example. I do not think anyone has a crystal ball for biology.

Susan Bewley: Why is all the research on eggs and sperm and not on the other difference between men and women, which is gestation? What about the artificial uterus, placenta and breastfeeding? But there is no time …

David Barlow: I want to try to understand the biology of derivation of gametes from embryonic stem cell lines. If you develop an embryonic stem cell line from a female blastocyst, you will only be able to generate X carrying sperm and not Y carrying sperm?

Peter Braude: It is to do with whether they have got SRY, and the germ cell going into the genital ridge. The factors that impinge on it decide whether it is going to go down the line of making sperm or making an egg and that is in fact engendered by the fact that the tissue surrounding it is XX or XY. So, in respect of making it in a dish you can only make X-bearing sperm. But I don't know about a Y-carrying egg.

References

1.   Palermo G, Joris H, Devroey P, Van Steirteghem AC. Pregnancies after intracytoplasmic injection of single spermatozoon into an oocyte. *Lancet* 1992;340:17–18.
2.   Clark AT, Bodnar MS, Fox M, Rodriquez RT, Abeyta MJ, Firpo MT, *et al.* Spontaneous differentiation of germ cells from human embryonic stem cells *in vitro*. *Hum Mol Genet* 2004;13:727–39.

Chapter 33
Managing expectations and achieving realism: the individual journey from hope to closure

Kate Brian

Childlessness is becoming more common and it is estimated that around one in five women of childbearing age will not have children in the UK.[1] The average age of a woman giving birth is 29 years[2] and, as more women delay motherhood, either until they feel ready or until they meet the right partner, the risk of leaving it too late to conceive grows.

Fertility treatment is often seen as a solution for older women who want children of their own. Of course, no one wants to have treatment in order to conceive but, if getting pregnant naturally is not easy, fertility treatment is seen as a way to overcome this. It is too frequently assumed that anyone who can afford treatment and who perseveres will eventually have a child of their own.

We hear very little about *in vitro* fertilisation (IVF) failure. The Human Fertilisation and Embryology Authority publishes IVF success rates and there is rarely any focus on the fact that the current average success rate, which is not far above 20% per cycle,[3] means that more than 75% of cycles will fail. Cumulative success rates suggest that many more couples will succeed if they can continue with treatment but not everyone will be able to afford this financially or emotionally.

Unrealistic expectations

Despite the figures, the idea that IVF can beat the biological clock remains, and fertility treatment is often seen as a solution for having left it 'too late' to conceive naturally. We know that the average age of fertility treatment patients is increasing, having increased from 33.6 years in 1991 to 34.9 years in 2005,[3] and this means that more women will be having IVF at an age when it is less likely to work. In some areas, the funding situation exacerbates this problem. Where NHS treatment is only available to younger women, older women have to self-fund. However, in some parts of the country, NHS treatment is only available for older women.[4] This means women are not able to access treatment when they are younger and have a greater chance of getting pregnant.

There is a lack of awareness about the age-related decline in IVF success rates. Successful patients are more vocal about their treatment than those who have not succeeded, while the media focuses on positive stories of 'miracle babies' conceived against the odds and celebrity mothers having babies in their 40s and even in their 50s, with the unspoken assumption that these women are getting pregnant naturally with their own eggs.

Access to treatment

In the UK at present, financial restraints make it impossible for some couples with fertility problems to consider assisted conception. Despite the recommendation by the National Institute for Health and Clinical Excellence (NICE) that three cycles of IVF should be funded for those who need treatment where the female partner is aged under 40 years,[5] the provision is at best patchy. In some areas, there is no NHS treatment available at all; in other areas, access is restricted by eligibility criteria.[4] This 'postcode lottery' means that couples who cannot afford to pay may never get the treatment they need. It can be particularly hard to cope with involuntary childlessness for those who know they might have been able to have a family if they'd just had the finances to pay for the treatment they needed.

Giving up on treatment

Making the decision to give up on treatment is not easy. Generally, patients will always be able to find a new clinic, or a new doctor, willing to treat them if they have the money to pay, and many cling to stories of exciting new developments in the field, hoping that this will give them one last opportunity to become parents. Although patients find it painful at the time, it may help if doctors are blunt about their chances of success,[6] as continued false hope will cost them more money and heartache. For some, the decision to stop is precipitated by financial restraints but others borrow in order to be able to afford more treatment.

Once patients have made the decision not to continue with treatment, the initial reaction is often a sense of loneliness and abandonment. Most do not have any support from the fertility clinic that has been their focus once they stop treatment. There is no longer a clear avenue for them to seek help from the medical profession and many feel they are not offered any advice or assistance to deal with their situation.[7] They can feel completely deserted at this point and often have feelings of grief to deal with which is not always understood or appreciated. Couples may experience a sense of bereavement for the loss of a future that they have long anticipated and it can be hard to come to terms with the fact that this is not to be.

Many of the emotional responses at this time are common to those who have been through infertility and treatment: people may feel guilty and blame themselves for what has happened, they may feel a sense of failure, that they are inferior to those who can conceive easily and that their role in society is somehow diminished by their childlessness.[8] Generally, these emotions will slowly fade with time but some people will continue to experience them for the rest of their lives.[6]

The social isolation and sense of exclusion at this time is particularly acute. Couples often say that they have lost friends during their fertility journeys, as they no longer find it easy to socialise with friends who have young children. At the same time, they believe their friends can sometimes find the almost obsessive nature of the desire to continue with fertility treatment difficult to comprehend.

Once people decide to stop treatment, they have to accept that their childlessness is now a reality for the rest of their lives. Friends and family may not understand their emotional reactions and former patients often say they sense that others feel they have not 'tried hard enough', believing that fertility treatment inevitably works for those who put in the effort. Family members may have their own disappointment to cope with about not being aunts and uncles or grandparents, and about the abrupt ending of one part of the family line.

Most people experience sadness at this time and, for many, this becomes full-blown depression. Some will have other health problems that they may attribute to their childlessness. Despite this, the sadness is often accompanied by some degree of relief. One of the difficulties of going through fertility treatment is the way that everything gets put on hold as couples put their lives in the hands of their clinic and find themselves constantly waiting for appointments, for treatment and for results. Couples often report that they feel they've lost control of their own lives: giving up on treatment means they can take control back again and can finally make plans for the future, albeit a different future to the one they had imagined. They may be able to rediscover an enjoyment in life that has been submerged during their treatment.

Long-term problems

Infertility is generally a lifelong problem and the consequences of coping with involuntary childlessness are long term. The experience may change with time but will not disappear, and many people find that the pain can return suddenly and sharply at certain times and in certain situations. Christmas is known to be a difficult period for couples with fertility problems and this can remain hard even for those who are some way down the line. Mothering Sunday and Father's Day can be painful[8] and there may be a whole variety of catalysts that can cause difficulties.

Many couples report that their relationship is altered by the experience and one study showed a higher rate of separation among couples that had been through treatment unsuccessfully.[6] We know that timing intercourse often damages the sex lives of those going through fertility treatment, and this problem is not automatically solved once couples decide to stop treatment. It has been found that some women feel their sexual lives have been irreparably damaged by their experience.[6]

The sense of being 'less worthy' that people often report during their fertility treatment may blight the lives of those who find themselves involuntarily childless, at least in part because our society is family orientated in ways that may only be really clear to those who find themselves outside society's norms. Those without children often feel they experience discrimination and prejudice, not just socially but also in the workplace and through government family-friendly policies.[9] The childless are often assumed to be career orientated, cold or selfish, while having a family is inevitably a 'good thing'. This can be particularly hard to deal with for those who have longed for a child of their own and who are struggling to come to terms with involuntary childlessness.

There may be renewed waves of emotion about childlessness as couples go through different stages of their lives. For women, this can happen when they reach the menopause or when they approach retirement and see their friends becoming grandparents. Once again, the focus of their lives is different and there may be a renewed sense of isolation.[6]

The after-effects of their involuntary childlessness follow people right to the end of their lives, when they can feel cut off from younger generations and socially isolated. Having a family means there are more likely to be people around who will take care of elderly parents or grandparents, and those who are childless often worry about who will be there to look after them in their old age.[6] These fears may be borne out by the statistics that show that childless women generally suffer more ill health and die earlier than their counterparts with children.[10]

Dealing with involuntary childlessness

During fertility treatment, many couples use a passive form of coping by trying to avoid situations that they know will be difficult. They may not talk about the issue and may attempt to keep away from babies and young children as much as they can. This may be a perfectly adequate way of coping during treatment but it does not do anything to relieve the problem. In the long term, it is not likely to be a practical or achievable way of managing involuntary childlessness. Active coping, which involves finding other positive aspects of life to focus on, is usually a more successful strategy as it involves moving forwards, away from the problem.[11]

There are some gender differences in coping strategies and it has been found that women find infertility more stressful, experience more anxiety and depression, and use passive coping strategies more often.[11] Men may find it easier to move onwards and seem to be better at closing down an aspect of life that is causing a problem. Some of these gender differences in dealing with infertility and childlessness may be related to the biological clock. Men know that they could in theory continue to father children well into their 50s and even their 60s, while women have to live with the reality of their rapidly declining fertility. They may hope against all the odds for some kind of miracle conception even when they have stopped treatment and the menopause can be a difficult phase, bringing with it the knowledge that even this last faint dream is now an impossibility.

Dealing with a lifetime of involuntary childlessness is about adapting to a different lifestyle and finding a way of making a fulfilling life for the future. Some people never really achieve this[6] but those who do it successfully manage to see new possibilities in a life without children and concentrate on the positive points of the experience. They have more time and money, and may focus on work, travel, further education or other aspects of life that they find rewarding. Some find that they can become more genuinely interested in other people's children once they have stopped trying to have their own and may devote time to caring for them.[6]

For many couples, part of the closure is knowing that they have done everything they possibly could before they finally gave up on treatment, This may be harder to achieve for those who have had to stop treatment, or who could not ever access it, because they did not have the money to pay for it.

For those who already have a child or children and cannot have another, the difficulties of not being able to conceive and having to live with this can still be very acute. In such cases, people do have something positive to focus on but they are also more aware what they are missing by not having another child. There are additional stresses for this group as it may be impossible for them to use passive coping strategies and avoid situations where they will have to face babies and small children when they are trying to conceive. There is also less understanding or sympathy for those living with secondary infertility. There are no support groups that deal specifically with this problem and couples may feel it would not be right for them to try to access the support that is available for the involuntarily childless.

It can also be harder to move on for women who have experienced a previous miscarriage or a termination. Women who have had a termination often end up blaming themselves for their infertility and this can be difficult to get over. Women who have had a miscarriage have had a glimpse of the future they might have had but this has been snatched away and it can be hard to let go of this. Some find they feel a sense of betrayal towards the child or children they have lost if they give up on treatment,[12] while others may take solace from the fact that they have at least at some point been able to achieve a pregnancy.

Those who have become step-parents but have not ever had children of their own can perhaps find comfort in their stepchildren but they still have to come to terms with their involuntary childlessness. Once again, funding can be a problem here as it can be particularly difficult to cope if the presence of a stepchild is what stands between a couple and access to NHS treatment.[4] There is a support network and website for childless stepmothers.[13]

Counselling

At present, couples who give up fertility treatment are not routinely offered help or counselling. Support counselling is available to couples having fertility treatment and implications counselling is available to those using donor gametes. Some clinics will suggest counselling after unsuccessful treatment but there is no obligation to offer help to couples at this time although it may be particularly beneficial.

Of course, there are some people who are sceptical about the value of counselling, or who will not want to talk at all at this stage, and others may simply drop off the clinic's radar when their treatment has not worked if they are not planning to return for another attempt. It would be helpful for couples to know in advance that there would be support available if the treatment did not work, as even those who have refused counselling in the past may find it useful after unsuccessful treatment. Initially, some kind of support counselling to help them through the immediate problems would be beneficial but there is likely to be a need for longer-term therapeutic counselling as couples reassess their lives and their priorities for the future.

Support

The involuntarily childless do not necessarily form a cohesive group and may not share the same concerns and goals in the way that people do when they have fertility problems or are going through treatment. Those living without children may have got to this point through a variety of different routes and the way they move forwards will vary from person to person. Many do not feel able to talk about their experiences or the way they are feeling and this can make it harder for them to look to one another for support, although it may help them if they do manage this.

In the UK, we have More to Life, a national support group for the involuntarily childless run under the auspices of Infertility Network UK. More to Life has a website with forums and chat rooms for discussion and members receive a quarterly newsletter. It has a regional network of contacts and arranges meetings and events. More to Life also runs a lending library and members have access to all the support services offered by Infertility Network UK. Infertility Network UK and More to Life staff and volunteers are constantly looking for new ways to increase membership and heighten awareness of what More to Life can offer but it is sometimes difficult to get media coverage as many members are understandably reluctant to come forward and discuss their personal experiences of involuntary childlessness. More to Life is an important resource but couples do not always know how it can help when they find themselves involuntarily childless and health professionals should endeavour to try to promote the charity, especially among those who are stopping treatment.

There is little else in the way of support for the involuntarily childless, although there are excellent networks for the childfree, who have dozens of websites, support networks and blogs to choose from. The childfree obviously share many of the same issues that the involuntarily childless have to deal with, and childfree websites discuss the ways that family-friendly policies discriminate against those without children and rally against assumptions that they must all inevitably be selfish, uncaring and career orientated. However, many childfree websites and support groups would be an anathema to the involuntarily childless. The childfree have made an active decision not to have children and some of the websites are quite militantly anti-children and anti-parent. Many involuntarily childless people would find some of the material on these websites upsetting and/or offensive.

One often-overlooked possibility of support for those who are facing involuntary childlessness may be complementary therapies. More and more couples are turning to complementary therapies as they search for a miracle solution to their infertility but such treatments may prove far more useful for their relaxing properties and the counselling element involved in talking at length to a complementary therapist about problems. When couples need time to talk and help readjusting to involuntary childlessness, this may prove beneficial.

Box 33.1 lists a number of childlessness and childfree websites that may be useful.

Books

There are a number of books that may be helpful to couples facing involuntary childlessness, particularly around the time of giving up treatment. *Pink for a Girl* by Isla McGuckin[14] can be thoroughly recommended as a positive story of actively coping with involuntary childlessness. Isla McGuckin and her partner changed their lives as a result of their fertility problems and the book tracks their experiences, providing a lesson in learning how to find positive aspects of the situation and move forwards.

Beyond Childlessness by Rachel Black and Louise Scull[8] is another excellent book that gives an extremely comprehensive picture of women's experiences of childlessness from a sympathetic viewpoint. *Sweet Grapes, How to Stop Being Infertile and Start Living Again* by Jean Carter and Michael Carter[15] is a US book that considers how to turn the negative experiences of infertility into a positive way of life without children and contains self-help tips for coping with the emotions involved in the process. Caroline Gallup's *Making Babies the Hard Way*[16] is about the journey towards stopping treatment and will be useful for those who are approaching this stage rather than those further down the line who are trying to cope with involuntary childlessness.

Box 33.1	Websites of childlessness and childfree support organisations, message boards and blogs

Childlessness websites:
Infertility Network UK: www.infertilitynetworkuk.com
More to Life: www.moretolife.co.uk
Miscarriage Association: www.miscarriageassociation.org.uk
Childless Stepmums: www.childlessstepmums.co.uk
A childless blog: www.childlessbymarriage.blogspot.com/

Childfree websites:
Kidding Aside (The British Childfree Association): www.kiddingaside.yuku.com
Childfree Living UK: www.childfreelivinguk.yuku.com
www.thecfcouple.proboards37.com
www.childfree.net
www.happilychildfree.com
www.childfreebychoice.com
www.child-free.com

Conclusion

The effects of infertility continue long after people have stopped fertility treatment and there is insufficient support for those who have to come to terms with involuntary childlessness. Many couples do manage to adapt their expectations and lifestyles and to lead fulfilling lives without children but the involuntarily childless are an often-overlooked sector of society who would benefit from more help and understanding.

References

1. McAllister F with Clarke L. *Choosing Childlessness*. London: Family Policy Studies Centre; 1998.
2. Office for National Statistics. *Birth and Fertility*. London: ONS; 2006 [www.statistics.gov.uk].
3. Human Fertilisation and Embryology Authority. *A Long Term Analysis of the HFEA Register Data 1991–2006*. London: HFEA; 2008 [www.hfea.gov.uk].
4. Department of Health. *Primary Care Trust PCT Survey – Provision of IVF in England in 2007*. London: Department of Health; 2008 [www.dh.gov.uk/en/Publicationsandstatistics/Publications/PublicationsPolicyAndGuidance/DH_085665].
5. National Collaborating Centre for Women's and Children's Health. *Fertility: Assessment and Treatment for People with Fertility Problems*. Clinical Guideline 11. London: RCOG Press; 2004.
6. Wirtberg I, Möller A, Hogström L, Tronstad SE, Lalos A. Life 20 years after unsuccessful fertility treatment. *Hum Reprod* 2007;22:598–604.
7. Peddie VL, van Teijlingen E, Bhattacharya S. A qualitative study of women's decision-making at the end of IVF treatment. *Hum Reprod* 2005;20:1944–51.
8. Black R, Scull L. *Beyond Childlessness*. London: Rodale; 2005.
9. Smith Squire A. The last great taboo: why are childless women treated like second-class citizens? *Daily Mail* 24 July 2008 [www.dailymail.co.uk/femail/article-1038090/The-great-taboo-Why-childless-women-treated-like-second-class-citizens.html].
10. Grundy E, Butterworth S, Henretta J, Wadsworth MEJ, Tomassini C. *Partnership and Parenthood History and Health in Mid and Later Life*. London: Economic and Social Research Council; 2006 [www.esrcsocietytoday.ac.uk/ESRCInfoCentre/ViewAwardPage.aspx?AwardId=2978].
11. Lechner L, Bolman C, van Dalen A. Definite involuntary childlessness: associations between coping, social support and psychological distress. *Hum Reprod* 2007;22:288–294.
12. The Miscarriage Association. *When the Trying Stops*. Wakefield: The Miscarriage Association; 2008 [www.miscarriageassociation.org.uk/ma2006/information/fclick.php?026].
13. Childless Stepmums Forum [www.childlessstepmums.co.uk].
14. McGuckin I. *Pink for a Girl*. London: Hay House; 2006.
15. Carter JW, Carter M. *Sweet Grapes; How to Stop Being Infertile and Start Living Again*. Indianapolis: Perspectives Press; 1998.
16. Gallup C. *Making Babies the Hard Way*. London; Jessica Kingsley Publishers: 2007.

Chapter 34
Managing expectations and achieving realism: the 'realpolitik' of reproductive ageing and its consequences

Zoe Williams

In 2006, the Institute of Public Policy Research (IPPR) produced a document, written by Mike Dixon and Julia Margo, detailing the consequences of the way we choose, *en masse*, to reproduce.[1] Their striking finding was that the timing, as much as the methods, of starting families has a number of impacts. First, late maternity drives fertility down and sparks a pension and overall welfare crisis if there are fewer citizens of working age than there are either side of it. Second, while childlessness is of course a personal issue, if women are finding themselves involuntarily childless at the age of 45 years through a lack of public health information, this raises questions about governmental duty and dereliction thereof. Third, if middle-class women are having children progressively later while women in lower social brackets are having children much earlier, the social divide that predates the maternity ossifies into alarmingly iniquitous outlooks for those children. The link between early motherhood and poverty is pronounced and any government with a stated interest in reducing child poverty would have to start here.

So, a number of questions remain. What are the predictions for population and how much should we trust them? Is there a European or another developed world model that we could usefully follow and which examples should we be avoiding? If population is being driven downwards, what are the driving factors? If, conversely, population might, through the mitigating factor of migration, remain static, does this mean that we have nothing to worry about, or will the social disparities persist regardless? What are the government's responsibilities towards fertility? Is a public health message enough, or should it be prosecuting an actively pro-natal policy? What would be the political ramifications of so doing and is it possible to pursue these aims without becoming embroiled in skirmishes between conservative moralising and leftist social engineering?

In July 2006, Tony Blair told a House of Commons Liaison Committee that the Government had no policy on population. It was said ruefully enough, but not without an edge of pride: it seemed to convey a liberal, open-minded flexibility about family planning, it sounded honest and self-aware about the limitations of Government, it was hands off, modern, a third way. And yet this is the same Prime Minister who said in 1999, 'our historic aim [is] that ours is the first generation to end child poverty forever'. As the memory of Blair's enthusiastic self-belief recedes, the incompatibility of these two statements becomes increasingly obvious. Dixon and Margo[1] showed conclusively that any government with an interest in social justice must address itself, with some urgency, to the politics of population and fertility.

Population decline in perspective

The situation in the UK is nothing like as bad as it is in Italy and Japan. These countries are two object lessons in what happens when you leave it too late to develop a population strategy and adopt the wrong tone when you finally do. In 2000, there were 1.61 people in Italy aged 15–59 years for every person aged 0–15 years or 60 years or over and 1.64 in Japan, but United Nations predictions give us 0.86 and 0.82, respectively, by 2050,[2] which will have a devastating impact on these countries' welfare systems, not to mention creating the negative feedback where the steady diminution of government welfare funding will potentially act as a disincentive to having children. The same set of predictions puts the UK at 1.04 by 2050, which is not a catastrophic dependency ratio but certainly is not buoyant. The various factors that brought Italy and Japan to this pass are too complicated to go into in full here but it is salutary to note that political inertia significantly compounded existing trends. Nothing was done in the early 1980s, which was when policy could have made most difference. Instead, Italy, in particular, started making strident and slightly panicky policy early in this century, paying women a one-off €1000 for having a second child. This was in no way enough to offset swingeing childcare costs and did nothing to alter the fiscal penalties of having children in a country with such unsophisticated maternity leave legislation. Consequently, it made little difference to the birth rate.

The other useful lesson is how conservative rhetoric damages the birth rate, while clearly intending to promote it. The emphasis on marriage, in both Italy and Japan, appears to have the effect of putting greater pressure on women to create the perfect, lasting family unit before they consider having children. The strong anti-abortion voice in mainstream Italian politics (abortion services are hard to access and, in 2005, there was a popular movement in Parliament to pay women not to have abortions) has fostered a very efficient approach to contraception: this is technically a good thing but, given that one in three babies in the UK are unplanned,[3] clearly it boosts population growth if some people feel able to leave it to chance.

Nevertheless, the UK is not in a position to feel smug. It is interesting that 2.4 children has always been the cliché when that has not been the birth rate in this country for 50 years. In 2001, the birth rate hit the all-time low of 1.63, since when it has climbed to 1.91 by 2007. The Government Actuary's Department,[4] whose work was taken over in 2006 by the Office for National Statistics, gave population projections at three possible fertility rates: static at 1.91 (or rather, at 1.74, as it stood in 2005 – the increase was unexpected); high at 1.94; and very low at 1.54. Under none of these conditions would we see replacement levels of fertility (which, at 2.1 children per woman, this country has not seen since the 1970s) but, of course, the dependency ratios are much better under the highest fertility rate. Dixon and Margo[1] pointed out, furthermore, that those ratios do not tell the whole story since they look static and mask the fact that the nation's dependency is all back-loaded. The fiscal dependency upon the state of a retired person is much greater, and is usually for longer, than that of a person aged under 16 years.

The IPPR report[1] also highlighted various trends that point to ever-decreasing fertility: greater student costs, high property prices and an overall increase in the amount of debt accrued by the average graduate compels them to delay starting a family. To these late starters, conditions affecting biological fertility – obesity, low sperm counts, sexually transmitted infections – become more problematic. (Bill Ledger, at a European Fertility Conference in Copenhagen in 2005, seized the popular imagination, albeit briefly, with his description of an 'infertility time bomb'. He predicted that, by 2015, one in seven couples would need treatment to conceive.) However, it should be noted that these have all been factors over the past 7 years and fertility has nevertheless increased.

Furthermore, not even a government-sponsored statistical analysis has total control over the future, and European projections are rather different. Eurostat, the 'numbers' arm of the European Commission, predicts that, by 2060, the UK population will increase by 25% from the current figure of just over 61 million to almost 77 million, making it the largest in Europe. How do they account for this curve, which runs counter to all similar nations? It is partly due to our relatively low average age (39 years at the moment and predicted to be 42 years by 2060, by which time it will be lower than anywhere but Luxembourg), but mainly it would be a result of migration. Now, immigration is no silver bullet: although migrant populations enter the workplace immediately and tend to be younger than the indigenous population, offsetting the fertility trends of this population would take far more immigrants than would be politically viable, at least in the current climate. You could argue that, were dependency ratios to look seriously unmanageable, opposition to immigration might evaporate but such on-the-hoof, fingers-crossed thinking is no way to map out a population policy. Furthermore, long-term macroeconomic forecasts are not the full extent of the fertility conundrum. Late maternity is the principal driver of low birth rates and it creates economic conditions that are as serious as a pensions crisis and more immediate.

The baby gap

The IPPR report[1] describes the number of children that women say they want in their 20s as a 'baby gap', compared with the number they have had by the time they are aged 45 years. Astonishingly, these 'missing babies' number 90 000 a year. The largest single impact factor for population is women remaining childless. In 2005, 9% of women aged 60 years were childless and the projection for women aged 35 years in the same year was 22%. There is no definitive study of how much of this is voluntary; the number of women who deliberately intend to remain childless is certainly growing but nothing like as fast as the numbers who find themselves childless at the age of 45 years. Although this will have a devastating effect on care provision when these childless women (and, of course, the corresponding men who remain childless) reach pensionable age, that is less pressing, from the point of view of governance, than the simple failure of public information regarding fertility. There is an abundance of tabloid static about this but it lacks rigour in its presentation and is contradictory and excitable. From the Department of Health, there is almost nothing. Reminders of diminishing fertility, having become associated with right-wing anti-feminist rhetoric, are greeted with hostility, even when solidly founded and well meant. Of course, at the coalface are the infertility doctors who have to deliver news that devastates when it should be common knowledge.

Those women who do have children have them later. In 2005, fertility among women in their 30s outstripped that among women in their 20s for the first time. Generally speaking, the older a woman is when she has her first child, the fewer children she will have. Even if her family size is the same as it would have been, there is a Doppler effect:

the gaps between the generations get larger so the population diminishes anyway.[5] There is also a downturn in the number of women having four children or more, but this is the least statistically significant trend. However, a more immediate problem than straight numbers is the social inequality that builds up around these trends.

The IPPR report[1] details a stark and growing economic environment for younger parents that the authors describe as the 'fertility poverty trap'. Part of the drift towards later maternity must be the biting financial penalties attached to having children at a younger age. Both fathers and mothers are affected but, given that women are still suffering from a gender pay gap (that is most punitive for part-time workers) and that single parents suffer most and are overwhelmingly female, this can, perhaps unhelpfully but not unreasonably, be presented as a woman's issue.

It is rare for anyone to be established in a career by the age of 25 years, so anyone becoming a parent at this age is likely to be in low-paid employment, or at best, low on the ladder of a higher paid profession. Katherine Rake, head of the Fawcett Society, has produced a set of figures for a woman's income expectations depending on her fertility choices.[6] The average mid-skilled woman who has her first child at 24 years of age foregoes £564,000 in earnings over her lifetime. If she waits until she is aged 28 years, the amount falls to £165,000. Economically, the later the better as far as childbirth is concerned and a US study found the economic advantages of late maternity so pronounced that they fostered better health among older mothers. In a study of 3000 US women,[7] the best age overall for a woman to have her first child was found to be 34 years. It is a high-risk strategy, though, to aim for a bull's eye so far into one's 30s. A couple encountering problems, having started trying when the woman was aged 34 years, might find themselves advised to not seek medical advice for 2 years, whereupon it is not unreasonable to assume another 3 years between diagnosis and waiting lists. So a woman's IVF treatment could be delayed until she is aged 39 years, by which time the chances of success have dropped from 25% to 15% and she is at the outer limit of the NHS cut-off point. Even if all the intentions are realised, a woman having her first child when she is aged 34 years will probably not have her second until she is 37 or 38 years old, by which age even a family of two will be a blessing not a certainty. Well, children are never certainties, of course, but some are likelier than others.

The poorer you are to start with, the higher the penalty for having children.[6] A low-skilled mother will earn an average £334,000 less over her lifetime, which is a stunning 53% of her earnings overall. A mid-skilled worker will lose out on £164,000 and a highly skilled woman will lose only £19,000 over a lifetime. Naturally, while the low skilled are not always young, the young are mainly low skilled. Perhaps we could look at this from another angle: since childcare costs are high, it often makes financial sense for mothers well into the middle-income brackets to look after their own children. Many skilled, professional women describe their work as fiscally neutral: it costs them so much to set up the childcare structures that allow them to go out to work that the work itself becomes a vanity project. If that's the case even for reasonably well-paid women, it would be doubly true for the low skilled: so talking about 'lost earnings' in the first 3 years of a child's life is a red herring. We could just as well term it 'money saved on childcare'. Perhaps as the Government addresses itself to preschool care, it could consider paying mothers or funding childcare swaps between parents.

Problems persist long after the first 3 years of parenthood and women who have children early find themselves beset from a number of angles. When returning to the workplace once the children have started school, women find themselves underskilled and out of the loop. Young mothers may have had their education interrupted by childbirth, and returning to education can prove to be even less flexible than returning to the workplace. Childcare tax credits are only paid to those who work and yet they are not enough to actually cover childcare so that shortfall might force a low-income mother back out of work, whereupon her tax credits are removed completely: so, even if she is minded to return to the workplace, she will not be able to afford childcare when it comes to applying and interviewing. If this sounds like a diatribe against the current government's policy on parenting, it is not: amazing strides have been made in both maternity and paternity leave over the past 10 years. When this government was elected in 1997, paid maternity leave was 13 weeks, which sounds almost inhuman; 12 years on, it is now 9 months, with plans to extend it to a year. Paternity leave was invented, certainly as part of UK policy, by this Government and stands at 2 weeks, with a possible 6 months mooted before the last election but not yet legislated. It should always be with a nod to these achievements that we point out how much more there is to do: Gordon Brown's announcement of proposed free childcare for children aged 2 years[8] was heartening, but only to a degree. Purportedly 'free' nursery places for those aged 3 years are only for 2–3 hours a day, which, at the very best, allows mothers to pursue only part-time work but realistically does not even cover that. Furthermore, while both Government and opposition parties are happy to address the feel-good issues of childcare generally, nobody is talking explicitly about this clear and causal link between early motherhood and child poverty. Indeed, the only audible political voice on any aspect of fertility has been the Conservative Party's emphasis on the traditional family, with tax breaks for married couples emerging as one of David Cameron's flagship policies. We will have to address ourselves another day as to whether or not this seriously promotes stability within families: in terms of population and fertility, this emphasis on old-fashioned respectability tends to discourage the very mothers who are cutting it rather fine already.

The flip side to this poverty trap is the trap at the other end of a woman's fertility span: involuntary childlessness, at worst, or the lesser but still meaningful baby gap due to starting too late and only being able to have one child. To deal with childlessness first, the hardboiled approach is to concentrate on the care burden on the state when the projected 22% of women that will remain childless reach pensionable age. Research solicited by the IPPR from the London School of Economics[9] showed that, for 43% of the 2 million older people receiving informal care in this country, that care came from their children. *Ergo*, childless women will take some looking after two decades hence and, factoring in possibly unfavourable dependency ratios, this leaves us with an extremely expensive welfare system. I would counter here that these childless non-mothers would have saved so much money by not having children, as we've just shown, that we must not presume them to be an enormous financial burden. They might make very substantial provision for themselves. I take much more seriously the emotional impact of involuntary childlessness, which has been eloquently described by Kate Brian.[10]

Governments tend to shy away from this area, thinking that it is, one assumes, too personal for state interference. Furthermore, it is a thin line between warning women of the dangers of late maternity and prosecuting an actively pro-natal policy and this latter is riven with ethical dilemma. It is a hard fit for a progressive government – how does one justify spurring on the reproduction of one's own populace? Why not encourage migration instead or, at the very least, slacken the barriers to migration, which would then, one imagines, take care of itself? In a gripping account of the pro-natal policy in Israel, Sarah Martha Kahn[11] points out that the basis for the policy was often, rhetorically and tacitly, underpinned by loss: either the loss of ancestors in the Holocaust or the loss of today's Israelis in the current fighting. This traumatic landscape is almost a necessary component of such an extreme policy, which otherwise sounds anachronistic and borderline eugenicist. But the problem, essentially, is that no progressive government has so far found the language to talk about this issue without being seen to bully women or harry couples into starting families, and thus falling foul of the women's movement. A solution must be found: there is a public health duty, besides anything else, to ensure that childlessness is an intended result or, at worst, the result of insurmountable barriers and has not just been slipped into accidentally by a populace that was not kept informed.* Even more importantly, the issue must be reframed as an integral element of progressive politics. Before the trend towards late motherhood became so marked, this family territory could with reason be written off as Tory ground, interesting only to those with a marriage agenda, not to social liberals or indeed any other element of the left wing. Now, however, the economic disparities created by it are too striking to ignore: younger mothers must be better supported in their return to the workplace and women must see conditions improve for earlier maternity before they will be tempted into it. Failure in this will lead to greater child poverty, deeper social fissures and an unacceptably uneven playing field for the coming generations.

The Dutch provide an excellent template for ideal maternal age: they give birth neither very early nor terrifically late. The percentage of deliveries to women in the Netherlands aged under 25 years is 11%; in the UK, that figure is 25%. Pregnancies are concentrated between the ages of 25 and 35 years, with the mean age at first delivery being 29 years.[13] Their conditions are not radically different to ours: certainly, none of their policies would seem fanciful to us. They are known to have a more open, evolved attitude to sex and to talk about it more freely, and this is held to reduce teen pregnancies as well as sexually transmitted infections.† They have similar numbers in higher education and similar ages of entry to the workplace (it is actually, at 27 years of age, somewhat higher than it is in the UK) but their university funding is better so graduates do not emerge with such high levels of debt and can start their families sooner. Their provision of preschool care is exemplary – a number of formalised structures, from state nurseries to communal childminding undertaken by groups of parents, are all eligible for means-tested grants. It has passed into accepted truth in the UK that means-testing is no longer a viable way of supplying benefits; it is too complicated to administer, it is stigmatising, it is unpopular. I think this has to be revisited in the area of childcare. Better state-funded preschool care could absolutely revivify people's prospects at the bottom of the financial pile but it would be too expensive to offer to all parents. Having said that, the cost of providing care at this stage could be balanced against the money saved by the NHS if better options for women drive down the mean age for first-time maternity and obviate (or reduce, at least) the need for fertility treatment. It should be noted at this point that the

---

* It could be argued that this is common knowledge but the Department of Health document on this issue, the NICE clinical guideline on fertility,[12] expressly states: 'The recommendations do not cover how fertility problems can be prevented in the first place'. Susan Seenan, from Infertility Network UK (INUK), says: 'There are no government guidelines for when a woman should start a family. It would not be appropriate, since every woman's circumstances are different, and many women are not ready to start trying for children in their twenties.' The upshot of this, however, is that INUK is often the first point of government advice on when and how fertility drops off; that is, there is no public health message until problems have already been encountered.

† This proposition is hard to test, but a useful counterpoint is the USA, where there is a direct correlation between the avoidance of safe-sex messages and the promotion of sexual abstinence as part of school syllabuses, and unwanted teen pregnancies and sexually transmitted infections. It is ironic, although not in a very amusing way. With the USA's often staunchly anti-abortion environment and limited access to adult education, prospects for pregnant teenagers are awfully bleak.

Netherlands has the highest perinatal mortality rates in Europe;[14] they may be a good role model in some respects but maternal age is clearly not the only factor in play here.

It is an oversimplification to try to put together a cost–benefit analysis on preschool care versus fertility treatment. The causal link is not well-enough established – what if women are delaying childbirth because men are reluctant to have children young? What if it is simply a function of a society that emphasises the individual over any other unit? The numbers are too hazy – how many preschool places should be provided? How much is fertility treatment forecast to cost the NHS over the coming years? The funding does not even come from the same budgets. The impetus to provide this all-important early-years care must, I believe, come from an ethical more than fiscal position. It should not be acceptable to any evolved society that women walk this tightrope between exclusion from the workplace and exclusion from family life.

Other suggested solutions centre on improving the nation's fertility generally, by well-worn means of fighting obesity and providing better sexual health care. While of course both these ends are worth pursuing for their own sake, from a social policy point of view, no great boon is wrought by enabling women to have children later and later. If maternal age is to creep up, so be it. If it can be forced down, all to the good, medically speaking. The crucial thing is that mothers cluster around the same age bracket and are not directed down very different paths according to pre-existing factors of class and education.

I am also often struck by how much bad publicity there is surrounding maternity provision in the UK. Ironically, considering this chest-beating about our falling birth rate, the recent mini-boom has put such pressure on the maternity services that both midwifery and neonatal units are understaffed, and this, if not driving down the birth rate, certainly gives many would-be mothers pause.

Overwhelmingly, though, governments need to tackle the 'opportunity cost' of having children. There are problems to be tackled within families – specifically the 'chores gap', identified by the Equal Opportunities Commission (now part of the Equality and Human Rights Commission). Women will continue to delay parenthood while they perceive, quite rightly, that the burden of it will fall mainly on them. That is a matter for a subtly evolving culture more than the jackhammer of legislation. Other encouraging features, such as the end of the pay gap between the genders and more flexible working practices so that part-time work does not necessarily have to be menial, are things that government and society are working towards anyway, as pleasing goals in their own right. Most urgently, this leaves us with birth-to-school care: solve that and the impediments to motherhood are radically reduced. If women still procrastinate, new models for welfare and benefit and redistribution of wealth will have to be found, but we will not know until this critical experiment has been undertaken, and with gusto.

References

1. Dixon M, Margo J. *Population Politics*. London: Institute for Public Policy Research; 2006.
2. United Nations. *World Population Ageing: 1950–2050*. New York: United Nations; 2002 [www.un.org/esa/population/publications/worldageing19502050/].
3. Lakha F, Glasier A. Unintended pregnancy and use of emergency contraception among a large cohort of women attending for antenatal care or abortion in Scotland. *Lancet* 2006;368:1782–7.
4. UK Government Actuary's Department. *Projected Cohort Expectations of Life (Years) Based on Assumed Calendar Year Mortality Rates from the 2004-Based Principal Projections and Historical Rates*. London: TSO; 2005 [www.gad.gov.uk/Demography_Data/Life_Tables/Period_and_cohort_eol.asp].

5. Smallwood S, Chamberlain J. Replacement fertility, what has it been and what does it mean? *Popul Trends* 2005;119:16–27 [www.statistics.gov.uk/downloads/theme_population/PT119v2.pdf].

6. Rake K. *Women's Incomes over the Lifetime: A Report to the Women's Unit, Cabinet Office*. London: The Stationery Office; 2000.

7. Mirowsky J. Age at first birth, health, and mortality. *J Health Soc Behav* 2005;46:32–50.

8. Wheeler B. Brown reveals free childcare plan. BBC News website, 21 September 2008 [news.bbc.co.uk/1/hi/uk_politics/7627625.stm].

9. Malley J, Wittenberg R, Comas-Herrera R, Pickard L, King D. *Longterm Care Expenditure for Older People: Projections to 2022 for Great Britain*. Report to IPPR. PSSRU Discussion paper 2252. London: Personal Social Services Research Unit (PSSRU), London School of Economics (LSE); 2005.

10. Brian K. *In Pursuit of Parenthood*. London: Bloomsbury; 1998.

11. Kahn SM. *Reproducing Jews: A Cultural Account of Assisted Conception in Israel*. 2nd ed. Durham, NC: Duke University Press; 2000.

12. National Institute for Clinical Excellence. *Fertility: Assessment and Treatment for People with Fertility Problems*. Clinical Guideline 11. London: NICE; 2004.

13. Sheldon T. Perinatal mortality in Netherlands third worst in Europe. *BMJ* 2008;337:a3118.

14. Mohangoo AD, Buitendijk SE, Hukkelhoven CW, Ravelli AC, Rijninks-van Driel GC, Tamminga P, et al. [Higher perinatal mortality in The Netherlands than in other European countries: the Peristat-II study]. *Ned Tijdschr Geneeskd* 2008;152:2718–27.

Chapter 35
The future: waking up

Discussion

Siladitya Bhattacharya: Thanks for two excellent presentations. So, what we are getting clearly is that the message needs to go out to people that there is a finite time over which women are able to reproduce. But how can that message be transmitted to the population without government support?

Zoe Williams: It would have to be with government support because you need some kind of neutrality. The way the media presents it is very overheated. A lot of people in the left-wing press present this (and I have been guilty myself) as a conspiracy against women, to pressurise them into early childbearing. It is not a conspiracy against women, but that is what if feels like when being constantly badgered. It has to come from a neutral body. What do you think?

Kate Brian: I think that is true, but at the moment people are really not aware of it. There are a lot of people who still think that it is vaguely 'made up'. People are not really aware of the realities, partly because there is still this idea that 'if I leave it too late I can still go and have fertility treatment'. People do still think that is a kind of safety net.

Stephen Hillier: I wonder to what extent government policy on population development takes into account or relies upon the wave of new manpower or womanpower from the European Union accession states?

Zoe Williams: There is scope within government to make policy on migration and demographics but it has not been done.

Roger Gosden: I wonder whether there has been any resurgence in birth rate in Scandinavia or Germany and other countries where there has been better social provision for childcare and financial incentive to promote childbearing at younger ages? Is there evidence that such government policy intentions actually work?

Zoe Williams: If you are talking about simple financial handouts, those do not seem to work, but if you are talking about better provision of full-time childcare then that does seem to have an effect. At least, where you see excellent childcare you also see a workable birth rate, but whether or not those two things are linked as cause and effect is hard to prove.

Susan Bewley: Australia has seen a bit of a birth rate boom with their change of policy and the Dutch data are also very interesting as they have decreasing birth rates both in the under-20s and over-40s. However, Stijn has looked into all these questions and has not been able to answer them, he just says it is impossible to tease out. I think it is difficult to prove cause and effect, and different cultures and subsets within different cultures have different approaches to childbearing. It must be very difficult for a government ever to implement a truly evidence-based policy, even though they all do have policy and claim some sort of a beneficial outcome as a result.

Zoe Williams: I think you have to look at the moral choices as well as the expedience. It is all very well to decide that full-time childcare should be available freely to people in order to increase the birth rate, but this is secondary really because the ethical position is that this provision helps people who need money.

Roger Gosden: But if you have two arguments it is better than one.

Zoe Willams: Yes, that is true too.

David Barlow: You mentioned the left-wing view of the agenda of the Government on this issue; what is the right-wing agenda?

Zoe Williams: The right-wing agenda, generally speaking, is to promote marriage and to be seen to be promoting marriage, so an awful lot of spending on families goes into tax breaks for married couples, for example. The Tories were talking about a one-off windfall payment to get married of £2000. There tends to be a lot of tub-thumping because there are easy votes in saying that we would like to help everybody to stay together. But these conditions are quite hard to create if you can make people who are not married feel really bad about it because then they do not clamour so much for tax breaks and social help because they feel this is their fault.

Peter Braude: You are being very honest. As a journalist in the field, clearly you wanted to postpone your own childbearing. Why did you not heed the message and what changed your mind?

Zoe Williams: Well I did heed the message because I only interviewed them [Susan Bewley and Melanie Davies] a year and a half before I became pregnant. I could have left it for years. Otherwise I probably would have left it until I was 39, or older.

Peter Braude: What were you searching for, what was missing?

Zoe Williams: I honestly thought that you start to worry at 38 and then you go to doctors at 39 and then you would have treatment to help you get pregnant. You don't get a close statistical reading from newspapers. You get big headlines.

Peter Braude: How do you get an intelligent person to decide that at 35? We actually put the facts down and it was unpleasant. When you write something in the media about getting pregnant at an earlier age, there is a backlash and allegation of a conspiracy.

Zoe Williams: I agree with you. Believe me, I was intending to be part of that backlash. There is no way of changing the fact that some people are ill-informed and don't want to listen. You have just got to keep saying it. Perhaps in the end you have to look at it like global warming. Twenty years ago it was almost unheard of. There were a few people saying then what everybody is saying now, and far more people using language like 'doom-mongering'.

Kate Brian: You just have to keep saying it.

Gita Mishra: I would like to talk about the dilemma of women in their late 20s and 30s. Women that age are finding it really difficult to get a partner. Their age range, I think, puts the men off because they feel that women are really only interested in them as a source of sperm, basically. What can we do to encourage people back into serious relationships?

Kate Brian: There are more single women now and the HFEA [Human Fertilisation and Embryology Authority] statistics show there are more single women having IVF. When I did my last book[1] we interviewed lots of single women about the reasons for having assisted conception and found that they had all thought about the implications of their decision really carefully. This was not a snap decision. They had not delayed having children because of their career; rather, it was because they had not met the right person. They finally decided that they had to face a stark choice: either I do it now by myself or it may never happen. Then, of course, once you are in that situation, how are you going to meet anyone when you are a single mother?

Zoe Williams: I can sit here and think that people are just too picky, but what is interesting is that this is one area in which the Government really cannot legislate. You have to let common sense prevail. One thing to really stress is how long a career is. People forget. It is years and years and years and years. You do not have to rush. If you are at the top by your mid-30s, what are you going to do with the rest of your life?

Maya Unnithan: Many people describe how the elements of their decision to go for treatment were triggered by social events in their lives, such as friends having children or entering menopause, etc. If one is counselling infertility patients who have been unsuccessful then it seems to me that there is much more needed than just to see them once after it is over.

Kate Brian: It is very difficult. They cannot carry on in therapeutic counselling for the rest of their lives. Most people do find a way of getting over it, but the reality is that it does not disappear. The rest of your life is not going to be how you thought it was going to be. People in this position do say that however much they have managed to find other positive things, it does still come back to them and it does still hurt. One woman I interviewed said that she felt worse in her early 60s, when all of her friends started having grandchildren, than she did at the age that she was experiencing not being able to have a child in her 30s. I thought that was shocking.

Melanie Davies: I was the other co-author of the *BMJ* article[2] and I am still recovering from the backlash. It was very hard after 30 years of considering myself a feminist to be accused of being anti-women! The education which I received from all of this is just how difficult it is to put out a message that is hard for people to hear. As an anecdotal comment, I went to Sweden about 10 days ago as part of a meeting with Medical Women and thought it would be nirvana with its social legislation, but of course it was not. Even though it is provisioned for prolonged maternity and parental leave, to actually take up the rights would be career suicide. So this shows that implementation is important even in the best legislative environment. The Government must be involved, but it is implementation that we must be working on.

Sean Kehoe: Well, I think on that note we have probably reached exactly the right time to stop. This is the time where I thank all participants, speakers and discussants.

References

1.   Brian K. *The Complete Guide to Female Fertility.* London: Piatkus; 2007.
2.   Bewley S, Davies M, Braude P. Which career first? *BMJ* 2005;331:588–9.

Section 10

Consensus views

Chapter 36

Consensus views arising from the 56th Study Group: Reproductive Ageing

Introduction

■ Reproductive ageing in women is caused by declining number and quality of oocytes. There is little immediate prospect of reversing the underlying biological phenomena and determinants of reproductive ageing. Male reproductive ageing also occurs and is associated with adverse effects, though to a lesser degree.

■ There is a steady continuing rise in age at childbirth. Women may face personal, social or economic constraints to earlier childbearing and these may also vary cross-culturally.

■ Sexually transmitted infections are rising in older women.

■ Early ovarian ageing affects around 10% of women in the general population. There is no evidence to support the use of screening for early ovarian ageing or ovarian response tests.

■ Infertility is a time of great emotional and social stress for women and couples. Reproductive outcome in fertility treatment depends mainly on the woman's age. Assisted reproductive technologies, including *in vitro* fertilisation (IVF) with the woman's own fresh oocytes, cannot compensate for the effect of reproductive ageing. The purported benefits of oocyte banking either by cryopreservation or by vitrification for postponing pregnancy to a later age are unproven.

■ Delay in childbirth is associated with worsening reproductive outcomes: more infertility and medical co-morbidity, and an increase in maternal and fetal morbidity and mortality. Women who start their family in their 20s or complete it by age 35 years face significantly reduced risks.

■ Multiple pregnancies are associated with poorer fetal and maternal outcomes.

■ The 2004 National Institute for Health and Clinical Excellence (NICE) clinical guideline on fertility[1] has not been fully implemented.

Recommendations for the RCOG

1. The RCOG should work closely with the Department of Health, the NHS and other groups to contribute to public debate and policy by increasing

public awareness of the effects of deferred childbirth on fertility and pregnancy outcome, and by alerting society to the public health implications so that the incentives and barriers to earlier reproduction are examined.

2. The RCOG should promote the view of a shared responsibility in addressing the problems associated with reproductive ageing and encourage an acknowledgement that personal and social circumstances play a role rather than placing 'blame' on individuals.

3. The RCOG should provide more information, modules and examinations about 'fertility facts' for: (a) medical school curricula, (b) DRCOG, (c) MRCOG, (d) continuing professional development.

4. The RCOG should promote information and education through schools, colleges, contraception and sexual health clinics and general practices to ensure women are aware that, biologically, the best age for childbearing is 20–35 years. It should work with the Consumer's Forum and in liaison with general educationalists and Government departments to publish simple information for use by the general public. Socio-cultural factors need to be taken into account to make the educational messages more relevant.

5. The RCOG should continue to strongly advocate that the 2004 NICE recommendations[1] should be rapidly and fully implemented with regard to the funding of fertility treatment.

6. The RCOG should consider working with the UK Obstetric Surveillance System (UKOSS) to generate reliable UK-wide data on obstetric outcome at the extremes of maternal age.

7. Interventions in pregnant women aged 40 years or over should be based on evidence of known risks and proven benefits. Women should be counselled regarding risks in terms of absolute rather than relative risks. An RCOG Green-top Guideline on the management of pregnancy in women aged 40 years or over could inform women and practitioners of the evidence and thus guide practice.

8. The RCOG should urge greater transparency and accuracy in depicting assisted reproductive technology success rates, including the cost and clinical efficiency of full cycles (full cycle implies cryopreservation of embryos).

Clinical practice

9. There are no contraceptive methods contraindicated by age alone. Older women may use combined hormonal contraception unless they have co-existing diseases or risk factors.

10. Amenorrhoea does not signify ovarian failure in older women using hormonal contraceptive methods.

11. Healthcare professionals and users should be aware of the contraceptive choices available in the UK, particularly the benefits of long-acting methods such as levonorgestrel intrauterine system.

12. Doctors should be ready and comfortable to ask about sexual problems or concerns whatever the age of the patient and be able to refer promptly to local sources of psychosexual help. Safe-sex campaigns and funding for sexual health clinics for over-45s should be supported.

13. Women aged 30 years or over should have their attention drawn to age-specific outcome data when discussing and making decisions about their fertility management.

14. Couples, and especially older women, seeking fertility advice and treatment should have prompt, or accelerated, access to fertility specialists, investigations and treatment plans in view of the reduced and worsening treatment outcomes in women aged 40 years or over.

15. Guidelines to women and clinicians should incorporate medical, anthropological and cultural understandings of how women (whether mainstream or minority) conceptualise and experience fertility and fertility treatment so as to enhance their effectiveness.

16. From the outset, patients should be offered counselling and support after unsuccessful fertility treatment. Their attention should be drawn to the existence of patient help organisations such as More to Life.

17. Single-embryo transfer should be discussed and encouraged in all women. Recipients of donor oocyte treatment should have single-embryo transfer if the donor was aged under 35 years at the time of donation. To reduce multiple pregnancies, there is a need to discourage excessively high numbers of embryos being replaced in donor cycles for women aged 40 years or over.

18. Sperm donors should not be older than 45 years.

19. No consensus is currently available about the optimal protocols for oocyte freezing or vitrification and the woman's age and ovarian reserve are key factors affecting the chances of a successful outcome. Oocyte banking technologies are no guarantee of success, and clinics that offer oocyte freezing and vitrification should report standardised data on live birth per oocyte frozen to the Human Fertilisation and Embryology Authority.

20. Advanced paternal age is not an indication for performing prenatal diagnosis. Neither advanced maternal nor paternal age is an indication for performing preimplantation genetic screening.

Research priorities

21. Further research is needed into the mechanisms controlling human gamete development *in vivo* and technologies for their derivation *in vitro*.

22. Further research is needed into age changes in gametes, including their abundance, developmental competence and the risks of congenital abnormality.

23. Further research is needed into characterisation of existing and novel ovarian biomarkers to provide clinically useful prediction of current and future fertility.

24. Further research is needed into the development and validation of existing and novel technologies for gamete preservation in patients at risk of premature fertility loss.

25. Further research is needed into the mechanisms mediating the decline in uterine and placental function with advancing maternal age.

26. Further research is needed into the effects of parental ageing and associated use of assisted reproductive technologies on the development, health and welfare of the child.

27. Further research is needed into the nature and determinants of reproductive behavioural trends, including both voluntary and involuntary childlessness, and their economic and health consequences for the population, and cultural data related to childbirthing and reproductive practices.

Data collection priorities

28. National data collection covers live births and terminations of pregnancy but should be expanded to include information about miscarriage.

29. There is a need for long-term coordinated follow-up of children born following new assisted reproductive technologies and, specifically, for births following oocyte freezing and vitrification, preimplantation genetic screening, preimplantation genetic diagnosis and intracytoplasmic sperm injection to record the short- and long-term medical and psychosocial outcomes for these children.

30. Inter-generational data on reproductive health and behaviour are required nowadays to predict the future health prospects for women.

Reference

1. National Collaborating Centre for Women's and Children's Health. *Fertility: Assessment and Treatment for People with Fertility Problems.* London: RCOG Press; 2004 [www.nice.org.uk/nicemedia/pdf/CG011fullguideline.pdf].

Index